BIOTEST®

Study Aids

Tina S. Haynes

Pediatrics

Biotest Publishing Company, Inc.
Ventura, California

About the Author

Tina S. Haynes, M.D. graduated from Texas Tech Health Sciences Center School of Medicine in 1991 where she was honored as the recipient of the annual Gold Headed Cane award. This award is presented to the graduate that best exemplifies the ideal of commitment and compassion expected in clinical medicine. She completed a residency in Pediatrics at Wilford Hall USAF Medical Center in San Antonio, Texas, followed by a tour of duty at Tinker AFB in Oklahoma City, Oklahoma. At Tinker AFB she rose to the military rank of Major. She served initially as a staff pediatrician, and then as the Director for the Maternal Child Health Flight and the Chief of the Pediatric Department. In 1999 she received the Air Force Commendation Medal for meritorious service. After completion of her military commitment, Dr. Haynes accepted a position as an Assistant Professor of General Pediatrics at the University of Oklahoma Health Sciences Center. She is an active medical staff member at The Children's Hospital at OU Medical Center, and an attending physician in the outpatient, inpatient, and emergency departments. Recently she became the Medical Director of the OU Physicians Pediatric Care Center. She thoroughly enjoys her work with the medical students and residents, and at this point, cannot imagine a career without teaching.

Contents

PREFACE **3**

ABOUT THE AUTHOR **5**

USER GUIDE **10**

1 THE HEALTH MAINTENANCE VISIT **11**

1.1 THE HEALTH SUPERVISION VISIT 11
1.2 SPECIAL CONSIDERATIONS 15
QUESTIONS 16

2 THE NEWBORN **19**

2.1 PRENATAL LIFE 19
2.2 BIRTH 19
2.3 ABNORMAL CONDITIONS OF THE NEWBORN 20
QUESTIONS 26

3 ADOLESCENT DISORDERS **29**

3.1 ADOLESCENT MEDICINE 29
3.2 MENSTRUAL DISORDERS 29
3.3 BREAST DISORDERS 32
3.4 SCROTAL DISORDERS 33
3.5 REPRODUCTIVE ISSUES 34
3.6 MENTAL HEATH ISSUES 37
3.7 LEGAL ISSUES OF ADOLESCENCE IN THE UNITED STATES 37
QUESTIONS 39

4 RECURRENT NONEMERGENT PROBLEMS **43**

4.1 GENERAL CONCEPTS 43
4.2 PROBLEMS OF ELIMINATION 43
4.3 RECURRENT PAIN SYNDROMES 45
4.4 RECURRENT INFECTIONS 46
4.5 CONDITIONS SEEN IN EARLY CHILDHOOD 46
4.6 ATTENTION DEFICIT DISORDER (ADD) 47
QUESTIONS 48

5 GENETICS, ENDOCRINE, AND METABOLISM **49**

5.1 GENETICS 49
5.2 ENDOCRINOLOGY 51
5.3 METABOLIC DISEASE 57
QUESTIONS 59

6 IMMUNOLOGY **63**

6.1 HOST DEFENSE 63
6.2 MANIFESTATIONS OF IMMUNE SYSTEM DEFECTS 64
6.3 DISEASE PROFILES 64
QUESTIONS 67

7 Infectious Disease **69**
7.1 GENERAL CONCEPTS 69
7.2 DIAGNOSIS 69
7.3 DISEASE PROFILES 70
QUESTIONS 82

8 RHEUMATOLOGY **87**
8.1 GENERAL CONCEPTS 87
8.2 DISEASE PROFILES 87
QUESTIONS 91

9 RESPIRATORY DISORDERS **93**
9.1 GENERAL CONCEPTS 93
9.2 DISEASE PROFILES 95
QUESTIONS 100

10 CARDIOVASCULAR DISORDERS **105**
10.1 CIRCULATORY EMBRYOLOGY 105
10.2 DIAGNOSTIC MODALITIES 106
10.3 HEART MURMURS 107
10.4 CONGENITAL HEART DISEASE 109
10.5 DISEASE PROFILES 111
10.6 ACQUIRED CARDIAC DISEASE 116
QUESTIONS 119

11 HEMATOLOGY **125**
11.1 GENERAL CONCEPTS 125
11.2 DIAGNOSTIC MODALITIES 125
11.3 DISEASE PROFILES 126
QUESTIONS 138

12 NEOPLASTIC DISORDERS **145**
12.1 GENERAL CONCEPTS 145
12.2 DISEASE PROFILES 146
QUESTIONS 151

13 GASTROENTEROLOGY **157**
13.1 GENERAL CONCEPTS 157
13.2 CONGENITAL MALFORMATIONS 157
13.3 PATHOPHYSIOLOGIC MANIFESTATIONS OF GASTROINTESTINAL DISORDERS 159
13.4 DISEASE PROFILES 160
13.5 SURGICAL GASTROINTESTINAL DISEASE 164
QUESTIONS 167

14 RENAL DISORDERS **173**
14.1 GENERAL CONCEPTS 173
14.2 DISEASE PROFILES 176
QUESTIONS 181

15 ELECTROLYTE AND ACID-BASE DISORDERS **185**
15.1 GENERAL CONCEPTS 185
15.2 FLUID AND ELECTROLYTE DISTURBANCES 185
15.3 ACID-BASE DISTURBANCES 188
QUESTIONS 190

16 NEUROLOGIC DISORDERS **193**
16.1 GENERAL CONCEPTS 193
16.2 DISEASE PROFILES 195
QUESTIONS 204

17 MUSCULOSKELETAL DISORDERS **211**
17.1 DEVELOPMENTAL CONSIDERATIONS 211
17.2 DISEASE PROFILES 211
QUESTIONS 216

18 DERMATOLOGY **221**
18.1 GENERAL CONCEPTS 221
18.2 VASCULAR MALFORMATIONS 221
18.3 CUTANEOUS NEVI 222
18.4 HYPERPIGMENTED LESIONS 223
18.5 HYPOPIGMENTED LESIONS 223
18.6 VESICULOBULLOUS DISORDERS 224
18.7 ECZEMA 224
18.8 DISORDERS OF THE EPIDERMIS 225
18.9 DISORDERS OF THE DERMIS 226
18.10 DISORDERS OF SWEAT GLANDS 227
18.11 DISORDERS OF THE HAIR 227
18.12 SKIN INFECTIONS 227
18.13 MISCELLANEOUS SKIN DISEASE 229
QUESTIONS 231

19 EYE DISORDERS **237**
19.1 GENERAL CONCEPTS 237
19.2 DISEASE PROFILES 237
QUESTIONS 243

20 PEDIATRIC EMERGENCIES **247**
20.1 GENERAL CONCEPTS 247
20.2 SELECTED PEDIATRIC EMERGENCIES 251
QUESTIONS 254

21 CHILDHOOD POISONINGS **257**
21.1 GENERAL CONSIDERATIONS 257
21.2 DISEASE PROFILES 259
QUESTIONS 264

22 CHILD ABUSE AND NEGLECT **267**
22.1 GENERAL CONCEPTS 267
22.2 ABUSE CLASSIFICATION 267
QUESTIONS 272

INDEX **273**

User Guide

64. Infants with which of the following abnormalities on chromosome analysis have a cat-like cry

B
5.1.3

- **A.** 47,XX (13^{+})
- **B.** 46,XY (5 p^{-})
- **C.** 46,XX, 45,XO
- **D.** 47,XXY

65. All of the following conditions are associated with tri... ...quences except

- **A.** spinocerebellar ataxia
- **B.** Huntington's disease

Answer conveniently placed adjacent to the question!

Answers are cross-referenced to the relevant subchapter!

B
5.1.3

- **C.** a complete extra chromosome 21
- **D.** an absent chromosome 13

67. Color blindness occurs with what type of inherita...

Biotest ruler stores neatly on the inside front cover and is ideal for concealing answers during self-testing!

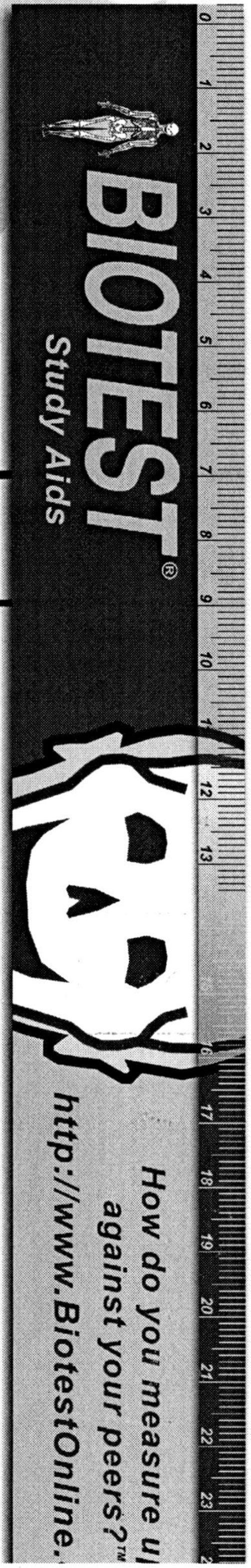

1 THE HEALTH MAINTENANCE VISIT

1.1 THE HEALTH SUPERVISION VISIT

1.1.1 Medical History

A. The pediatric interview is unique in that until the child is developmentally mature enough to actively participate in the process, the parents or guardians provide the majority of the historical information.

B. The interview should be conducted at every health supervision visit.

1. Obtain prenatal and birth history including events or maternal illnesses during pregnancy, prenatal drug, cigarette, or alcohol exposure, gestational age at birth, difficulties with delivery, and newborn nursery course.
2. Identify acute and/or chronic medical conditions including duration and attempted treatments.
3. Review the family history for evidence of heritable diseases.
4. Perform a complete review of systems. Inquire about sexual behavior, tobacco, drug, and alcohol use if age appropriate.
5. Investigate the social history including passive smoke exposure, daycare, school performance, and peer group interactions.
6. Record the parental observations of the child's developmental level.

C. The medical interview provides an opportunity to observe the parent-child interaction.

1.1.2 Physical Examination

A. **Growth Curve Measurements**. Height or length, weight, and head circumference (until 2 years old) should be measured and plotted on age and sex appropriate growth curves at each visit. Whether or not the child is following his growth curve is more important than any single measurement.

1. Height is recorded in inches or centimeters. It is measured as crown to heel length until the child is able to stand independently.
2. Weight should be recorded in kilograms to facilitate drug dosing if necessary. Infants are expected to double their birth weight by 4 to 5 months and triple by 1 year of age.
3. Head circumference is measured in centimeters at the level of the frontal and occipital bones. The head should grow 2 cm per month for the first 3 months, 1 cm per month from 3 to 6 months, then 0.5 cm per month until 1 year of age.

B. The physical exam additionally encompasses systematic inspection, palpation, and auscultation of all body systems.

C. Examination findings unique to the infant and young child.

1. **Anterior fontanelle.** This 2 by 2 cm structure generally closes between 9 and 18 months of age. Early closure implies premature fusion of cranial sutures or poor brain growth. Delayed closure or larger size than normal is associated with several conditions

Table 1.1.3 Developmental milestones

Age	Highlights of Developmental Milestones	Developmental Warning Signs
2 weeks	Lifts chin when prone Lies in a flexed position Fixates to close objects and light	Femoral click or hip instability (through 12 months) Undue maternal anxiety (true for all ages)
2 months	Smiles Coos Listens to voice Follows objects with eyes past midline Head steady while held sitting	Persistent heart murmur Absent response to noise Failure to fix gaze on face
4 months	Lifts head and chest from prone, holds vertically Rolls over front to back No head lag when pulled to sitting Reaches for object, brings to mouth Excited at sight of food Laughs out loud	Lack of bonding (a concern at any age) Nystagmus
6 months	Sits without support Transfers objects hand to hand Babbles Rolls over back to front	Failure to follow objects 180°

(continued)

Table 1.1.3 Developmental milestones (continued)

Age	Highlights of Developmental Milestones	Developmental Warning Signs
10 months	Crawls Pulls to stand and cruises Thumb and finger grasp Uncover hidden toy Voluntary release of object Says nonspecific "Mama" or "Dada" Plays peek-a-boo waves bye-bye	Absence of babble Unable to sit alone
12 months	Stands alone Walks alone or with one hand held Says specific "Mama" or "Dada" Three words in addition to "Mama" or "Dada" Fine pincer grasp Plays simple ball game	Unable to transfer objects hand to hand Absence of weight bearing while held
15 months	Walks backwards Crawls up stairs Inserts pellet into bottle Eats with a spoon Hugs parents	Unable to pull self to stand Abnormal grasp or pincer grip
18 months	Walks up stairs with one hand held Runs stiffly Dumps pellet from bottle Stacks four cubes Feeds self Knows 10 words Names pictures Kisses parents with pucker	Open anterior fontanel Inability to walk alone Absence of constructive play Lack of spontaneous vocalization
24 months	Runs well Walks up and down stairs one step at a time Opens doors Scribbles Combines three words into basic sentence structure Kicks a ball forward on request Listens to stories	Absence of recognizable words
3 years	Rides tricycle Briefly stands on one foot Alternates feet up stairs Builds bridge of 3 cubes Copies a circle Knows age and sex	Speech unintelligible to strangers
4 years	Hops on one foot Throws ball overhand Climbs well Copies cross and square Goes to toilet alone Cooperative play Tells a story	Inability to perform self-care tasks: hand washing, simple dressing, daytime toilet

(continued)

including hydrocephalus, hypothyroidism, rickets, achondroplasia, osteogenesis imperfecta, and numerous genetic syndromes.

2. **Posterior fontanelle**. This fingertip sized structure is present at birth in most infants but is usually no longer palpable after 6 weeks of age.
3. **Deciduous teeth**. Primary teeth have a predicted order and age of eruption. However, there is wide variability in what is considered normal teething sequence in individual children.
   - **a.** Lower central incisors erupt between 5 and 7 months and are shed at 6 to 7 years.
   - **b.** Upper central incisors erupt between 6 and 8 months and are shed at 7 to 8 years.
   - **c.** Lateral incisors erupt between 7 and 11 months and are shed at 7 to 9 years.
   - **d.** First molars erupt between 10 and 16 months and are shed at 10 to 12 years.
   - **e.** Cuspids (canines) erupt between 16 and 20 months and are shed at 9 to 11 years.
   - **f.** Second molars erupt between 20 and 30 months and are shed at 10 to 13 years.

1.1.3 Developmental Screening

A. The child's developmental level should be assessed by history and examination at each visit. The Denver II is a widely used formal screening tool for ages 0 to 6 years.

B. Table 1.1.3 is a summary of highlights in age appropriate developmental progression.

1.1.4 Cardiovascular Risk Screening

A. Blood Pressure (BP)

1. Measure BP routinely in children 3 years of age and older.
2. Compare result to age related norms.

B. Cholesterol Levels

1. Measure total cholesterol levels in children with a parental history of hypercholesterolemia >240 mg/dl.
   - **a.** Children with cholesterol levels <170 mg/dl require no intervention except retesting in 5 years.
   - **b.** In children with cholesterol levels >200 mg/dl perform a fasting lipid profile.
   - **c.** If the value is between 170 and 200 mg/dl, repeat the total cholesterol level. If the average value of the two tests is >170 mg/dl, perform a lipid profile.
2. Measure a lipid profile in children with a family history of premature (less than age 55 years) coronary artery disease in parents or grandparents.
3. Drawback. This screening protocol may miss greater than 50 percent of children with hypercholesterolemia.

1.1.5 Sensory Screening

A. Vision screening is subjective until the child is able to cooperate with standard mechanisms to measure visual acuity.

Table 1.1.3 Developmental milestones (continued)

Age	Highlights of Developmental Milestones	Developmental Warning Signs
5 years	Skips Copies a triangle Names 4 colors Counts 10 pennies Dresses and undresses Domestic role playing	Inability to distinguish colors or count Lack of organized complex play
Early school years	Is able to take formal tests to assess developmental level of achievement Concrete logical thinking predominates Puberty begins as early as 8 years in girls and 9 years in boys	School failure Aggressive behavior such as fire setting
Adolescence	Formal assessment tools can be used to quantitate level of functioning Transition to abstract thought Idealism Development of stable body image Cliques Dating Career decisions	School absenteeism or school failure Social isolation Distorted body image

1. The most important thing to be learned from anthropomorphic measurements at well child visits is — D 1.1.2

A. height
B. head size
C. weight compared to height
D. how well the child's measurements are following standard growth curves

2. Which of the following would make you suspect developmental delay — C 1.1.3

A. a 1-year-old child does not walk
B. a 6-month-old child does not sit alone
C. a 2-month-old child does not fixate or follow
D. a 4-month-old child does not transfer objects

3. The head circumference of a 5-month-old increases at what rate — B 1.1.2

A. 0.5 cm per month
B. 1 cm per month
C. 1.5 cm per month
D. 2 cm per month

4. Which of the following prompt more than routine screening — D 1.1.4 1.1.6 1.1.7

A. child lives with tuberculous parents
B. father with a history of heart attack at age 50 years
C. the child has been fed homogenized milk since 1 month of age
D. all of the above

5. A 20-month-old child has an open anterior fontanelle. What condition should you be worried about in this child — A 1.1.2

A. hypothyroidism
B. decreased brain growth
C. craniosynostosis
D. this is normal

6. A child can stand alone, says "mama" and "dada," and has a fine pincer grasp. What is his developmental age — C 1.1.3

A. 6 months
B. 10 months
C. 12 months
D. 15 months
E. 18 months

7. This child can ride a tricycle and build a bridge with 3 cubes. He knows how old he is. Do you? — B 1.1.3

A. 2 years
B. 3 years
C. 4 years
D. 5 years

8. The child with human immunodeficiency virus should not be vaccinated with which of the following agents — B 1.1.7

A. any live vaccine
B. varicella vaccine
C. measles-mumps-rubella vaccine
D. hepatitis B vaccine
E. diphtheria-tetanus-acellular pertussis vaccine

9. Which of the following is an absolute contraindication to vaccination with diphtheria-tetanus-acellular pertussis A 1.1.7

A. onset of encephalopathy within 7 days of a previous dose
B. seizures within 3 days of a previous dose
C. inconsolable crying associated with a previous dose
D. Guillain-Barré syndrome within 6 weeks of a previous dose

10. A 10-month-old child has an anaphylactic response to neomycin. Which vaccine should not be administered D 1.1.7

A. diphtheria-tetanus-pertussis vaccine
B. *Haemophilus influenzae* type b conjugate vaccine
C. hepatitis B vaccine
D. measles-mumps-rubella vaccine
E. hepatitis A vaccine

11. Who should receive annual skin testing for tuberculosis D 1.1.7

A. children exposed to residents of nursing homes
B. children whose parents immigrated from an area endemic for tuberculosis
C. children exposed to intravenous drug abusers
D. children with human immunodeficiency virus
E. all of the above

12. The infant who weighed 7 pounds at birth should weigh how much at 6 months of age C 1.1.2

A. 9 pounds
B. 10 pounds
C. 14 pounds
D. 21 pounds

2 THE NEWBORN

2.1 PRENATAL LIFE

2.1.1 Intrauterine Development – General Concepts

A. Normal gestation is 40 weeks.
   1. Infants born less than 37 weeks gestation are considered premature.
   2. Infants born greater than 42 weeks gestation are considered post-term.

B. The **embryonic phase** consists of the first 12 weeks of development postfertilization.
   1. Organogenesis occurs.
   2. Development occurs by hyperplasia (an increase in the number of cells).

C. The **fetal period** refers to the remainder of intrauterine life.
   1. This is the period of somatic growth and differentiation of organ systems.
   2. Early in fetal life, hyperplasia continues. However, growth in the second half of gestation is characterized by hypertrophy (an increase in individual cell size).

D. **Placental Function**
   1. Maintains the pregnant state by production of hormones.
   2. Selectively transfers nutrients and metabolic byproducts between the mother and the fetus. It does not prevent the passage of many bacteria, viruses, and drugs.
   3. Carries out the primary function of gas exchange.

E. **Fetal Respiration**
   1. The fetus begins making respiratory efforts during the first half of gestation.
   2. Alveolar development sufficient to maintain extrauterine respiration does not occur until approximately 24 weeks gestation, the age at which most providers consider the fetus viable with intensive care support.
   3. Surfactant, the substance that aids lung expansion and protects against atelectasis, is present as early as 20 weeks gestation. Adequate levels are usually not present until 35 weeks gestation.

2.2 BIRTH

2.2.1 Circulation

A. Prenatal Fetal Circulation
   1. Before birth, only 10% of fetal circulation perfuses the lungs.
   2. Oxygenated blood from the placenta flows to the right atrium via the inferior vena cava and then to both ventricles because the foramen ovale (an opening between the atria) is present.
      a. The left ventricle perfuses the brain and the heart.
      b. The right ventricle perfuses the lower body via the ductus arteriosus.
   3. Pressures are approximately equal in both sides of the circulatory system.

B. Normal Transition to Extrauterine Life
   1. Pulmonary blood flow increases 8- to 10-fold due to functional closure of the foramen ovale and the ductus arteriosus resulting in the circulatory flow pattern that will persist for the remainder of life.
   2. Left-sided circulatory pressure is higher than right-sided pressure, thus maintaining closure of the foramen ovale

2.2.2 Perinatal Complications

A. The greatest risk to the fetus is from interruption of fetal blood flow from the placenta. This can occur with umbilical cord compression or rupture, or with placental abruption with resultant hypoxemia and/or hypovolemia.

B. Maternal anesthesia may cause depression of newborn respiration.

C. Prolonged rupture of membranes (PROM) may predispose the infant to sepsis, as can maternal colonization with bacteria such as group B streptococcus or viruses such as herpes simplex virus (HSV).

2.2.3 Delivery Room Management

A. Prior to delivery, the newborn team assures availability of any equipment needed for resuscitation includ-

Table 2.2.3 Apgar score

Score	0	1	2
Appearance	blue, pale	body pink, acrocyanosis	no cyanosis
Pulse	absent	<100/minute	>100/minute
Grimace	no response	grimace	sneeze or cough
Activity	flaccid	weak flexion	strong flexion
Respiratory effort	absent	weak, irregular	strong, regular

ing an oxygen source, suction, a warming bed or warm towels and blankets, equipment for definitive airway management, medications, and personal protective gear.

B. In most cases, resuscitation proceeds easily. The infant requires only suctioning of the mouth, then the nose, drying, and warming.

C. Resuscitation efforts are assessed using the Apgar score shown in Table 2.2.3.
   1. Scores are assigned at minute of life 1 and 5. If the 5-minute Apgar score is less than 7, scores continue to be reported every 5 minutes until 2 consecutive scores are 7 or better.
   2. The Apgar score is determined by tabulating the points assigned for 5 activities.

2.2.4 Immediate Post-Resuscitation Management

A. Silver nitrate or erythromycin ointment is instilled into the eyes as prophylaxis for gonococcal ophthalmia neonatorum.

B. Intramuscular vitamin K is administered to facilitate the synthesis of coagulation factors to prevent hemorrhagic disease of the newborn.

C. Blood glucose is measured in infants with symptoms of hypoglycemia or risk factors for hypoglycemia, such as intrauterine distress or maternal diabetes. A blood glucose level below 40 mg/dl is considered hypoglycemia.

D. Additional activities are accomplished depending upon maternal history, intrapartum course, or newborn exam.
   1. Obtain blood type and Coombs status in infants born to mothers who are type O or Rh-.
   2. Infants who are small or large for gestational age may have polycythemia or hypocalcemia Therefore, a complete blood count (CBC) and calcium level are indicated.
   3. Infants of mothers with hepatitis B should receive hepatitis B immune globulin and their first hepatitis B vaccination in separate sites.
   4. Infants at risk for sepsis, such as when maternal intrapartum fever occurs, should have blood cultures drawn and may have urine and cerebrospinal fluid (CSF) collected as well, prior to initiation of antibiotic treatment.

E. The infant is presented to the mother as soon as possible to initiate infant-maternal bonding.

2.2.5 Neonatal Feeding

A. Breast-Feeding
   1. May begin in the delivery room.
   2. **Colostrum** is produced for the first 48 to 72 hours in a much lower volume than breast milk but is higher in protein content and contains immunologic factors.
   3. Mothers of premature infants who are unable to nurse may express breast milk which can be fed to their infants by gavage or bottle.
   4. Mothers who are human immunodeficiency virus (HIV) positive should not breast-feed due to the presence of viral particles in the breast milk. Other maternal viral infections such as hepatitis C are not considered absolute contraindications for breast-feeding.

B. Formula-Feeding
   1. The first feeding usually consists of sterile water. Thus infants with tracheoesophageal fistula or neurologic impairment of swallowing will demonstrate these abnormalities before a milk feeding. Formula is more irritating to lung tissue if aspirated.
   2. The average term infant will consume 30 to 60 ml of formula every 3 hours.

C. Feeding Facts
   1. The term infant requires 100 to 120 kcal/kg/day for normal growth.
   2. Infants usually lose weight during the first week of life. They should have regained this weight by 14 days of age.
   3. Failure of the infant to demand breast- or formula-feeds at regular intervals should prompt a search for sepsis, metabolic abnormalities, maternal prescribed and illicit drug effects, and nervous system abnormalities.

2.3 ABNORMAL CONDITIONS OF THE NEWBORN

2.3.1 Respiratory Distress

A. Respiratory distress is one of the most common problems encountered in the newborn infant.

B. Physical findings of respiratory distress include a sustained respiratory rate over 60 breaths-per-minute, nasal flaring, chest wall retractions, cyanosis, expiratory grunting, or persistent cough.

C. Common etiologies include:
   1. Respiratory disorders such as upper airway obstruction (choanal atresia, vocal cord paralysis), transient tachypnea of the newborn (TTN), neonatal respiratory distress syndrome (RDS), meconium aspiration, pneumonia, pneumothorax, pleural effusions, and structural lung abnormalities (hypoplasia, cystic adenomatoid malformation).
   2. Cardiac disorders such as hypoplastic left heart, aortic stenosis, coarctation of the aorta, cyanotic congenital heart disease (transposition of the great vessels, total anomalous pulmonary venous return, tricuspid atresia, truncus arteriosus, Tetralogy of Fallot).
   3. Miscellaneous conditions such as sepsis, hypothermia or hyperthermia, hypoglycemia, polycythemia, metabolic acidosis, neuromuscular diseases, phrenic nerve palsy, brain abnormalities, and diaphragmatic hernia.

2.3.2 Neonatal Seizures

A. General Considerations
   1. Neonatal seizures are not a single disease entity. Metabolic disorders, infection, hypoxemia, central nervous system (CNS) hemorrhage, and congenital CNS anomalies may all manifest with seizure activity.
   2. Neuronal development of the neonatal brain is incomplete, so generalized tonic-clonic seizures are difficult to generate. Therefore, they are the least common variant.
   3. Seizure activity may be associated with tachycardia and hypertension.
   4. Seizure activity cannot be suppressed by physical restraint.
   5. Telemetric electroencephalogram (EEG) monitoring may be useful in identifying seizure activity.

B. Types of Neonatal Seizures
   1. **Focal seizures** are unilateral rhythmic movements most commonly localized to the face or extremities and are associated with structural lesions, infection, and subarachnoid hemorrhage.
   2. **Myoclonic seizures** are brief jerking movements primarily of distal muscle groups that may be focal or generalized.
   3. **Tonic seizures** are associated with rigid posturing of the trunk and/or extremities. Eye deviation may be present as well.
   4. **Clonic seizures** are rhythmic motions of multiple muscle groups.
   5. Seizures may also be subtle, manifested by lip smacking, tongue thrusting, blinking, bicycling of extremities, apnea and/or color changes.

C. Evaluation
   1. A careful history, paying particular attention to prenatal drug use, injury, infection, perinatal fetal distress, and family history of neonatal seizures, syndromes, or childhood death, should be obtained.
   2. Physical examination should be performed looking for skin manifestations of neurocutaneous disorders, chorioretinitis seen in TORCH infection, along with a careful neurologic exam to define the extent of deficits. Note, **TORCH** is an acronym for toxoplasmosis, other agents, rubella, cytomegalovirus (CMV), and herpes simplex virus (HSV).
   3. Laboratory studies should include a lumbar puncture, serum electrolytes, serum glucose, magnesium, calcium, phosphate, and a urine drug screen if toxin exposure is suspected. If an inborn error of metabolism is suspected, serum ammonia, lactate, plasma amino acids, and both urine and plasma organic acids should also be drawn.
   4. Neuroimaging by computed tomography (CT) scan or magnetic resonance imaging (MRI) is indicated.

2.3.3 Hyaline Membrane Disease (HMD)

A. HMD occurs primarily in premature infants due to a deficiency of **pulmonary surfactant**, reduced number of alveoli, and increased chest wall compliance resulting in hypoxemia, hypercarbia, and acidosis.

B. Alternate terminology is RDS of the newborn.

C. Immature levels of pulmonary surfactant lead to alveolar atelectasis, hyaline membrane formation, and interstitial edema.

D. Prematurity, maternal diabetes, multiple gestations, cesarean section delivery, asphyxia, precipitous delivery, cold stress, and family history of other affected infants are recognized risk factors.

E. Previously described symptoms of respiratory distress occur. Affected infants may become apneic as well.

F. On physical examination, breath sounds may be normal or decreased. Crackles may be heard with inspiration.

G. Arterial blood gas reveals respiratory acidosis, or mixed respiratory and metabolic acidosis, and hypoxemia.

H. Differential diagnosis includes group B streptococcal sepsis, congenital pneumonia, TTN, and persistent fetal circulation with pulmonary hypertension.

I. Complications include pulmonary interstitial emphysema, pneumothorax, CNS hemorrhage, and bronchopulmonary dysplasia.

J. Diagnosis is based upon physical, laboratory, and radiologic findings. The classic finding on chest x-ray is the "ground glass" appearance of the lung fields.

K. RDS is treated by administration of pharmaceutical surfactant directly to the lungs, oxygen, and supportive care of other organ systems.

2.3.4. Neonatal Sepsis

A. Sepsis refers to bacteremia in conjunction with any of the following: apnea, cyanosis, hypotension, and disseminated intravascular coagulation (DIC).

B. Pathogens gain entry through breaches in the skin, umbilical cord, lungs, gastrointestinal, and urinary tracts, or via prenatal transfer across the placenta.
   1. Group B streptococcus is the most common causative agent.
   2. Gram negative bacteria such as *Escherichia coli* and *Klebsiella* species also cause disease.
   3. Enterococci species are frequent isolated pathogens.
   4. *Listeria monocytogenes* is less common than other bacterial species but causes overwhelming disease.

C. Neonates are relatively immune compromised.
   1. They have relative or absolute deficiencies of immune globulin.
   2. Neutrophil function is impaired and granulocytopenia may occur.

D. Low birth weight, maternal fever during labor, chorioamnionitis, prolonged rupture of membranes, congenital anomalies, immune deficiency disorders, galactosemia, male sex, and multiple gestation are known risk factors.

E. Symptoms vary from mild to severe and include temperature instability, poor feeding, apnea, respiratory distress, and irritability.

F. Physical examination reveals abnormalities related to specific organ dysfunction.

G. Laboratory findings include the presence or absence of pathogens on body fluid culture, elevated white blood cell (WBC) count or neutropenia, and a left-shift (elevated neutrophil and band counts) on manual differential.

H. Differential diagnosis includes RDS, hypothyroidism, drug withdrawal, cardiac disease, and infections of single organ systems.

I. Mortality rate varies from 10 to 70% based on etiology and severity at the time of diagnosis and may be due to shock-related end organ dysfunction.

J. Treatment with broad spectrum antibiotics should be initiated prior to laboratory confirmation of the causative agent. Ampicillin and either gentamicin or a 3rd generation cephalosporin are the drugs of choice. Double drug therapy is necessary as *Enterococcus* and *Listeria* are susceptible only to ampicillin in this treatment regimen.

2.3.5. Hyperbilirubinemia

A. Almost 50% of all newborn infants will develop clinically evident hyperbilirubinemia by the third day of life.
   1. Jaundice is usually detectable with a serum bilirubin of 7 mg/dl or greater.
   2. Approximately 3% of all newborns will have a serum bilirubin >15 mg/dl. Six to 7% will have levels over 13 mg/dl.
   3. Most neonatal jaundice is not considered pathologic.

B. General Concepts
   1. **Bilirubin** is produced primarily from the breakdown of red blood cell (RBC) hemoglobin.
   2. The newborn has a greater red cell mass with a 25% shorter life span than older children leading to increased bilirubin production.
   3. Most of the released bilirubin is bound to albumin. It is transported on albumin to the liver for conjugation by glucuronyl transferase. The newborn liver is not an efficient conjugator of bilirubin.
   4. After conjugation into a water soluble form, **conjugated (direct) bilirubin** is excreted into the bile.
   5. Gut bacteria would normally inhibit the reabsorption of bilirubin into the blood. However, the newborn gut is sterile, thus bilirubin reenters the blood stream via enterohepatic circulation.

C. **Physiologic Jaundice**
   1. All of the factors listed in the preceding section contribute to increased levels of serum bilirubin in the normal newborn infant.
   2. Normal infants have an **indirect (unconjugated) bilirubin** level less than 3 mg/dl at birth. Their serum bilirubin level increases at a rate of <5 mg/dl/24 hours and peaks by day of life 4. It decreases again to less than 2 mg/dl by 7 days of age.
   3. Risk factors for indirect hyperbilirubinemia include prematurity, race (Japanese, Korean, and Native American), family history of hyperbilirubinemia in siblings, maternal diabetes, altitude, polycythemia, bruising, cephalohematoma, dehydration, and delayed stooling. Greater numbers of risk factors imply a higher level of indirect bilirubinemia in an individual infant.

D. **Breast-feeding Associated Jaundice**
   1. Infants who are breast-fed may have higher levels of indirect hyperbilirubinemia in the first week of life attributed to decreased calorie and fluid intake.
   2. A small percentage of breast-fed infants will have elevations of indirect bilirubin as high as 30 mg/dl after the first week of life. This "**Breast Milk Jaundice**" is thought to be due to the presence of glucuronidase in some breast milk. Untreated, breast milk jaundice resolves slowly over a period of a few weeks. Cessation of breast-feeding results in rapid resolution, but is not routinely recommended or necessary.

E. **Pathologic (Nonphysiologic) Jaundice**
   1. Clinically evident jaundice present within the first 24 hours of life or appearing after the third day of life should be considered pathologic, as is jaundice that is prolonged for several weeks.
   2. A direct bilirubin level that is greater than 20% of the total bilirubin level is abnormal and warrants investigation of hepatic function.
   3. ABO and Rh incompatibility can result in a Coombs positive hyperbilirubinemia.
   4. Other common causes of pathologic jaundice include sepsis, single site infection (specifically, urinary tract infections), polycythemia, congenital hepatitis, congenital infection, galactosemia, spherocytosis or other heritable conditions associated with increased RBC turnover such as glucose-6-phosphate dehydrogenase (G6PD), maternal diabetes, enclosed hemorrhage, prematurity, and hypothyroidism.

F. Laboratory Investigations
   1. Total serum bilirubin is elevated with >80% being unconjugated (indirect) bilirubin.
   2. If pathologic jaundice is suspected, a CBC with reticulocyte count and Coombs test should be obtained to rule out a hemolytic process. Examine a peripheral smear for abnormal RBC cell types.
      a. The hematocrit on the CBC can identify poly-

cythemia or anemia secondary to hemolysis, hemorrhage, or red cell defects.
   b. The reticulocyte count may be elevated in the presence of hemolysis.
3. If sepsis is suspected, obtain appropriate cultures.
4. A urine reducing substance determination may be positive in galactosemia.
5. Additional testing may be based upon the suspected diagnosis in an individual patient.

G. Treatment – **Phototherapy**
1. Term infants with bilirubin levels peaking at 20 mg/dl on day 3 of life usually do not need medical treatment.
2. Phototherapy involves exposure of the infant to blue or cool white light (420 to 470 nm range is most effective). This causes reversible photoisomerization of unconjugated bilirubin in the skin tissue to a nontoxic isomer form that is more readily excreted in the bile. An irreversible reaction resulting in lumirubin also occurs. Lumirubin is excreted through the kidneys.
3. Complications of phototherapy include diarrhea, rashes, hyperthermia, hypothermia, dehydration, and bronze baby syndrome (grayish-brown skin discoloration).
4. The infants eyes must be occluded to protect them from the light.

H. Treatment – **Exchange Transfusion**
1. This procedure is reserved for infants with potentially toxic levels of serum bilirubin.
2. It can correct anemia and lowers the serum bilirubin to approximately one-half the pre-exchange level.
3. It usually requires placement of both an umbilical artery and umbilical vein catheter.
4. A single exchange replaces 72% of the blood volume, while a double exchange replaces 87% by infusing fresh blood and removing the infant's blood in small aliquots.
5. Complications include electrolyte and serum calcium abnormalities, hypervolemia, hypovolemia, coagulation defects, exposure to infection through blood products, and complications of umbilical line placement.

I. Special Considerations – **Kernicterus**
1. Kernicterus is a disease characterized by the presence of marked jaundice with bilirubin deposition in the basal ganglia, globus pallidus, putamen, and caudate nuclei of the brain.
2. Infants present with jaundice, hypotonia, vomiting, poor feeding, and a high pitched cry.
3. The disease may progress to include seizures, fever, rigidity, opisthotonos, and paralysis of upward gaze, then death.
4. Survivors develop spasticity, athetosis, deafness, mental retardation, and paralysis of upward gaze.
5. Historically, this disease was seen most frequently in infants with Rh- incompatibility induced hemolysis (erythroblastosis fetalis). It can be seen in any condition that results in significant indirect hyperbilirubinemia (generally >25 mg/dl).

2.3.6 Hypoglycemia

A. Hypoglycemia in a newborn less than 24 hours old is defined as a serum glucose level less than 40 mg/dl.

B. Hypoglycemia may have multiple etiologies.
1. Hyperinsulinemia lowers serum glucose levels and may be due to maternal diabetes with poor glucose homeostasis, exchange transfusion, pancreatic islet cell hyperplasia, Beckwith-Wiedemann syndrome, insulin producing tumors, or maternal drug therapy with sympathomimetics or chlorpropamide.
2. Decreased glucose stores due to prematurity or intrauterine growth retardation (IUGR) are common causes.
3. Disorders of metabolism such as galactosemia, adrenal insufficiency, hypopituitarism, shock, asphyxia, and hypothermia lower serum glucose, as do sepsis and polycythemia (RBC's are capable of glycolysis).

C. The infant may be asymptomatic or may have irritability, lethargy, tremulousness, apnea, cyanosis, weakness, hypotonia, or seizures as manifestations.

D. Early and frequent screening of heel stick glucose measurements are indicated for any symptomatic or "at risk" infant.

E. Complications include permanent neurologic injury or death.

F. Treatment includes early feeding of at risk infants or rapid intravenous infusion of 2 to 3 ml per kg of 10% dextrose solution followed by a continuous glucose infusion calculated to provide a glucose infusion rate of 7 mg/kg/minute.

2.3.7 Galactosemia

A. Galactosemia occurs in 1 out of 60,000 live births.

B. Classic disease is due to a deficiency in the enzyme **galactose-1-phosphate uridyl transferase**, resulting in elevated concentrations of galactose in the blood, urine, and body tissues. **Galactokinase**, which phosphorylates galactose, and uridine diphosphate galactose 4-epimerase may also be deficient, resulting in galactosemia.

C. Symptoms include vomiting, hypoglycemia, lethargy, poor feeding, poor weight gain, and convulsions.

D. The infant may have hepatosplenomegaly, jaundice, cataracts, and ascites on exam.

E. Laboratory studies reveal positive urine reducing substance, elevated serum galactose, and deficient galactose-1-phosphate uridyl transferase activity in RBC hemolysates.

F. Since breast milk and standard formula preparations may contain significant amounts of lactose (glucose-galactose), treatment involves feeding with a non-lactose containing formula at an early age.

G. Complications include hepatic cirrhosis, cataracts, and mental retardation if the condition is not treated. Infants are also at a higher risk for *Escherichia coli* sepsis. Because mothers may be heterozygous for the condition, some injury may be apparent at birth due to transplacental passage of galactose.

2.3.8 Necrotizing Enterocolitis (NEC)

A. NEC is necrosis of the bowel wall seen primarily in premature infants. It usually occurs in the first two weeks of life, but can be seen in infants up to 2 months of age.

B. The etiology of NEC is unclear.

1. Prematurity, polycythemia, early enteral feeding, and shock predispose infants to this condition.
2. Any other condition that is associated with hypoperfusion of the intestinal tract such as sepsis, perinatal asphyxia, or hemorrhagic shock is also a risk factor.
3. Clustering of cases of NEC suggests a potential infectious etiology.

C. The distal ileum and proximal colon are the sites most often involved with varying degrees of mucosal and transmural necrosis. Gas accumulates in the submucosa which may be visible on plain x-ray (**pneumatosis intestinalis**). Perforation of the bowel wall may occur.

D. The symptoms of NEC are abdominal distention, emesis or delayed gastric emptying, apnea, shock, and stools with either occult or frank blood.

E. Findings on physical exam vary with the severity of illness.

1. The most common early symptom is abdominal distention. Bowel sounds may be absent and evacuation of the stomach may reveal retained feedings.
2. As the disease progresses, the infant may develop apnea and show signs of poor perfusion progressing to shock.

F. Laboratory findings reveal metabolic acidosis, hypoxemia, and hypercapnia. A CBC may show leukocytosis or leukopenia as well as thrombocytopenia.

G. Radiologic Examination

1. Bowel wall thickening with dilated bowel loops are early findings.
2. If present, pneumatosis intestinalis is diagnostic.
3. Air may be visible in the portal vein or biliary tree and is a poor prognostic indicator.
4. Free air may be seen in the abdomen if perforation has occurred.

H. Differential diagnosis includes sepsis, intestinal obstruction, and volvulus.

I. Complications include peritonitis, perforation, sepsis, shock, intestinal stricture, and short gut syndrome. Death occurs in 5% of affected infants.

J. Therapy

1. Feeds should be discontinued if NEC is suspected.
2. Provide vigorous fluid resuscitation if shock is present.
3. Cultures of blood, stool, and CSF should be obtained.
4. Antibiotic therapy with an anti-pseudomonal penicillin, aminoglycoside, and clindamycin should be started.
5. Fluids and hyperalimentation should be instituted early to maintain adequate nutrition and fluid balance.
6. If the infant is seriously ill or apneic, intubate.
7. Monitoring of serial blood gases, serum electrolytes, and CBC's is essential, correcting abnormalities as they are identified.

2.3.9 Hemorrhagic Disease of the Newborn

A. This is a condition characterized by life threatening hemorrhage primarily in the intestinal tract, nares, scalp, and central nervous system. It occurs usually in the first week of life.

B. The etiology is due to a transient decrease in the levels of the vitamin K-dependent clotting factors II, VII, IX, and X in the presence of vitamin K deficiency.

1. Infants do not receive vitamin K by the transplacental route due to lack of free vitamin K in the mother.
2. Infants do not have the intestinal bacterial flora necessary for the synthesis of vitamin K.
3. The clotting factor levels generally return to normal by 7 to 10 days of age.
4. Late presentations, beyond 1 week of age, can occur with vitamin K malabsorption from the intestinal tract. Neonatal hepatitis and biliary atresia are examples of conditions associated with vitamin K malabsorption.
5. Infant boys who undergo circumcision may develop hemodynamically significant post procedural bleeding.

C. Predisposing conditions include:

1. Prematurity.
2. Maternal use of phenobarbital or phenytoin which interferes with vitamin K function.
3. Breast-feeding, as breast milk is a poor source of vitamin K.
4. Home births when vitamin K prophylaxis is not provided.

D. Laboratory studies show decreased levels of vitamin

K-dependent clotting factors and prolonged prothrombin, partial thromboplastin, and bleeding times.

E. The differential diagnosis includes factor VIII and factor IX deficiency, DIC, and ingested maternal blood (when blood is noted in the gastrointestinal tract).

F. The complications of the condition are hypovolemic hemorrhagic shock, intracranial hemorrhage, and death.

G. Therapy

1. Prophylactic administration of 1 mg of vitamin K intramuscularly at birth prevents the natural transient decrease of vitamin K-dependent cofactors.
2. Premature infants or infants born to mothers treated with phenytoin or phenobarbital, if symptomatic, may require continuous intravenous infusion of vitamin K. They can also be treated by transfusion with fresh frozen plasma or whole blood.

2.3.10 Neonatal Hepatitis

A. This is a disorder of multiple etiologies that presents as hepatic inflammation.

B. Etiology

1. Common causes are congenitally acquired hepatitis B, CMV, syphilis, toxoplasmosis, HIV, neonatal sepsis, HSV infection, and indirect hyperbilirubinemia.
2. Hepatitis A, D, and E rarely cause transplacentally acquired hepatitis.
3. Perinatal transmission is rare with hepatitis C but is increased in infants of mothers with HIV infection or mothers with high titers of hepatitis C virus.

C. Symptomatic infants can present with vomiting, poor feeding, jaundice, or signs of disseminated infection with HSV, syphilis, HIV, or toxoplasmosis.

D. Physical examination reveals jaundice, hepatomegaly, and alteration of consciousness.

E. Laboratory findings include elevated hepatic enzyme levels, elevated serum bilirubin, and with severe hepatic dysfunction, elevated serum ammonia and decreased levels of coagulation factors.

F. The differential diagnosis is biliary atresia, cystic fibrosis, galactosemia, tyrosinosis, α_1-antitrypsin deficiency, choledochal cyst, drug exposure, and disorders of bile acid metabolism.

G. Hepatic cirrhosis, hepatocellular carcinoma, development of a carrier state, shock, and death are recognized complications.

H. Prevention and Treatment

1. Routine prenatal care for expectant mothers may help prevent some cases of hepatitis.
   a. Maternal hepatitis B surface antigen (HBsAg) status should be determined during pregnancy, as should HIV if allowed, so that the infant can receive prophylactic therapy for these conditions.
   b. Infants of mothers who are HBsAg positive should receive hepatitis B immune globulin and the first in a series of hepatitis B vaccinations at separate sites of the body within 12 hours of birth.
   c. Mothers infected with HIV can be treated with zidovudine (ZDV) to help prevent intrauterine transmission of the virus.
   d. Infants of HIV positive mothers should undergo serial blood testing for viral load and be treated with ZDV for 6 weeks if their mothers did not receive prenatal ZDV. These infants should take sulfamethoxazole plus trimethoprim for *Pneumocystis carinii* prophylaxis once they turn 6-weeks-old until they are confirmed negative for HIV.
2. Famciclovir and foscarnet can be used to treat CMV.
3. Acyclovir is used to treat HSV and varicella viruses.

13. A young Asian woman presented to the hospital in labor. On her last prenatal checkup, she had a positive test for hepatitis B surface antigen. How will you treat her baby — A 2.2.4

A. hepatitis B immune globulin and hepatitis B vaccine at separate sites within 12 hours of birth
B. hepatitis B vaccine at 2 months of age
C. hepatitis B immune globulin at birth with hepatitis B vaccine at 1 month of age
D. hepatitis B immune globulin and hepatitis B vaccine at 2 months of age
E. none of the above

14. Most full-term infants will regain their birthweight by what age — C 2.2.5

A. 48 hours
B. 4 days
C. 14 days
D. 30 days

15. You attend the delivery of a newborn. At one minute of life, his pulse is 60, he has no respiratory effort, he is cyanotic, flaccid, and does not respond to suctioning. What is his Apgar score — B 2.2.3

A. 0
B. 1
C. 2
D. 3
E. 4

16. An infant has a one minute Apgar score of 1. At 5 minutes, he has acrocyanosis, a heart rate of 120, decreased flexor tone, a good cry, and grimaces with nasal suctioning. His Apgar score is now — B 2.2.3

A. 7
B. 8
C. 9
D. 10

17. Each of the following statements about breast-feeding is true except — C 2.2.5

A. breast-feeding can be initiated in the delivery room for healthy full-term infants
B. colostrum is present in the breasts for 2 to 3 days and is nutritionally complete
C. mothers with human immunodeficiency virus may breast-feed, as there is a low likelihood that the disease will be transmitted to the infant
D. mothers of premature infants may express breast milk to be fed to their infants by gavage

18. Each of the following suggests respiratory distress in the newborn except — B 2.3.1

A. nasal flaring
B. respiratory rate of 46
C. cyanosis
D. persistent cough
E. intercostal space retractions

19. A term infant weighed 3.2 kg and was delivered vaginally by low forceps after 28 hours of labor. She is now 1-day-old and her nurse reports to you that she has a rectal temperature of 35.9° C and is not feeding well. You elect to — C 2.3.4

A. have the nurse recheck her temperature and feeding effort in an hour
B. examine the baby and reassure the nurse that she is "fine"
C. perform a sepsis work-up and start antibiotics pending results
D. send the infant out to her mother for the night

20. Which of the following is associated with neonatal seizures — E 2.3.2

A. sepsis
B. hypoglycemia
C. maternal drug use
D. family history of neonatal seizures
E. all of the above

21. Respiratory distress syndrome of the newborn is caused by — D 2.3.3

A. respiratory acidosis
B. poor chest wall compliance
C. increased alveoli
D. deficient surfactant
E. interstitial emphysema

22. The most common causative agent for neonatal sepsis is — A 2.3.4

A. group B streptococcus
B. *Escherichia coli*
C. group A β-hemolytic streptococcus
D. enterococcus
E. *Listeria*

23. Risk factors for neonatal sepsis include — D 2.3.4

A. relative deficiency of immunoglobulins
B. low birthweight
C. maternal fever
D. all of the above
E. A and C

24. Jaundice is clinically detectable on visual exam at what serum level — C 2.3.5

A. 3 mg/dl
B. 5 mg/dl
C. 7 mg/dl
D. 9 mg/dl

25. What factor predisposes the newborn to jaundice — A 2.3.5

A. greater red blood cell mass
B. red blood cell life span is greater than that of older children
C. bilirubin is poorly bound to albumin, limiting processing by the liver
D. gut bacteria promote reabsorption of excreted bilirubin

26. How much of the fetal circulated blood volume perfuses the fetal lungs — A 2.2.1

A. 10%
B. 20%
C. 5%
D. 15%

27. An infant presents with a bilirubin level >30 mg/dl, irritability, vomiting, and seizures. He dies within 2 days of admission. The finding on autopsy that supports the diagnosis of kernicterus is — D 2.3.5

A. jaundice of the skin
B. normal hematocrit for age
C. muscle flaccidity
D. staining of the basal ganglia by bilirubin
E. evidence of hepatitis

28. All of the following statements regarding physiologic jaundice are true except — A, 2.3.5

A. it is generally evident within the first 24 hours of life
B. bilirubin levels peak on the fourth day of life
C. affected infants may have a family history of jaundice in older siblings
D. bilirubin levels increase at a rate of <5 mg/dl/24 hours
E. infants may have a cephalohematoma

29. Signs of hypoglycemia in the newborn include all of the following except — B, 2.3.6

A. normal exam
B. heel stick glucose of 50 mg/dl
C. seizures
D. irritability
E. hypotonia

30. Infant's with galactosemia are at risk for — E, 2.3.7

A. *E. coli* sepsis
B. hypoglycemia
C. hepatic cirrhosis
D. mental retardation
E. all of the above

31. In an infant with necrotizing enterocolitis, the indicator with the worst prognosis is — C, 2.3.8

A. abdominal distention
B. acidosis
C. air within the biliary tree
D. leukopenia
E. bowel wall thickening

32. Which of the following clotting factors transiently decrease in the newborn who does not receive prophylactic vitamin K — B, 2.3.9

A. II, V, VII, IX
B. II, VII, IX, X
C. V, VII, IX, XII
D. V, VII, IX, X

3 ADOLESCENT DISORDERS

3.1 ADOLESCENT MEDICINE

3.1.1 General Considerations

A. Adolescents are not a homogenous group.

B. "**Adolescence**" is a period of life beginning with puberty and terminating with cessation of somatic growth.

C. It is also a biopsychosocial process that may begin before puberty and extend well beyond the end of somatic growth, in which case, it is culturally defined.

3.1.2 Developmental Considerations

A. Physical Development

1. **Puberty** is the period during which secondary sex characteristics begin to develop.
2. Hypothalamic-pituitary changes include:
   - **a.** Nocturnal sleep-related augmentation of pulsatile leuteinizing hormone (LH) secretion secondary to an increase in pulsatile gonadotropin-releasing hormone (GnRH) release.
   - **b.** Decrease in hypothalamic and pituitary sensitivity to estradiol and testosterone.
   - **c.** Increase in LH and follicle-stimulating hormone (FSH).
   - **d.** In females, the development of a positive ovulation feedback system: increases in estrogen lead to increased GnRH which in turn leads to LH secretion and subsequently ovulation.
3. Adrenal Gland Changes: increased secretion of sex hormones occurs. However, these are not necessary for development of secondary sex characteristics.
4. Insulin secretion, plasma somatomedin C levels, and growth hormone-releasing hormone (GHRH) also rise in puberty.

B. Pubertal Developmental Highlights

1. Female
   - **a.** Puberty starts between 8 and 13 years and lasts for 3 to 4 years.
   - **b.** **Breast development** typically precedes pubic hair development.
   - **c.** Adult height is reached in mid-puberty.
2. Male
   - **a.** Puberty begins between ages 9.5 and 13.5 years with a duration of 3 years.
   - **b.** **Testicular enlargement** is the first change.
   - **c.** Adult height is reached in the latter half of puberty.

C. Sexual Maturity Rating (Tanner) Stages

1. Female Breast Development
   - **a.** Stage I – No glandular tissue and the areola conforms to the chest line.
   - **b.** Stage II – Breast bud forms and the areola widens and elevates.
   - **c.** Stage III – Continued enlargement of the breast bud with further elevation and enlargement of the areola. There is no separation in breast contours.
   - **d.** Stage IV – Areola and papilla form a mound projecting from the breast contour.
   - **e.** Stage V – Breast is adult size with the areola and breast in the same plane and the papilla (nipple) projecting above the areola.
2. Male Genitalia Development
   - **a.** Stage I – Prepubertal with testes <1.5 cc in volume.
   - **b.** Stage II – Testes enlarge. The scrotum is larger with skin that is thinner and reddish in color.
   - **c.** Stage III – Testes and scrotum continue to grow. Penile length increases.
   - **d.** Stage IV – Testes and scrotum continue to grow. The scrotum darkens. The penis grows in width and length and the glans develops.
   - **e.** Stage V – Testes, scrotum, and penis are adult size and shape.
3. Male and Female Pubic Hair Development
   - **a.** Stage I – No pubic hair.
   - **b.** Stage II – Small amount of long, slightly pigmented hair along the base of the scrotum and penis in the male or the labia majora in females.
   - **c.** Stage III – Moderate amount of more curly, pigmented and coarser hair that begins to spread laterally and over the mons pubis.
   - **d.** Stage IV – Resembles adult hair in coarseness and curliness. Does not extend over medial surface of thighs.
   - **e.** Stage V – Adult type and quantity of pubic hair extending to medial thigh and in 80% of males, along the linea alba.
4. Height Growth
   - **a.** Pubertal growth accounts for 25% of final adult height.
   - **b.** Timing of the growth spurt is highly variable and usually lasts 24 to 36 months.
   - **c.** Peak height velocity occurs 18 to 24 months earlier in females than males and averages 2 cm/year less than in males.
5. Weight Gain
   - **a.** Pubertal weight gain accounts for 50% of an individuals ideal adult body weight.
   - **b.** Peak weight and height velocities coincide in males.

3.1.3 Psychosocial Development

A. General tasks of Adolescence (Table 3.1.3)

1. Achieve independence from parents.
2. Adopt peer codes and lifestyles.
3. Assign increased importance to body image and accept one's own body image.
4. Establish sexual, ego, vocational, and moral identities.

3.2 MENSTRUAL DISORDERS

3.2.1 Amenorrhea

A. **Primary Amenorrhea** is the lack of episodes of spontaneous uterine bleeding by 14 to 16 years of age with absent secondary sexual characteristics, or by 16 to 18 years of age when normal secondary sexual characteristics are present.
   1. Evaluation is directed toward determination of pubertal maturation and the presence or absence of internal genitalia.
   2. A bimanual pelvic exam or ultrasound should be done to establish the presence or absence of a uterus and ovaries. The results can then be used to focus on a cause of the amenorrhea as depicted in Table 3.2.1.

B. **Secondary Amenorrhea.** After previous uterine bleeding, there is no subsequent menses for 6 months or a length of time equal to 3 previous normal cycles.
   1. Always consider pregnancy as a cause even if the history given does not suggest the diagnosis. Once pregnancy has been ruled out, the evaluation focuses on the hypothalamic-pituitary-ovarian axis.
   2. Evaluate for the presence of hypothyroidism and hyperprolactinemia.
   3. If hirsutism is present, check testosterone and dehydroepiandrosterone (DHEA) levels.
      a. If testosterone and DHEA are elevated, rule out adrenal hyperplasia or tumor.
      b. If levels are normal, consider a progesterone challenge
   4. Progesterone Challenge
      a. Menses should occur if the endometrium is estrogen primed. If menses is the result and other laboratory studies are normal, the adolescent is anovulatory.
      b. If withdrawal bleeding does not occur, cycle with estrogen and progestin.
         (1). If bleeding still does not occur, refer to a gynecologist for evaluation for uterine synechia.
         (2). If withdrawal bleeding occurs, perform an LH and FSH assay.
            (a). If levels are high, the adolescent has ovarian failure and treatment consists of cycling with estrogen and progesterone. These patients are generally sterile.
            (b). If levels are normal or low, perform a brain scan via computed tomography (CT) or magnetic resonance imaging (MRI) to rule out a central nervous system (CNS) lesion. If no lesion is present, the patient has hypothalamic amenorrhea and should be cycled with oral contraceptive pill's (OCP's). If the study is

Table 3.1.3 Tasks to be accomplished at each stage of adolescence

Task	Early Adolescence	Mid-Adolescence	Late Adolescence
Independence	Less interest in parental activities	Conflict with parents peaks	Reacceptance of parental values
Body image	Preoccupation with self and pubertal changes	General acceptance of body	Acceptance of pubertal changes
Peers	Intense relationships with same-sex friends Conformity to peer group values	Peak peer group involvement More time spent in sharing intimate relationships	Peer group less important Increased sexual activity and experimentation
Identity	Increased ability to reason abstractly Increased need for privacy Idealistic Test authority	Increased scope of feelings Increased creative and intellectual activities Feelings of omnipotence and immortality	Rational and realistic conscience Sense of perspective Ability to delay, set limits Practical vocational goals Refinement of moral, religious and sexual values

abnormal, refer for definitive treatment of the lesion.

3.2.2 Dysmenorrhea

A. Painful menstruation is the most common gynecologic problem in adolescence occurring in 75% of menstruating women.

B. **Primary dysmenorrhea** occurs without identifiable pelvic pathology. The symptoms can be explained by the action of uterine prostaglandins ($PGF_{2\alpha}$, $PGE_{2\alpha}$, and cyclic endoperoxidases).

C. Treatment of Primary Dysmenorrhea
1. Oral contraceptives reduce growth of endometrium and therefore decrease uterine prostaglandin production.
2. Prostaglandin inhibitors block production of prostaglandins. Examples include naproxen and ibuprofen.

D. **Secondary Dysmenorrhea**
1. This is pain from malformation, endometriosis, infection, or uterine fibroids.
2. Abnormal uterine position or shape suggests a uterine malformation since fibroids are rare in adolescents.
3. Treatment is by correction of the underlying pathology if possible, OCP's, or prostaglandin inhibitors.

3.2.3 Dysfunctional Uterine Bleeding (DUB)

A. DUB is abnormal endometrial bleeding in the absence of structural pelvic pathology. It is usually associated with anovulation.

B. Estrogen stimulation of the endometrium by corpus luteal progesterone causes overgrowth of the endometrium with patchy desquamation and sloughing.

C. The approach to the adolescent with DUB should include queries regarding a family history of bleeding disorders, a personal history of easy bleeding or bruising, contraceptive use including intrauterine device

Table 3.2.1 Primary amenorrhea

	UTERUS ABSENT	**UTERUS PRESENT**
BREASTS ABSENT	Conclusion: Genetic males; gonads produce Müllerian-inhibiting substance but do not produce enough testosterone to induce normal male internal and external genitalia. Karyotype (XY): Gonadal enzyme deficiency Agonadism	Conclusion: Lack of ovarian estrogen production. Müllerian system developed normally. FSH low: Hypogonadotropic hypogonadism Central nervous system lesion Kallmann syndrome Pituitary gonadotropin deficiencies (chronic disease, anorexia nervosa) FSH high: Gonadal dysgenesis 45,XO (Turner syndrome) Other X chromosome variants Pure XX or XY dysgenesis Gonadal enzyme deficiency
BREASTS PRESENT	Conclusion: Genetic male with androgen insensitivity or genetic female with uterine agenesis. Karyotype: Female (XX) Müllerian agenesis or hypoplasia Mayer-Rokitansky-Küster-Hauser syndrome Male (XY) Androgen insensitivity (testicular feminization)	Conclusion: Normal phenotypic female with normal Müllerian and pubertal development. Absent menses is due to outlet obstruction or lack of endometrial development and shedding. Cyclic pain present: Vaginal obstruction Imperforate hymen Transverse vaginal septum Cyclic pain absent: Hypothalamic-pituitary-ovarian axis disturbance (evaluate as secondary amenorrhea)

(IUD), sexual history, and possibility of pregnancy.

D. Immediate goal during exam is to assess hemodynamic stability and identify the site of bleeding.

E. Laboratory evaluation includes a complete blood count (CBC), pregnancy test, wet prep of vaginal discharge, cervical cultures for gonorrhea and chlamydia, thyroid studies, liver enzymes, and clotting studies if indicated.

F. The differential diagnosis is extensive and includes:

1. Complications of pregnancy such as ectopic pregnancy, abortion, or placental polyp.
2. Infections such as pelvic inflammatory disease (PID), endometritis, vaginitis, or cervicitis.
3. Cervical or endometrial cancers.
4. Vaginal pathology including polyps, foreign body, or trauma.
5. Polycystic ovarian syndrome or ovarian tumors.
6. Iatrogenic bleeding from IUD's, OCP's, or some tranquilizers.
7. Blood dyscrasias, hepatic cirrhosis, or endocrine dysfunction.

G. Management is based on the severity of bleeding.

1. Mild, inconvenient, and unpredictable bleeding with a normal hemoglobin (Hgb) can be treated with reassurance, a menstrual calendar, and/or OCP's. Reevaluate in 3 months.
2. Moderate, irregular, prolonged, heavy bleeding, or bleeding with mild anemia (Hgb >10 mg/dl) should be treated with iron supplementation, a menstrual calendar, and medroxyprogesterone acetate or OCP's. Reevaluate in 1 to 3 months.
3. Severe bleeding associated with anemia (Hgb <10 mg/dl).
   - **a.** If not actively bleeding, provide iron supplementation and OCP's with reevaluation every 1 to 3 months.
   - **b.** If actively bleeding, hospitalize for intravenous therapy with conjugated estrogens, oral norgestrel, and transfusion if needed. OCP's should be continued on an outpatient basis for 6 to 12 months. If bleeding continues, refer to a gynecologist for dilatation and curettage. Reevaluate monthly.

3.3 BREAST DISORDERS

3.3.1 Asymmetry

A. Initial breast development may be asymmetric.

B. Asymmetry may be due to congenital absence of breast tissue or pectoral muscles, rib defects, or iatrogenic causes such as scarring from chest wall procedures performed in infancy or childhood.

C. After puberty, when growth is finished to allow for full development and equalization, surgery can be performed to repair the defect.

3.3.2 Accessory Breast Tissue

A. This is the most common breast anomaly, occurring in 1 to 2% of females.

B. The tissue is usually located on the fetal nipple line, most commonly below the normal breast on the chest or upper abdomen.

3.3.3 Breast Masses

A. **Fibroadenomas** are benign neoplasms of the mammary gland.

1. They are the most common breast lesion (76 to 90% of benign lesions) in early and middle adolescent females.
2. They are firm, smooth, discrete, mobile masses, usually located on the lateral portion of the breast.
3. They generally are less than 5 cm in diameter.
4. In 10 to 15% of adolescents with this condition, the lesions are multiple.

B. **Fibrocystic Disease** (FD)/change

1. FD is proliferation of stromal and epithelial elements of breast tissue with subsequent ductal dilatation and cyst formation occurring in many individuals.
2. These changes are induced by excess estrogen in relation to progesterone. Some studies implicate methylxanthines in this process.
3. Fibrocystic changes can result in tenderness that is increased in the late menstrual cycle.
4. The cysts are small, bilateral, firm, and mobile.
5. Breast nodules are hard and painful to palpation and may be up to 1 cm in size.

C. Management of Breast Masses in Adolescents

1. Reassure the adolescent that the lesion is most likely benign.
2. If a breast mass feels cystic, aspiration can be done.
3. Consider surgical removal of solid masses greater than 2 to 3 cm in diameter.
4. Observe most masses for at least 2 to 3 months before intervention. Resolution may occur following a menstrual cycle.
5. Mammography is not helpful in most cases.
6. Never biopsy or excise a possible breast bud.

D. **Gynecomastia** is excessive development of male mammary glands.

1. The etiology is unknown but is possibly due to an increase in biologically active estrogen or increased sensitivity to estrogen.
2. Ductal proliferation and lobule formation or stromal changes with fibrosis are the pathologic findings.
3. An affected adolescent may have tenderness on palpation of the affected breast.
4. Peak incidence is 64% at 14 years of age.
5. Classification System
   - **a.** Type I – One or more freely mobile subareolar nodules.

b. Type II – Breast nodules beneath the areola and extending beyond the areolar perimeter.
c. Type III – Resembles the breast development in sexual maturity rating (Tanner) stage 3 females.

6. On exam, look for signs suggestive of hypogonadism, thyroid dysfunction, or liver disease, as well as the presence of testicular masses or atrophy.
7. Differential Diagnosis. Gynecomastia may be caused by drug exposure (estrogen, testosterone, anabolic steroids, phenothiazines, digoxin, tricyclics, phenytoin), renal failure, liver disease, recovery from malnutrition, endocrine disease (hyperthyroidism, hypothyroidism, hypergonadotropic hypogonadism — i.e. Klinefelter's syndrome), tumors (testicular, bronchogenic, pituitary, adrenal, Hodgkin lymphoma, hepatoma), and pseudogynecomastia secondary to adipose tissue in obese males or increased muscle tissue in athletes.
8. Diagnostic Plan
   a. In healthy pubertal males with normal growth, no tests are indicated.
   b. If gynecomastia occurs before the onset or after the completion of puberty, consider performing a karyotype, chorionic gonadotropin (hCG) level (may be increased in various carcinomas), serum estradiol (feminizing adrenal tumors), prolactin level, thyroid or liver function tests, chest x-ray to rule out pulmonary tumors, and neuroimaging to rule out brain and pituitary tumors.
9. The therapeutic plan involves ruling out treatable causes, reassurance, and surgery if gynecomastia is massive or is causing severe psychological problems.

3.3.4 Galactorrhea

A. This is a milky or watery discharge from one or both sides in nonpubertal breasts.

B. Microscopic examination of discharge demonstrates fat globules.

C. Galactorrhea is due to disruption of hypothalamic-pituitary control of prolactin (PRL) secretion.

D. Differential Diagnosis
1. Drug use.
   a. Tranquilizers, reserpine, methyldopa, and opiates lead to decreased dopamine secretion resulting in increased PRL levels. Dopamine has an inhibitory effect on PRL secretion.
   b. Oral contraceptives increase baseline PRL and cause LH and FSH suppression.
   c. Hypothyroidism leads to elevated thyrotropin-releasing hormone (TRH) secretion. TRH increases prolactin secretion.
2. Pituitary adenomas (micro <10 mm, macro >10 mm) may secrete PRL. Other pituitary disorders, empty sella syndrome and acromegaly, have also been associated with galactorrhea. It is also seen with Cushing's disease.
3. Other causes are hypothalamic tumors, infections, infiltrative disorders (sarcoidosis, histiocytosis), chronic renal disease (decreased clearance of PRL), ectopic PRL production, and chest wall manipulation (manual, surgery, trauma).

E. Treatment is geared toward correcting the abnormality responsible for galactorrhea (discontinue offending drugs, treat thyroid disease, excise or suppress PRL secreting tumors).

3.4 SCROTAL DISORDERS

3.4.1 Painless Scrotal Masses or Swelling

A. Hydrocele
1. This is a fluid filled mass in the tunica vaginalis.
2. It transilluminates.
3. It is present in approximately 2% of male newborns, but less common in adolescents. If present, it may be communicating and should be treated as an inguinal hernia.
4. Therapy is usually not necessary for noncommunicating hydroceles unless the mass is uncomfortable or uncosmetic, or the tense fluid collection reduces blood flow to the testicle.
5. Definitive therapy is high ligation of the processus vaginalis.

B. Spermatocele
1. This is a cystic lesion containing sperm located on the upper pole of the testis.
2. It will transilluminate.
3. Treatment by surgical removal is only necessary if the lesion enlarges or is painful.

C. Varicocele
1. This condition is the abnormal dilatation of the pampiniform plexus due to incompetent valves in the spermatic vein.
2. The prevalence of this lesion is 5% in adolescents and 15% in adults.
3. It is commonly described on palpation as a "bag of worms."
4. It is more common on the left spermatic cord, bilateral 10% of the time, and only rarely seen as an isolated right scrotal lesion.
5. It is the most common etiology of correctable decreased fertility in men.
6. Surgical therapy in boys is necessary if the condition is painful, causes massive distention of the scrotum, when the involved testis is significantly smaller than the other, or when the opposite testis is diseased or absent.
7. If a varicocele is identified in a boy <10 years old or is located on the right side only, search for an

abdominal or retroperitoneal mass.

D. Inguinal Hernia

1. Inguinal hernia is the most common scrotal condition requiring operative repair in children.
2. The ratio of boys to girls is 4:1.
3. Indirect hernias are the most common type, with 60% on the right side, 30% on the left, and 10% bilateral.
4. An increased incidence of inguinal hernias is seen in children with a positive family history of hernias, cystic fibrosis, undescended testicle, hypospadias, epispadias, abdominal wall defects, ambiguous genitalia, developmental dysplasia of the hip, and connective tissue disorders such as Ehlers-Danlos syndrome.
5. Treatment is surgical repair.

E. Testicular Tumors

1. Testicular tumors are the most common solid tumors in males 15 to 35 years old, but can occur at any age.
2. They are firm masses that do not transilluminate.
3. Sixty-five percent are malignant.
4. **Cryptorchidism** (undescended testis) increases the incidence of testicular cancer by 4- to 10-times that of the general population. Risk is increased further if the condition is bilateral.
   a. Seminomas represent 65% of cancers in non-repaired undescended testicles.
   b. Orchiopexy does not decrease the overall risk of testicular tumors, but the incidence of seminoma declines to 35%.
5. Testicular tumors may not be a primary tumor. The testicular mass is a common presentation in relapse of leukemia.

3.4.2 Painful Scrotal Masses or Swelling

A. Testicular Torsion

1. This is the most common cause of testicular pain in adolescents.
2. It occurs due to the presence of a "bell clapper deformity" where there is redundant tunica vaginalis resulting in a highly mobile testis. This allows for twisting of the testis on the spermatic cord. The deformity is usually bilateral.
3. Testicular torsion is a surgical emergency. If it is not repaired within 6 hours of occurrence, testicular function may be lost.
4. Torsion can be distinguished from an incarcerated inguinal hernia due to the lack of swelling in the inguinal area in torsion.
5. Failure of pain to lessen with elevation and support of the affected scrotum when torsion is present (Prehn's sign) helps to distinguish torsion from epididymitis.

B. Torsion of the Appendix Testis

1. The **appendix testis** is a remnant of the Müllerian duct.
2. It is the most common cause of testicular pain in boys <11 years old, and rare in adolescents.
3. The torsed appendix may be visible through the scrotal skin ("**blue dot sign**").
4. Progressive inflammation of the testis and epididymis results in pain and scrotal swelling that may be difficult to distinguish from testicular torsion.

C. Epididymitis

1. Epididymitis is acute inflammation of the epididymis usually caused by migration of infectious agents from the urethra via the vas deferens.
2. After puberty, epididymitis is the primary cause of painful scrotal swelling in sexually active adolescents.
3. Testing for *Neisseria gonorrhea* and *Chlamydia* is indicated as they are organisms implicated in the development of epididymitis. However, many times, the infectious agent is not identified. It may be caused by viral agents such as mumps as well.
4. Treatment consists of bedrest and antibiotic treatment for the likely bacterial agent.

D. Orchitis is a complication of mumps (17 to 35%), enterovirus (up to 17%), and tuberculosis in adolescents.

E. Trauma may result in testicular rupture or hematoma formation.

3.5 REPRODUCTIVE ISSUES

3.5.1 Contraception

A. Over half of all adolescents have had sexual intercourse by the time they graduate from high school, yet fewer than 30% use any form of contraception.

B. Oral Contraceptive Pills (OCP's)

1. OCP's are the most common form of contraception used by adolescents.
2. The failure rate is 4 to 6% in this age group.
3. OCP's suppress ovulation, decrease the likelihood of implantation, and make cervical mucous hostile to sperm.
4. Side effects include bleeding, nausea, weight gain, headaches, and mood swings. Positive effects include improved acne and decreased dysmenorrhea.
5. Contraindications
   a. Absolute contraindications are hypertension, history of thromboembolic disease, and undiagnosed abnormal genital bleeding.
   b. Relative contraindications are migraine, diabetes, sickle cell disease, and borderline hypertension.
6. Before prescribing the pill, screen for contraindications, perform a physical exam including a pelvic exam, screen for pregnancy, sexually transmitted diseases (STD's), and perform a Pap smear.

Table 3.5.2 Sexually transmitted diseases

Disease/Organism	Clinical Presentation	Diagnosis	Treatment	Complication/Sequelae
Nongonococcal Urethritis: • *Chlamydia trachomatis* (40%) • *Ureaplasma urealyticum* (30%) • *Mycoplasma genitalium* (10%) • *Trichomonas vaginalis*	Males: Dysuria Frequency Mucoid to purulent urethral discharge Some asymptomatic	WBC's on gram stain of discharge +Chlamydia probe/culture -Gonorrhea probe/culture	Doxycycline, tetracycline, erythromycin, or azithromycin Treat partner Use condoms	Urethral strictures Prostatitis Epididymitis
Mucopurulent Cervicitis: • *Chlamydia trachomatis* • *Neisseria gonorrhoeae* • Herpes simplex virus	Females: Asymptomatic or yellow mucopurulent endocervical exudate	Exudate on endocervical swab >20 PMNs/HPF on gram stain of endocervical discharge +Chlamydia probe/culture +Gonococcal probe/culture	Ceftriaxone IM or cefixime PO PLUS Doxycycline, azithromycin, or erythromycin Treat partner Use condoms	Salpingitis PID Conjunctivitis and/or pneumonia in newborn.
Human Papillomavirus *Condyloma acuminata* (genital warts)	Single or multiple soft fleshy growths on perineum, perianally, on cervix, or intravaginally	Visual colposcopy Pap smear	Cryotherapy Podophyllin (not in pregnancy) Trichloroacetic acid Electrocautery Treat partner	Obstruction of vagina Infection of newborn (uncommon) Cervical cancer
Gonorrhea	Males: Dysuria, purulent urethral discharge Females: Vaginal discharge, abnormal menses, abdominal pain Look for pharyngeal or rectal infection	Microscopic identification of gram-negative diplococci on urethral exudate or endocervical material Positive culture or DNA probe	Ceftriaxone IM or cefixime and doxycycline, tetracycline, azithromycin, or erythromycin Spectinomycin IM for cephalosporin allergic patients Treat partner Use condoms	PID Epididymitis Sterility
Pelvic Inflammatory Disease (PID)	Females Pain and tenderness in lower abdomen, cervix, uterus, and adnexa Fever, chills, increased sedimentation rate, increased WBC's Hx: multiple sexual partners, past history of PID, or IUD	Definitive: Visualization of inflamed fallopian tubes and positive culture of tubal exudate at laparoscopy Presumptive: Clinical presentation +/- positive cultures	Outpatient: Cefoxitin with probenecid or ceftriaxone PLUS doxycycline or ofloxacin plus metronidazole Inpatient: doxycycline PLUS cefoxitin or clindamycin PLUS gentamicin Treat partner Use condoms	Ectopic pregnancy Abscess Involuntary infertility Recurrent PID Recurrent pelvic pain

(continued)

C. **Barrier Methods** (diaphragm, cervical cap, condom)
   1. These methods are used by <20% of adolescents with a failure rate of 10 to 20%.
   2. There are no contraindications for use.

D. IUD is not usually recommended for use in teenagers.

E. **Injectable Progesterone**
   1. Reliable method of contraception requiring intramuscular injection every 3 months.

Table 3.5.2 Sexually transmitted diseases (continued)

Disease/Organism	Clinical Presentation	Diagnosis	Treatment	Complication/Sequelae
Pediculosis *Phthirus pubis* (pubic louse)	Itching, erythematous papules, nits, or adult lice on pubic hairs	Exam demonstrates lice or nits on pubic hairs	Lindane, pyrethrins, or permethrin Clean linen in hot water Treat partner	Excoriation Lymphadenitis pyoderma
Herpes Genitalis Herpes simplex virus (HSV), types I & II	Single or multiple vesicles on genitalia Rupture leads to painful ulcers	Presumptive: History, typical lesions, multi-nucleated giant cells on Pap smear Definition: HSV tissue culture showing cytopathic effects or HSV shell viral antigen testing	No known cure Palliative: acyclovir with 1st episode Annual Pap smear Treat partner	Fetal wastage infection of newborn Urethral stricture
Syphilis *Treponema pallidum*	Primary: Classical chancre is painless and indurated Suspect syphilis in all genital lesions Secondary: Skin rash (palms and soles) *Condyloma lata* Lymphadenopathy Latent: No clinical signs	Presumptive: Primary– Typical lesion and newly positive serologic test or second titer for syphilis 4-fold greater than last titer Secondary– Presentation and strongly reactive serological test Definitive: Positive dark field examination of material from lesion	Primary, secondary, early syphilis <1 year: Benzathine penicillin OR if allergic to penicillin use doxycycline or erythromycin Treat partner	Congenital syphilis Cardiovascular syphilis Neurologic involvement
Chancroid *Haemophilus ducreyi*	Single, superficial painful ulcer, inguinal bubo (25-60%)	Presumptive: Clinical presentation (R/O syphilis) Definitive: Culture + for *H. ducreyi*	Erythromycin or ceftriaxone Treat partner	Secondary infection of ulcer Buboes may rupture causing fistula
Molluscum Contagiosum (DNA virus from poxvirus group)	1-5 mm smooth, rounded, shiny, firm papules with umbilicated centers	Presentation: Microscopic exam of material from lesion reveals molluscum inclusive bodies	Curettage Cryotherapy Treat partner	Secondary infection

2. Side effects include amenorrhea, DUB, and weight gain.

3.5.2 SEXUALLY TRANSMITTED DISEASE (Table 3.5.2)

3.6 MENTAL HEATH ISSUES

3.6.1 Depression

A. Sixty percent of teenagers surveyed said they experienced depression once a month to daily. It is more common in women than men.

B. Etiology
1. The adolescent may have a change in peer and/or dating relationships.
2. Problems with parents or other family members may cause negative stress.
3. The adolescent may report poor school experiences such as bad grades, conflict with teachers, and peer conflict.
4. The individual may have a poor self image.

C. Clinical Features include recurrent somatic complaints, mood swings, decline in school or work performance, and apathy.

D. Therapy usually includes family and individual counseling. Antidepressants can be used but should only be prescribed by those familiar with their use in children and adolescents.

3.6.2 Suicide

A. Suicide is the third most common cause of death in adolescents.

B. Suicide attempts outnumber successful suicides 50 to 200:1.

C. Females make more attempts but males more often succeed.

D. Of teenagers who commit suicide, 60% have made a previous attempt.

E. A teenager recovering from depression is more likely to commit suicide.

F. Suicide Prevention
1. All adolescents should be asked about suicidal thought.
2. If suicidal thoughts are present, assess risk.
   a. Review the adolescent's history of suicide/suicide attempts.
   b. Assess the level of family support and recognition of the problem.
   c. Look for signs of intent such as getting affairs in order, giving things away, and social isolation.
   d. Identify family histories of suicide or substance abuse.
   e. Identify precipitating events such as failed relationships, conflicts with peers or parents, and pregnancy.

G. Therapy
1. Utilize a team approach (physician, social worker, psychiatrist or psychologist).
2. Ambulatory treatment can be considered in the following situations.
   a. The adolescent has no past history of attempts.
   b. The method used was less lethal.
   c. The attempt occurred when help was available.
   d. The family recognizes the problem and is supportive of treatment.
   e. A mental health worker is available.
   f. The patient and the family are willing to participate in follow up care.
3. Hospitalization is necessary if the above conditions are not met, a safe environment is not available, there is a history of depression, or the event occurred without warning.

3.6.3 Substance Abuse

A. Stage I – Experimentation
1. This stage starts with peers. The adolescent succumbs to pressure to participate.
2. There are few behavioral changes.
3. The user experiences euphoria and guilt.

B. Stage II – Abuse to Relieve Stress
1. This stage involves more than occasional use.
2. Use occurs in nonsocial settings.
3. A supply of substance is maintained.
4. A peer group develops around substance abuse.

C. Stage III – Regular Abuse
1. The user is involved in drug-oriented culture.
2. Most of the peers use drugs.
3. May have trouble with the law.
4. User is depressed when not using drugs.
5. User needs to raise money to support the habit.

D. Stage IV – Dependence
1. The drug is used to prevent depression, not to produce euphoria.
2. The adolescent may drop out of school.
3. Physical changes such as weight loss, fatigue, blackouts, and chronic cough may occur.

E. Therapy
1. Stages I and II may be treated on an outpatient basis.
2. Stages III and IV require hospitalization and/or placement in a residential rehabilitation facility.

3.7 LEGAL ISSUES OF ADOLESCENCE IN THE UNITED STATES

3.7.1. A **mature minor** is an individual who appears to understand risks and benefits of services provided and who, in the opinion of the health care provider, is of sufficient intellect and maturity to have that understanding.

3.7.2. **Emancipated minors** are individuals aged 16 years

and older who are married, in the armed services, parents, or are living on their own and are managing their own financial affairs.

3.7.3. **State laws** vary in rights of adolescents to receive care without parental consent. Most allow mature minors to obtain treatment for drug abuse, physical and sexual abuse, STD's, and pregnancy-related issues without parental consent.

3.7.4. **Confidentiality** is a central part of adolescent care. It may be breached when life is at risk.

33. An 18-year-old female comes to your office for evaluation of failure to begin menses. On exam she has sexual maturity rating (Tanner) stage IV breasts and pubic hair. A pelvic exam reveals a vagina without a palpable cervix, uterus, or ovaries. The most likely diagnosis is — C 3.2.1

A. Turner's syndrome
B. hypothalamic-pituitary-ovarian axis disturbance
C. testicular feminization
D. XY karyotype with gonadal enzyme deficiency
E. Kallmann's syndrome

34. Which of the following changes does not occur in puberty — A 3.1.2

A. increase in hypothalamic and pituitary sensitivity to estradiol and testosterone
B. increased plasma somatomedin C
C. increased insulin secretion
D. increased gonadotropin-releasing hormone secretion
E. increase in follicle stimulating hormone

35. Which of the following is an absolute contraindication to oral contraceptive use — E 3.5.1

A. sickle cell disease
B. diabetes
C. migraine headaches
D. follicular ovarian cysts
E. hypertension

36. A 17-year-old female is in the clinic for evaluation of lower abdominal pain and fever. Laboratory studies reveal an increased white blood cell count and an increased erythrocyte sedimentation rate. On exam she has significant right adnexal tenderness and cervical motion tenderness. What is the most appropriate therapy for this disease — A 3.5.2

A. intramuscular ceftriaxone followed by doxycycline for 14 days
B. erythromycin orally for 7 days
C. intramuscular benzathine penicillin
D. metronidazole orally for 7 days
E. ciprofloxacin orally for 10 days

37. A child is noted to have pubic hair that is like adult hair but does not extend to the medial thighs. This corresponds to what sexual maturity rating (Tanner) stage — C 3.1.2

A. II
B. III
C. IV
D. V
E. VI

38. The following are emancipated minors except — B 3.7.2

A. married minors
B. a 13-year-old
C. military servicemen
D. a 16-year-old managing his own financial affairs
E. a 14-year-old parent

39. All of the following are considered tasks of adolescence except — C 3.1.3

A. achieve independence from parents
B. assign importance to one's own body image
C. ultimately reject parental values
D. acceptance of one's body image
E. establish a moral identity

40. A 14-year-old female comes to the clinic for evaluation of a breast mass. On exam, you note a single, firm, discrete 3 cm mass which seems mobile, located in the left upper quadrant of the breast. You diagnose — C 3.3.3

A. fibrocystic disease
B. accessory breast tissue
C. fibroadenoma
D. malignant tumor
E. gynecomastia

41. In evaluating a female patient (not sexually active by self-reporting) for secondary amenorrhea, the first test to perform is — A 3.2.1

A. pregnancy test
B. thyroid studies
C. prolactin level
D. dehydroepiandrosterone level
E. testosterone level

42. A 14-year-old male presents with mildly tender bilateral breast development. You should — E 3.3.3

A. send him to the plastic surgeon
B. give him steroids
C. image his brain
D. check his chromosomes
E. reassure him that he is normal

43 A 16-year-old presents with a urethral discharge. You should — D 3.5.2

A. give him intramuscular ceftriaxone and oral azithromycin
B. culture him for gonorrhea and chlamydia
C. examine his throat
D. all of the above
E. A and B

44. The following is true about adolescents with depression except — C 3.6.1

A. 60% of teenagers report experiencing depression
B. it can be precipitated by conflicts with peers or family members
C. antidepressant medications should always be prescribed
D. somatic complaints are common

45. A 15-year-old girl presents with an accidental drug overdose. She is not seriously ill. The girl feels ashamed over her actions. She states this is the first time she has ever "done drugs." Treatment should occur in which of the following settings — A 3.6.3

A. an outpatient clinic
B. jail
C. an inpatient hospital unit
D. a residential drug treatment facility

46. A 14-year-old male comes to the clinic for evaluation of testicular pain. The pain began abruptly. He has noticed no penile discharge but he is sexually active. On exam, the left testis is swollen and seems higher than the right. The pain is not relieved by scrotal elevation. You suspect — D 3.4.2

A. epididymitis
B. testicular tumor with hemorrhage
C. hydrocele
D. testicular torsion
E. varicocele

47. What stage of substance abuse does the patient, with no previous drug experience and embarrassment or remorse over drug use, represent A 3.6.3

A. I
B. II
C. III
D. IV

48. A mother brings her 9-year-old daughter in for an examination of a lump noted under her right nipple. You should B 3.1.2 3.3.1

A. send her for biopsy of the lesion
B. reassure the parent that the child is normal
C. aspirate the mass
D. draw blood for hormone level testing

49. The most common gynecologic problem in adolescence is D 3.2.2

A. primary amenorrhea
B. secondary amenorrhea
C. dysfunctional uterine bleeding
D. dysmenorrhea
E. fibroids

4 RECURRENT NONEMERGENT PROBLEMS

4.1 GENERAL CONCEPTS

4.1.1 The Social Dynamic

A. Multiple perplexing problems will tend to surface over and over again in the pediatric clinic setting. Many of these visits are simply due to the parent's or child's need to know if they need to worry and just how much they should worry.

B. The clinician's role is to sort through the parent's and patient's frustrations and fears in order to find out what are their real concerns.

1. Attempts should then be made to systematically evaluate whether there is a need for concern. If so, where do we go from here?
2. If not, give parents permission to quit worrying or at least decrease their fears. Do not be trapped into making a diagnosis by becoming fixated on the parent's or patient's perception of the problem.

4.1.2 The Rational Approach

A. Remember that not all problems need to be solved in a single visit.

B. Most of these problems have more than one method of treatment.

C. Some of these problems may never be totally cured.

4.2 PROBLEMS OF ELIMINATION

4.2.1 Diurnal Enuresis (Daytime Wetting)

A. **Diurnal Enuresis** is the lack of bladder control during waking hours in a child old enough to maintain bladder control.

1. **Primary Enuresis**. Child remains untrained after 2.5 years even though otherwise developmentally normal.
2. **Secondary Enuresis**. The child was previously toilet trained, then regresses.
   - **a.** Usually the void empties the entire bladder contents (occasional seepage of a few drops is probably normal).
   - **b.** Sporadic wetting during the first 2 years post training is not abnormal. It is usually associated with postponement of voiding.

B. Organic Causes

1. This accounts for 5% of children with diurnal enuresis.
2. The primary cause is urinary tract infection (UTI) associated with frequency, urgency, and dysuria.
3. Females who take bubble baths or use soaps in the genital area may develop daytime wetting in association with urethritis.
4. If the child is continually wet, search for an ectopic ureter.
5. Neurogenic bladder is associated with incontinence and usually poor bowel control. A common example is the child with spina bifida. This condition can be occult, so always examine the back of a child with diurnal enuresis.
6. Lower urinary tract obstruction leads to bladder distension and overflow incontinence. The history is that of straining at urination, dribbling, or a small caliber stream.
7. Pelvic masses such as presacral teratoma, hydrocolpos, or fecal impaction lead to pressure on the bladder with resultant stress incontinence during running, coughing, or lifting.

C. Physiologic Causes

1. Urine refluxes into the vagina during voiding. After voiding is complete, the refluxed urine seeps out. This is most common in obese girls.
2. Giggle incontinence is due to detrusor instability (>90% female).
3. Bladder spasms may lead to abrupt voiding. Many children have associated nocturnal enuresis.
4. Dysfunctional voiding may be seen in children who, due to a history of delaying voiding, do not consciously recognize the urge to empty the bladder and subsequently experience incontinence.

D. Psychogenic Causes

1. Stress related incontinence is common between ages 2 and 6 years. It is associated with fear or anxiety as might be experienced with the birth of a sibling, loss of a relative, school related problems, or abuse. It tends to be irregular and infrequent. These children may also experience increased urinary frequency.
2. Refusal to potty train in a child greater than 2.5 years is most often seen in boys. It is frequently associated with a high pressure approach to toilet training including physical punishment.

E. The incidence of diurnal enuresis is approximately 1% in 7 to 12 year olds. Up to 60% of those affected have associated nocturnal enuresis.

F. Evaluation

1. History to elicit includes dysuria, frequency, hematuria, continuous dampness vs intermittent flow, previous UTI, precipitating events, use of punishment or coercion, and associated nocturnal enuresis or encopresis.
2. Physical Exam is performed to rule out bladder distension or fecal impaction, assess perianal sensation, anal tone, quality of urine stream, and identify low back abnormalities.
3. A urinalysis and urine culture are necessary laboratory exams.
4. If the child has a history of recurrent UTI's or abnormal findings on physical exam, refer to a urologist for consultation.

G. Treat daytime incontinence before nocturnal enuresis.

1. Relieve identified stressors.
2. Practice stream interruption exercises, scheduled voiding, and double voiding.
3. Discontinue the use of punishment in the resistive child. Offer positive reinforcement for success. Encourage positive interaction between the caregiver and the child.

4.2.2 Nocturnal Enuresis

A. The involuntary passage of urine during sleep occurring greater than one time per month in a developmentally normal child older than 3 years.

B. The incidence is 30% at age 4 years, declining to 3% at age 12 years. One percent of 18 year olds may experience enuresis.

C. Numerous risk factors exist and include familial predisposition, male sex, small functional bladder capacity, and coexisting UTI.

D. Spontaneous cure rate is 15% per year.

E. Since the condition resolves spontaneously, aggressive intervention is not warranted.

1. Offer reassurance to the parents and the child. Decrease family friction.
2. Encourage the child to take an active role in management (get up and change wet clothes, put soiled linens in a laundry hamper).
3. Provide positive reinforcement for dry nights.
4. Decrease oral fluids 3 hours before bedtime and encourage voiding just prior to bedtime.
5. At 6 to 8 years old, employ bladder stretching exercises, stream interruption, and increase early morning fluid intake.
6. Enuresis alarms may be used in children over 8 years old. The alarm should awaken the child and not the family when the first few drops of urine hit the sensor device. Alternatively, the child may set an alarm to arouse him to void 4 hours after retiring to bed.
7. Medications are only used in children greater than 8 years old if all other methods have failed and the condition is significantly emotionally disturbing to the child or parents. Recurrence is common upon cessation of treatment.
   a. Imipramine is a tricyclic antidepressant that can be used with care. It has a high incidence of side effects and, if taken in excess, is deadly. It must be kept under lock and key out of children's reach.
   b. Ditropan, an antispasmodic, may be used if an unstable bladder or bladder spasm is suspected.
   c. Desmopressin, an antidiuretic, is effective but expensive. Electrolyte abnormalities are a possible side effect.

4.2.3 Encopresis

A. Encopresis is deposition of formed or semiformed stool in the underwear or other abnormal places, occurring after the age of 4 years.

B. The prevalence is 1 to 3 % of school-aged children with boys (86%) most frequently affected.

C. Development of Encopresis

1. The child experiences intermittent stool retention leading to rectal distention.
2. As constipation increases, the rectal wall becomes stretched and unable to contract effectively. Sensory feedback also becomes impaired leading to further stool accumulation.
3. Stools become harder and larger leading to painful defecation and further retention.
4. Soft stool and mucus begins to seep around impacted stool.
5. Some children may pass large diameter stools as well.

D. Potential Etiologies

1. Toilet training resistance with development of stool withholding. The situation may be exacerbated by parental overreaction.
2. Some children may have an aversion or phobia related to the toilet.
3. Often, it may be related to situational toilet avoidance (children avoid defecation at school).
4. Incomplete defecation can lead to constipation.
5. Encopresis is common in children with attention deficit disorder or psychosocial stressors.

E. Other causes of chronic constipation include Hirschsprung disease (aganglionic megacolon), spinal cord lesions, anteriorly displaced anus, malnutrition, dietary indiscretions (lack of fiber, overindulgence in milk), disorders of voluntary muscle function (amyotonia congenita, cerebral palsy, infectious polyneuritis), and metabolic disorders (infantile renal acidosis, diabetes insipidus, idiopathic hypercalcemia).

F. Evaluation requires a thorough history, complete physical exam including a rectal, abdominal x-ray, barium enema when indicated by history or exam, and rectal biopsy if Hirschsprung disease is suspected.

G. The goal of management is to attain regular bowel habits and restore neuromuscular bowel function.

1. Demystify the condition. Reassure parents that many children have this problem and that the child often cannot feel a bowel movement coming on.
2. Catharsis is accomplished by an initial clean out procedure with enemas and laxatives followed by regular use of laxative agents (mineral oil, lactulose, MiraLax®).
3. Establish regular bowel habits by sitting on the toilet and attempting to defecate for 10 minutes at least two times per day after meals (gastrocolic reflex).
4. Increase dietary fiber.
5. Treatment requires long-term commitment as 20% of cases may have recurrence of symptoms. Encour-

age perseverance.

6. Enlist school cooperation to permit bathroom visits when needed. Provide a private bathroom if necessary.

4.3 RECURRENT PAIN SYNDROMES

4.3.1 Recurrent Abdominal Pain (RAP)

A. "The presence of at least three discrete episodes of debilitating (abdominal) pain occurring over at least a three month period during the year preceding the clinical examination." (Apley 1975)

B. RAP occurs in 10 to 15% of school-aged children.

C. Personality Profile. Two distinct personality types are associated with RAP.

1. Super achievers are verbal, obsessive-compulsive, sensitive, and "older than their years."
2. The second group consists of children of average intelligence who are immature in speech and behavior when compared to more productive siblings.

D. Family History. Often, many relatives will have a history of conditions such as irritable colon, spastic colitis, anxiety attacks, and mental illness. Positive family history of migraines is also common.

E. Differential Diagnosis

1. Organic Considerations
   a. Occult constipation of childhood (colonic distension leads to crampy abdominal pain).
   b. Lactase deficiency or malabsorption (including insufficiency and celiac disease).
   c. RAP is a well known side effect of chronic ingestions (lead) and medication.
   d. Chronic medical problems like peptic ulcer disease, Crohn disease, ulcerative colitis, rheumatic and collagen vascular diseases, hereditary angioneurotic edema, and Henoch-Schönlein purpura.
   e. Hematologic disorders such as sickle cell disease, hemolytic anemia, leukemias, lymphoma and other neoplasms.
   f. Parasitic infections. Giardiasis is a common painful infection. Please note, pinworms do not induce pain.
   g. Other miscellaneous causes of recurrent pain include trauma, gynecologic conditions (endometriosis, pelvic inflammatory disease, hematocolpos), and metabolic derangements (diabetic ketoacidosis, porphyria, hyperlipidemia).
2. Functional Considerations. RAP may be associated with an increased number of stressful or traumatic events in families. It is also often associated with school phobia and avoidance.

F. Evaluation includes a complete history and physical exam, laboratory studies (complete blood count, erythrocyte sedimentation rate, urinalysis, tuberculin skin test, stool for ova and parasites, and liver function tests at a minimum), and x-ray or ultrasound if indicated.

G. Management

1. Discuss family concerns and assure parents and child that no major illness is evident.
2. Alter the environment as necessary.
3. Discuss the fact that the emotional state can influence the gastrointestinal tract.
4. Keep a diary of episodes and related events.
5. Treat the underlying cause of the pain.
6. DO NOT feel pressured to make a diagnosis on the first visit.
7. Give follow-up and positive reinforcement, allowing time for both parent and child, separately.
8. Refer for psychological evaluation in confusing or refractory cases.

4.3.2 Headache (HA)

A. Incidence and Prevalence

1. Nonspecific, nonrecurrent HA's are noted in 40% of children by 7 years of age. By the time they reach 15 years, 75% report HA's.
2. Frequent recurring nonmigraine HA's are present in 15.7% of children by age 15 years, with the incidence of migraine being lower at 5.3%.
3. Under 15 years old, the male:female ratio is 5.5:4.3. Over 15 years, females are more commonly affected, 4.6:9.

B. Migraine

1. Migraine is defined as recurrent HA with symptom free intervals and at least 3 of the following symptoms: nausea, vomiting, abdominal pain, throbbing HA, unilateral location, aura, relief with sleep, photophobia or phonophobia, or a family history of migraine.
2. **Common migraine** without aura is the most prevalent migraine type in children.
   a. It is unilateral at onset but may become bilateral involving the frontal or temporal areas.
   b. It tends to be less severe in children than in adults.
3. In **classic migraine**, the aura is present. The aura is likely to be vertigo, image distortion, or paresthesias. Visual aura does occur but is less common than in adults.
4. **Complicated migraine** is a HA in which the child develops transient neurologic dysfunction that persists beyond resolution of the HA such as hemiparesis, blindness, or a confusional state.
5. Diagnosis is usually made based on a careful history and physical exam.
6. Treatment
   a. The child should avoid known triggers.
   b. Acute therapy with analgesics and antiemetics is indicated as soon as symptoms occur.
   c. Abortive therapies may be instituted in the case of infrequent HA's and include ergotamine (ex-

cept in the presence of hemiplegic migraine), chlorpromazine, or sumatriptan (5-hydroxytryptamine receptor agonist).

d. Prophylactic treatment is indicated for patients who have 2 or more episodes a month. Therapies include propranolol, calcium channel blockers, tricyclic antidepressants, anticonvulsants, biofeedback, and self-hypnosis.

7. Prognosis is good with 10% remittance per year until adolescence. Adolescent migraine HA's often persists into adulthood.

C. Nonmigraine Headache

1. **Tension HA** is often difficult to differentiate from migraine. It tends to occur most often during the school day and is exacerbated by anxiety. It is a dull ache, most often frontal in location, and is not associated with nausea and vomiting.
2. **Traction HA's** account for a small percentage of HA's in children but have serious implications.
   - **a.** Pain is holocephalic and occurs often in the early morning hours.
   - **b.** It is increased by any activity that raises intracranial pressure.
   - **c.** There is usually associated irritability and lethargy.
   - **d.** The most common etiologies are intracranial masses and pseudotumor cerebri. Other causes include arteriovenous malformation, cerebral aneurysm, hypertension, and collagen vascular disease.

D. HA's may be due to diseases of other head and neck structures (eyes, sinuses, teeth). However, these are rare causes of recurrent HA's in children.

E. Indications for Neuroimaging

1. Abnormal neurologic exam including focal neurologic findings occurring during the HA.
2. School failure or behavioral problems of recent onset.
3. HA's with associated seizure.
4. Early morning HA or HA that causes awakening from sleep.
5. Sudden increase in the frequency or severity of HA symptoms.
6. The presence of "cluster" HA.
7. Complaint of HA in a child <6 years old.
8. Brief cough HA in children or adolescents.

4.4 RECURRENT INFECTIONS

4.4.1 Causative Agents

4.4.1 Causative Agents. These infections occur in normal childhood and are not necessarily an indication of an immune deficiency.

A. Bacterial Infections. Meningitis, otitis media, pharyngitis, sinusitis, gastroenteritis, pneumonia (unless recurrent or caused by unusual organisms), cellulitis, impetigo, and urinary tract infection.

B. Viral Infections: Upper respiratory tract infections (colds), lower respiratory tract infections (bronchiolitis), gastroenteritis, and viral syndromes or exanthems.

C. Fungal Infections. Superficial fungal infections or thrush.

4.4.2 Evaluation

A. As with most medical encounters, the history and physical exam will play the largest role in determining whether a child's infection falls within normal limits or whether further work-up is desirable.

B. Underlying immune deficiencies can arise from defects in B cells and T cells, phagocytic defects, or complement defects. See Chapter 6 for a discussion of immune deficiency evaluation.

4.5 CONDITIONS SEEN IN EARLY CHILDHOOD

4.5.1 Infantile Colic

A. Paroxysm of irritability, fussing, or crying lasting a minimum of three hours a day and occurring on more than three days in any one week in an infant <3 months of age.

B. Colic occurs in approximately 10% of infants age 1 to 3 months. It usually resolves spontaneously by 3 to 4 months of age.

C. Possible Etiologies

1. Colic may be an intrinsic problem of temperamental predisposition and low sensory threshold.
2. Extrinsic problems such as an overstimulating environment and maternal anxiety may lead to excessive crying.
3. Feeding problems cause discomfort and subsequent crying (underfed/overfed, excessive air swallowed, inadequate burping, milk allergy).

D. Colic is a diagnosis of exclusion.

1. Include a detailed history, a narrative of the infant's typical day, and both occurrence and progression of symptoms.
   - **a.** Usually the crying time is late afternoon and evening.
   - **b.** There is a short-lived remission following any maneuver.
   - **c.** Babies usually have proper or even excessive weight gain.
2. Rule out organic causes for excessive crying.
3. Laboratory studies are seldom indicated.

E. Management

1. Counsel the parents, reassuring them that their infant is healthy. Empathize with their plight and discuss their anxiety and psychosocial stressors.
2. Observe parental handling of the infant and intervene appropriately (decrease overstimulation).
3. Discuss the option of NOT always picking up the

child if crying occurs when the child is dry and well fed.

4. Medication use is controversial and not recommended.
5. Provide close follow-up and continued reassurance.

4.5.2 **Failure to Thrive** (FTT)

A. FTT is a term used to describe infants or young children whose weights are persistently below the third percentile for age on standardized growth charts or crosses two percentile growth lines.

B. FTT is fairly common with 3% to 5% of infants under one year of age admitted to the hospital, 70% to 80% of those without an organic etiology.

C. Etiology

1. Nonorganic FTT is most common.
   - **a.** Inadequate intake of calories is the usual cause.
   - **b.** Underlying psychosocial issues may play a large part since psychologic stress can inhibit growth hormone production.
   - **c.** Emotional deprivation and/or physical abuse or neglect may be involved.
2. Organic FTT has many etiologies but is far less common than nonorganic FTT. Representative conditions are central nervous system abnormalities, malabsorption, cystic fibrosis, oral maxillofacial disorders, congenital heart disease, endocrine disorders, chromosomal abnormalities, renal disease, chronic infection, rheumatic disease, and malignancies.

D. Diagnosis and Evaluation

1. Obtain a thorough history including family history of growth patterns.
2. Obtain a detailed feeding history.
3. Observe the interactions between the parents and the child.
4. Prepare a detailed growth chart.
   - **a.** Has the growth been steady even though below the third percentile.
   - **b.** Was the growth normal and suddenly slowed.
5. Perform a careful physical exam.
6. Do a developmental assessment.
7. Collect a baseline complete blood count and urinalysis. Additional testing is based on history and examination findings.
8. Consider a period of observation in the hospital while ensuring adequate caloric intake.

E. Management

1. Address all medical problems.
2. If inadequate intake is identified, ensure adequate calories for maintenance and catch up growth.
3. Perform frequent weight checks.
4. Indications for hospitalization are severe malnutrition or dehydration, failure of outpatient management, evidence of abuse or neglect, or extreme parental anxiety.

4.6 ATTENTION DEFICIT DISORDER (ADD)

4.6.1 Characteristics of Affected Children

A. Short attention span with a high level of distractibility leads to inability to ignore extraneous stimuli and attend to task.

B. They are often impulsive and have difficulty regulating their actions to conform with social norms.

C. They are often hyperactive and have poor frustration tolerance.

D. Emotional and behavioral difficulties are common.

E. They often are socially ostracized.

F. They have poor self-esteem.

G. There is an increased incidence of learning disabilities.

H. They are often reported by caregivers to have been more active than normal from birth.

4.6.2 Diagnosis

A. History

1. Obtain a thorough past medical history and developmental history.
2. Review the parents' perceptions of their child's behavior.
3. Collect data regarding the teacher's perception of the child and the classroom performance.
4. Behavior rating scales (i.e. Conners Parent Rating Scale, Conners Teacher Rating Scale) should be sent with parents and teacher for rating over a period of several days.

B. Physical exam should include vision, hearing, and neurologic evaluation.

1. Be aware that the patient may not display his or her characteristic behavior in the physician's office.
2. Children with ADD may show increased numbers of "soft" neurologic signs (mixed hand preference, impaired balance, astereognosis, dysdiadochokinesia, and problems in fine motor coordination).
3. Laboratory examination is not generally helpful.
4. Consider referral for psychometric testing when learning difficulties are present.

4.6.3 Management

A. Family Counseling. Help the parents to understand the child's problems.

B. Behavior Modification. Necessary for both the parent AND the child.

C. Encourage a structured environment.

D. Stimulant Medication. Methylphenidate and similar medications can help the child modify his or her behavior.

E. Consider referral for psychiatric care if comorbid mental health disorders are suspected.

50. A 15-year-old girl presents with a 6 month history of recurrent pulsatile headache preceded by vertigo. Her diagnosis is — C 4.3.2

A. tension headache
B. school avoidance
C. classic migraine
D. common migraine
E. traction headache

51. The following statements about patients with failure to thrive are true except — D 4.5.2

A. the child's weight curve has fallen across two percentile lines on standard growth charts
B. the child is emotionally deprived
C. the child has poor caloric intake
D. growth is steady along the fifth percentile
E. the child may be developmentally delayed

52. A 7-year-old male wets the bed at least twice a week. Evaluation and management should include all of the following except — C 4.2.2

A. obtain a family history looking for bed wetting in parents
B. bladder exercises
C. punish for failure to stay dry at night
D. institute a system of positive reinforcement
E. decrease oral fluids before bedtime

53. A 4-year-old child presents having never been continent for urine. He has — D 4.2.1

A. ineffective parents
B. secondary enuresis
C. psychological problems
D. primary enuresis

54. Characteristics of children with encopresis include all of the following except — D 4.2.3

A. avoidance of defecation at school
B. may have attention deficit disorder
C. may have painful defecation
D. volitional defecation in inappropriate places
E. may have a diet low in fiber

55. A 10-year-old boy presents with a several month history of episodes of abdominal pain that interfere with school participation. He appears to be growing well and has no abnormal findings on examination. He has no other symptoms. He most likely has — C 4.3.1

A. inflammatory bowel disease
B. malingering
C. recurrent abdominal pain of childhood
D. lymphoma
E. Wilms' tumor

56. A child with a history of impulsivity, easy distractibility, poor self esteem, and school failure probably is afflicted with which of the following — D 4.6.1

A. bad teachers
B. a high intelligence quotient
C. obsessive compulsive disorder
D. attention deficit disorder
E. birth trauma

5 GENETICS, ENDOCRINE, AND METABOLISM

5.1 GENETICS

5.1.1 General Considerations and Terminology

A. A large portion of medically significant disease is genetically mediated through congenital malformations, metabolic disease, specific organ dysfunction, or abnormalities of sexual differentiation. Approximately 1% of all newborns manifest monogenic disease, 0.5% manifest a chromosomal abnormality, and 1 to 3% will have a multifactorial disease.

B. **Human Chromosome Complement**
   1. Each normal human somatic cell contains 23 pairs of chromosomes (22 pairs of autosomes and 1 pair of sex chromosomes).
   2. Genes responsible for defining tissue composition and function are present in two doses, one from each parent.

C. **Morphogenesis** refers to the growth of body and form.
   1. There are three general genetic causes of abnormal morphogenesis: mutant genes, gross chromosomal abnormalities, and polygenic determinants.
   2. **Malformations** represent abnormalities or incomplete development of tissue formation.
   3. **Deformations** are due to altered mechanical forces on normal tissue.
   4. **Disruption** is the result of breakdown of previously normal tissue.

D. Characteristics of genes are expressed through Mendelian inheritance patterns.
   1. **Autosomal Dominant**. A single mutant gene (allele) produces an abnormal characteristic. The person is heterozygous for the defect (only one of the two gene copies is abnormal).
   2. **Autosomal Recessive**. A mutant gene produces an abnormal characteristic only when present in a double dose. The person is considered homozygous for the defect (both of their genes carry the abnormality).
   3. **X-Linked Inheritance**. The mutant gene or genes are located on the X chromosome. It may be dominant or recessive.
      a. In dominant forms, affected males will have normal sons, but all daughters will be affected.
      b. Recessive forms carry a 50% risk for males to be affected and a 50% risk for females to be carriers.

E. **Syndromes** are patterns of human malformations and dysmorphic features. Not all of the features of a given syndrome need to be present to make the diagnosis.
   1. **Dysmorphisms** are abnormalities of physical features, form, or structure that vary objectively or subjectively from what is considered the norm for a population. They may be of no medical consequence.
   2. Syndromes have multiple causes, not limited to gene and chromosome defects. Teratogens are common causes of recognizable syndromes.
   3. **Teratogens** cause approximately 10% of all birth defects. They are environmental factors that interfere with prenatal development or cause disruption of tissue.
      a. Exposure prior to 10 days usually results in embryonic wastage.
      b. Exposure during the first 12 weeks of pregnancy causes defects in morphogenesis.
      c. Exposure after 12 weeks gestation generally results in central nervous system disturbance and poor growth.
      d. Some examples of teratogens are chemicals, drugs, prescribed medications, infections, radiation, and maternal metabolic factors.

5.1.2 Evaluation

A. Diagnostic Modalities
   1. Prenatal testing can be very safe or carry the risk of loss of the pregnancy, depending upon the method. Available tests include ultrasonography, amniocentesis, chorionic villus sampling, fetoscopy, α-fetoprotein analysis, deoxyribonucleic acid analysis, and enzyme assays.
      a. α-fetoprotein levels are increased in multiple gestation, neural tube defects, gastrointestinal obstruction, congenital nephrosis, and impending fetal demise.
      b. α-fetoprotein levels are decreased in trisomy 21.

B. The history is vital, especially any family history of heritable disease or consanguinity. Note the families ethnic background, as certain conditions are more prevalent in certain populations, such as cystic fibrosis in Northern and Central Europeans, and Tay-Sachs disease in Ashkenazi Jews.

C. Indications for Genetic Testing
   1. Presence of dysmorphic features on physical exam. If 3 or more minor abnormalities are present, the chance of diagnosing a genetic syndrome increases.
   2. Presence of multiple organ system malformations.
   3. Developmental delay or mental retardation.
   4. Short stature, especially in females, or very delayed menarche.
   5. Ambiguous genitalia.
   6. History of recurrent miscarriage or intrauterine fetal demise.
   7. Testing should be undertaken to confirm a suspected heritable disease or syndrome if a test method is available.

5.1.3 Representative Examples of Genetic Abnormalities (This is not an all inclusive list)

A. Autosomal Chromosome Disorders
   1. **Trisomy 21 (Down's Syndrome)**. Results when ex-

tra chromosome 21 material is present in the genome.

a. Findings on chromosome analysis reveal non-disjunction (complete extra 21 due to failure of chromosome pairs to separate during gametogenesis) in 95% of affected children. The non-disjoined chromosome is contributed by the mother in over 65% of the cases.
b. Extra genetic material can also occur as a result of unbalanced translocations between chromosome 21 and chromosomes 13, 14, or 15.
c. A mitotic division error early in embryogenesis can result in mosaicism (some cells affected with some normal) for the condition. Phenotypically, the children look like others with Down's syndrome.
d. Incidence is increased with very young maternal age or age >35 years.
e. Characteristics of children with trisomy 21 include developmental delay, hypotonia, single palmar crease, flattened face with upslanting palpebral fissures, medial epicanthal folds, small mouth, small ear canals, short hands and fingers, excess neck skin, and short stature. They may also have defects of internal structures. The most common are endocardial cushion defects followed by septal defects, duodenal atresia ("double bubble" sign on x-ray), and Hirschsprung's disease.
f. Children with trisomy 21 are at increased risk for leukemia, and if they survive into the fourth or fifth decade, a dementia syndrome much like Alzheimer's disease.

2. **Trisomy 18 (Edwards' Syndrome)**
   a. This syndrome is almost always caused by non-disjunction (90% meiotic and 10% mitotic).
   b. Increased risk exists with advanced maternal age but not as strong an association as that seen with trisomy 21.
   c. Characteristic features include intrauterine growth retardation, microcephaly with prominent occiput, central nervous system malformation with severe mental retardation, micrognathia (small jaw), hypertonia, overlapping fingers with fixed contractures, rocker bottom feet, and congenital heart disease.
   d. Ninety-five percent of affected patients die within the first year of life.
3. **Trisomy 13 (Patau's Syndrome)**
   a. Trisomy 13 is due to meiotic non-disjunction of chromosome 13 in 75% of the cases.
   b. Syndrome features include cleft lip, flexed fingers with polydactyly, hypertelorism, bulbous nose, small skull with central nervous system malformation (holoprosencephaly), microphthalmia, and cardiac, visceral and genital abnormalities.

B. Sex Chromosome Disorders

1. **Turner's Syndrome**. A condition in females who only have a single normal X chromosome.
   a. Fifty-five percent are due to complete absence of the second X chromosome. The others are due to structural alterations of one chromosome, or mosaicism (45,XO and 46,XX or 46,XY).
   b. Turner's syndrome can be confused with Noonan's syndrome. Children with Noonan's syndrome are phenotypically similar to Turner's syndrome patients but not genetically similar. Noonan's syndrome can also affect males.
   c. Features include lymphedema of the hands and feet at birth, shield-shaped chest with widely spaced nipples, neck webbing, short stature, gonadal dysgenesis, renal anomalies (40%), cardiac anomalies (20%; most common is bicuspid aortic valve followed by coarctation of the aorta and aortic stenosis), learning disability, and lack of pubertal development.
   d. Patients with Y chromosome material are at risk for developing gonadoblastoma.
2. **Klinefelter's Syndrome**
   a. These male children have an extra X chromosome (80%) or are mosaics (46,XY and 47,XXY).
   b. Characteristically, these children usually have tall statures compared to other family members. They tend to be sterile with decreased masculinization. They may have gynecomastia. Behavioral problems are common.
   c. Klinefelter's syndrome may not be diagnosed until adulthood during evaluation for sterility.

C. Syndromes Associated with Chromosome Deletion

1. These syndromes can occur due to de novo deletion of material from a chromosome or by unbalanced translocation.
2. **Cri du chat syndrome** is caused by deletion of material from the short arm of the fifth chromosome ($5p^-$). It is so named because of the characteristic cat-like cry. Although many patients survive to become adults, they are affected with severe mental retardation and central nervous system abnormalities.
3. Retinoblastoma is associated with a deletion of the long arm of chromosome 13.
4. Wilms' tumor with aniridia carries an association with deletions on the short arm of chromosome 11.
5. **Prader-Willi syndrome** is identified by an interstitial deletion on the long arm of chromosome 15 in 70% of affected patients. Uniparental disomy (both chromosomes of the pair come from the same parent) is present in 60% of affected individuals.
   a. In infancy, these patients are severely hypotonic

with feeding difficulties and failure to thrive. Later, they develop a ravenous appetite with resultant obesity if diet is not strictly controlled.
  b. Development is delayed and there are associated school and behavior problems.
  c. Males have hypogonadotropic hypogonadism and may have cryptorchidism at birth.

D. Fragile Sites
  1. Fragile sites are regions of chromosomes that tend to separate or break under deficient growth conditions.
  2. **Fragile X** is the most common cause of mental retardation in males and can occur in females as well.
    a. The fragile site is located on the distal long arm of the X chromosome, associated with allelic expansion (the presence of triplet nucleotide repeats, i.e. CAGCAGCAG, etc.), increasing the size of a deoxyribonucleic acid sequence. The presence and severity of the phenotype is based on the number of repeats present in a given individual.
    b. Typical features include mental retardation, macroorchidism, long face with prominent jaw, large ears, and behavior problems.
  3. Other syndromes associated with triplet repeats are spinocerebellar ataxia, myotonic dystrophy, and Huntington's disease.

E. Autosomal Dominant Diseases
  1. **Neurofibromatosis** (von Recklinghausen's Disease). A neurocutaneous autosomal dominant disease felt to arise as a result of neural crest differentiation and migration abnormalities. See section 16.2.5.
  2. **Achondroplasia**. A short-limbed chondroplasia.
    a. Affected children have a large head and normal sized trunk.
    b. They are at risk for spinal cord compression, obstructive and central apnea, bowing of legs, articulation disorders, and hearing loss.
    c. It is fatal in the thanatophoric form and in the homozygous offspring of two affected parents.
  3. **Marfan's Syndrome**. An autosomal dominant disorder associated with arm span greater than height, joint hypermobility, arachnodactyly, ocular lens subluxation, and cardiac abnormalities including mitral valve prolapse and dilatation of the aortic root. It is due to abnormalities in the synthesis of fibrillin.
  4. **Osteogenesis Imperfecta**. Caused by defects in type I collagen, leading to fragile bones, blue sclera, and deafness. Severity varies with the form of osteogenesis imperfecta, some being fatal in infancy and others improving as the patient ages.

F. Autosomal Recessive Diseases
  1. **α_1-Antitrypsin Deficiency**. This syndrome is responsible for some cases of neonatal cholestasis and childhood cirrhosis due to the absence of the serum protease inhibitor, α_1-antitrypsin.
  2. **Galactosemia**. See section 2.3.7.
  3. **Tay-Sachs disease**. A gangliosidosis that presents in initially normal appearing infants as loss of developmental milestones progressing to spasticity, seizures, blindness, and deafness, with death occurring in early childhood from aspiration or pneumonia.
  4. **Wilson's Disease** (Hepatolenticular Degeneration). A degenerative disorder of the brain and liver with associated corneal Kayser-Fleischer rings, due to accumulation of copper in these tissues. Serum ceruloplasmin (copper binding protein) is typically low. The disease does not present until after age 5 years and is fatal from liver, neurologic, renal, and hematologic failure if untreated by copper chelation.

G. X-Linked Disorders
  1. Hemophilia is a bleeding disorder due to deficiencies of various coagulation factors.
  2. Color blindness, or defective color vision, is common in males but rare in females.
  3. Bruton agammaglobulinemia is associated with decreased B-cell number and impaired function. It is associated with recurrent pyogenic infections, particularly severe hepatitis, and enteroviral infections. Other viral infections usually do not pose a threat.

5.2 ENDOCRINOLOGY

5.2.1 Insulin-Dependent Diabetes Mellitus ([IDDM]; Type 1 Diabetes Mellitus)

A. IDDM results when pancreatic β-islet cell function drops below 10%.
  1. Insulin secretion diminishes to a level that results in impaired glucose transport into cells.
  2. Counterregulatory hormone levels (glucagon, epinephrine, cortisol, growth hormone) increase, with resulting gluconeogenesis and glycogenolysis. This leads to increasing circulating glucose and lipolysis, which gives rise to increasing circulating fatty acids and ketones.
  3. When glucose levels exceed 180 mg/dl (renal threshold), glucosuria occurs.

B. The etiology of IDDM is not clear. It is suspected to be multifactorial. Known associations include viral infection, human leukocyte antigen (HLA) links resulting in genetic predisposition (HLA-B8, -B15, -DR3, -DR4), and autoimmunity with anti-islet cell antibodies detected in some patients and first degree relatives.

C. The classic symptoms of new onset IDDM are polyuria, polydipsia, and polyphagia with weight loss. The child may also have enuresis and a fruity breath odor.

D. Therapy
  1. Provide insulin to maintain near normal glycemia.
  2. Follow the child in a multidisciplinary clinic with a

dietitian, endocrinologist, diabetes educator, and psychologist, with periodic evaluations by an ophthalmologist.

3. Dietary management is shifting toward carbohydrate counting. The child or parent is taught to estimate insulin need per meal based on carbohydrate content.
4. Encourage regular exercise.

E. Complications of IDDM include neuropathy, retinopathy, nephropathy, and atherosclerosis.

F. **Diabetic ketoacidosis** (DKA) occurs when insulin secretion or exogenous insulin administration is insufficient, leading to the catabolic process described in section 5.2.1.A.

1. DKA may be a child's first presentation of IDDM.
2. Symptoms include the classic signs of IDDM, in addition to dry mouth, nausea, abdominal pain, and vomiting. The child may be lethargic or even comatose.
3. On exam, the child will have tachycardia, signs of dehydration (dry mucosa, poor perfusion, hypotension), Kussmaul's respirations (deep rapid breathing), and look significantly ill.
4. Laboratory evaluation reveals a metabolic acidosis (pH <7.3), concentrated hematocrit, leukocytosis, factitiously low sodium (low serum sodium measurement caused by the osmotic effect of hyperglycemia), elevated extracellular potassium (total body potassium is low), elevated glucose, glucosuria, ketonuria, ketonemia, low serum phosphate, low bicarbonate level, and elevated blood urea nitrogen.
   a. Na^+ measurement is decreased by 1.6 mEq/L for each 100 mg/dl rise in glucose over 150 mg/dl.
   b. Laboratory measurements should be repeated frequently (every one to two hours) to assess progress with therapy.
5. Therapy for DKA
   a. Assume dehydration and provide an initial 20 cc/kg bolus, replacing the remaining deficit over the next 24 hours. Be cognizant of ongoing fluid losses.
   b. Provide insulin as a continuous infusion. Because of its rapid metabolism, intermittent intravenous doses are of no benefit. Because subcutaneous or intramuscular insulin may have erratic absorption due to impaired perfusion, such routes of administration should be avoided in the acute management of DKA.
   c. Achieve a rate of fall in the glucose level of 80 to 100 mg/dl/hour. When the serum glucose approaches 250 mg/dl, add dextrose to the intravenous fluids.
   d. Replace potassium, if the patient is urinating, as KCl or KPO_4 when the levels decline to 5 mEq//L or less.
   e. Bicarbonate use to correct acidosis is controversial and generally not recommended due to the risk of worsening hypokalemia. It may also increase the incidence of cerebral edema.
6. Potential complications of DKA (and treatment) include hypoglycemia, hypokalemia, cerebral edema, and death.

5.2.2 Non-Insulin-Dependent Diabetes Mellitus ([NIDDM]; Type II Diabetes Mellitus)

A. NIDDM is usually thought of as an adult disease, yet the incidence is increasing significantly in childhood.

B. It is due to either resistance of insulin at the cell receptor level or a decrease in receptor sites.

C. Insulin levels may be normal or elevated.

D. NIDDM shows a familial predisposition.

E. Therapy consists of maintenance of ideal body weight, dietary moderation, exercise, and if needed, oral hypoglycemic agents or injected insulin.

5.2.3 Hypoglycemia

A. Hypoglycemia is a serum level <40 mg/dl in newborns, <60 mg/dl from 1 week to 16 years of age, and <70 mg/dl in individuals over 16 years of age.

B. Newborn transient hypoglycemia is addressed in section 2.3.6.

C. **Recurrent hypoglycemia**

1. Hypoglycemia can occur secondary to increased insulin secretion.
   a. Hyperplasia of β-islet cells or islet cell adenoma can result in refractory hypoglycemia.
   b. Nesidioblastosis is scattering of β-islet cells outside of the Islets of Langerhans with resulting increased insulin production.
   c. Maternal hyperglycemia with transplacental transport of glucose can result in sustained increased insulin production in infants for several days after birth.
   d. Hypoglycemia can also be seen as a function of excess exogenously supplied insulin in the treatment of diabetes mellitus or in child abuse (Munchausen syndrome by proxy).
2. Hypopituitarism can result in hypoglycemia due to the absence of counterregulatory hormones. These children show a decreased tolerance for fasting due to decreased glycogen stores and decreased ability to utilize substrate as seen in metabolic disease.

5.2.4 Disorders of Lipid Metabolism

A. Familial hypercholesterolemia is an autosomal dominant disorder with decreased low-density lipoprotein receptors.

1. Heterozygotes develop atherosclerotic heart disease by their third or fourth decade.
2. Homozygotes for the gene have cholesterol levels

between 600 and 1000 mg/dl and can experience myocardial infarction as early as the first decade of life.

3. Treatment is with lipid lowering agents and diet.

B. Familial hypertriglyceridemia is due to a deficiency of lipoprotein lipase with resultant hyperchylomicronemia.

1. Side effects are pancreatitis, hepatosplenomegaly, and cutaneous xanthomas.
2. Treatment is strict restriction of dietary fat.

C. Hyperlipidemia may develop as complications of other diseases such as IDDM, NIDDM, hypothyroidism, renal disease, or liver disease.

D. Universal screening of children for hyperlipidemia is not recommended. Screen based on family history (see section 1.1.4).

Table 5.2.5 Adrenal biosynthetic pathways

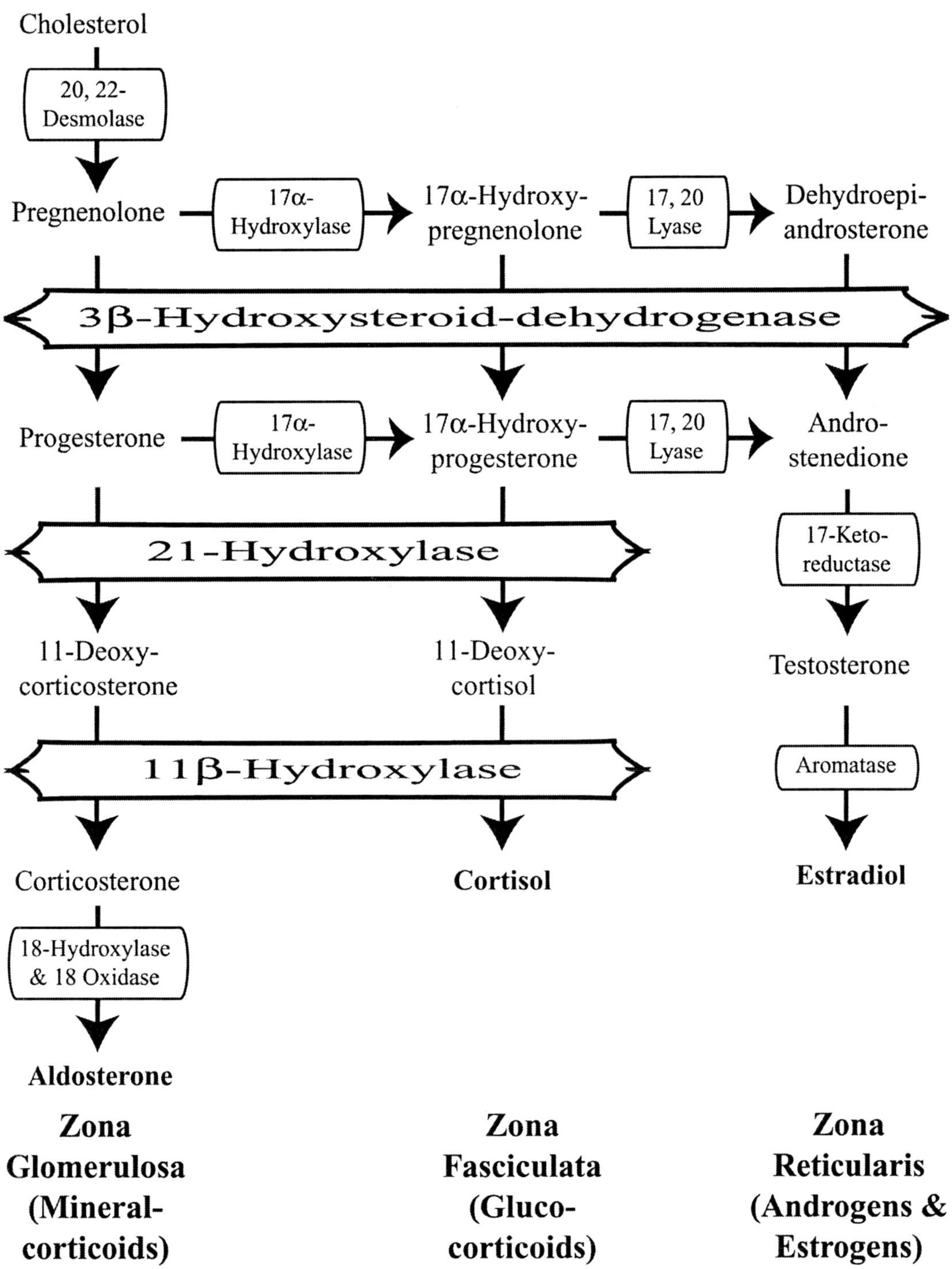

5.2.5 Adrenal Disorders

A. Table 5.2.5 is a summary of the adrenal biosynthetic pathways

B. **Congenital Adrenal Hyperplasia** (CAH); Adrenogenital Syndrome. A family of autosomal recessive deficiencies of the enzymes of adrenal cortisol synthesis.

1. The pathophysiologic abnormality is cortisol and aldosterone deficiencies with accumulation of precursors in blocked pathways that shunt through unaffected enzyme pathways, causing excess androgen and weak mineralocorticoid production. Knowing the enzyme defect allows prediction of the phenotypic presentation. (See table 5.2.5 to visualize synthetic pathways)
2. **21-hydroxylase deficiency** accounts for >90% of all cases of CAH.
   a. Classic salt-wasting 21-hydroxylase deficiency is associated with decreased cortisol, increased adrenocorticotropic hormone (ACTH), decreased aldosterone, and increased precursors to the catalyzed step.
   b. Female infants are born with ambiguous genitalia and males have no genital abnormalities. Both may have hyperpigmentation of the genitalia.
   c. Symptoms of salt-wasting, hyperkalemia, hypoglycemia, vomiting, dehydration, and shock develop within the first few weeks of life.
   d. Therapy is aimed at replacement of cortisol and mineralocorticoids, correction of genital abnormalities, and careful follow-up.
3. Simple virilizing 21-hydroxylase deficiency produces signs and symptoms due to androgen overproduction alone.
   a. Female infants have ambiguous genitalia and male infants look normal.
   b. Therapy is the same as with the salt-wasting form except that these infants may or may not require some mineralocorticoid supplementation.
4. **11β-hydroxylase deficiency** occurs in approximately 5% of infants with CAH.
   a. Signs and symptoms are due to overproduction of adrenal androgens and underproduction of cortisol as in 21-hydroxylase deficiency.
   b. Deoxycorticosterone (a precursor of this enzymatic step) is also increased. It has mineralocorticoid activity and results in hypertension and hypokalemia.
5. Other less common forms of CAH include 3β-hydroxysteroid-dehydrogenase deficiency, 17α-hydroxylase deficiency, and 20,22-desmolase deficiency.

C. **Adrenal Insufficiency (Addison's Disease)**

1. Addison's disease is caused by infectious, infiltrative, or autoimmune destruction of the adrenal glands.
2. Destruction of the gland leads to both glucocorticoid and mineralocorticoid deficiencies.
3. Predisposing conditions include autoimmune polyglandular syndrome, adrenal tumor or hemorrhage, inherited forms of CAH or adrenoleukodystrophy, and sepsis (Waterhouse-Friderichsen syndrome).
4. Symptoms include nausea, fatigue, weight loss, and increased skin pigmentation due to overproduction of ACTH (lack of negative feedback effects of cortisol).
5. Adrenal crisis may occur and is characterized by fever, vomiting, dehydration, shock, and ultimately death if not treated. It can be prevented by providing stress dose steroids to deficient individuals during times of illness or trauma.
6. Adrenal insufficiency is treated with oral corticosteroid replacement.

D. **Cushing's Syndrome**

1. **Adrenal Hyperplasia (Cushing's Disease).** Over production of ACTH by the pituitary gland, not responsive to the negative feedback effect of cortisol, or to the overproduction of cortisol by adrenal tumor or hyperplasia.
2. Evaluation includes serum cortisol levels, dexamethasone suppression testing of urine free cortisol, and imaging of the adrenal glands.
3. Cushing's syndrome can also be due to exogenous steroid use.
4. Treatment is removal of the offending agent, tumor, or pituitary adenoma.

E. Adrenal Medullary Tumors

1. The adrenal medulla is responsible for the production of epinephrine and norepinephrine.
2. **Neuroblastoma** is a tumor of neural crest cell origin that secrete catecholamines, vasoactive intestinal peptide, lactic dehydrogenase, and neuron specific enolase.
3. **Pheochromocytoma** is a tumor of chromaffin tissue that also results in an overproduction of catecholamines (epinephrine, norepinephrine, vanillylmandelic acid ([VMA];3-methoxy-4-hydroxy-mandelic acid). Side effects are related to catecholamine excess and resolve with surgical excision of the tumor.

5.2.6 Multiple Endocrine Neoplasia (MEN) Syndromes

A. These syndromes are a family of heritable disorders resulting in hyperplasia and tumors of various endocrine tissues in recognizable patterns.

B. MEN I:

1. Anterior pituitary adenomas with associated pituitary hyperfunction or hypofunction (secondary to

space occupying, nonfunctioning tumor).

2. Pancreatic islet cell tumors secreting insulin, gastrin (Zollinger-Ellison syndrome), or glucagon.
3. Parathyroid hyperplasia leading to increased parathyroid hormone (PTH) production and hypercalcemia.

C. MEN II:

1. Pheochromocytoma.
2. Parathyroid hyperplasia.
3. Medullary thyroid carcinoma.

D. MEN III includes:

1. Multiple mucosal neuromas.
2. Pheochromocytoma.
3. Medullary thyroid carcinoma.

5.2.7 Thyroid Disorders

A. Hypothyroidism

1. Congenital hypothyroidism results when the thyroid gland fails to develop, is underdeveloped, or ectopic.
   - **a.** Deficient thyroid hormone synthesis leads to prolonged neonatal jaundice, constipation, lethargy, large anterior fontanel, vocal hoarseness, coarse facial features, and decreased tone.
   - **b.** If untreated, the child will have growth delay, developmental delay, and mental retardation.
   - **c.** Skeletal age in children with hypothyroidism is decreased when compared to chronological age.
2. **Acquired Hypothyroidism**
   - **a.** This may be due to autoimmune phenomenon such as "burned out" Hashimoto's chronic lymphocytic thyroiditis, trauma, surgery, and radioactive ablation.
   - **b.** Symptoms include slow growth, delayed puberty, cold intolerance, decreased appetite, lethargy, and constipation.
3. Thyroxine (T_4) and thyroid-stimulating hormone (TSH) levels, antithyroid antibodies, bone age, and thyroid scanning are among the available diagnostic tests.
4. Treatment is with supplemental oral thyroxine for both congenital and acquired hypothyroidism.

B. Hyperthyroidism

1. Hyperthyroidism (Graves' disease, thyrotoxicosis) is an autoimmune disease mediated by thyroid-stimulating immunoglobulins (TSI), long-acting thyroid stimulator (LATS), and thyrotropin receptor-blocking antibody (TRBAb).
2. There is a genetic predisposition in association with HLA-B8 and -DR3.
3. Females are affected six times more often than males.
4. Symptoms include nervousness, increased appetite with weight loss, heat intolerance, palpitations, hyperactivity, increased sweating, sleep disturbance, and poor school performance.
5. Goiter, tachycardia, tremor, exophthalmos, thyroid bruit, and eyelid lag may be evident on physical exam.
6. Laboratory testing is the same as for hypothyroidism.
7. Complications are hypertension, cardiac arrhythmia, thyroid storm, and progressive ophthalmopathy.
8. Differential diagnosis includes Hashimoto's thyroiditis, thyroid nodule, and thyroid hormone resistance.
9. Three options for therapy are surgery, radioiodine injection, and antithyroid drug therapy (propylthiouracil or methimazole). Thyroid storm is treated with antithyroid medications and β-blockade.
10. Neonatal Graves' disease may occur due to transplacental passage of thyroid stimulating antibodies.

5.2.8 Disorders of the Anterior Pituitary Gland

A. Growth Hormone (GH) Deficiency

1. GH deficiency may be idiopathic or occur in association with other anterior pituitary hormone insufficiencies. It may be seen in septooptic dysplasia, central nervous system tumor, trauma, surgery, malignant infiltration, and infection.
2. Growth velocity in children with GH deficiency falls off between 6 and 12 months of age until it is less than 5 cm per year, with delayed skeletal maturation evident on bone age determination.
3. Provocative testing by inducing conditions that would normally stimulate GH release, such as hypoglycemia, is used to confirm the diagnosis.
4. Treatment is with subcutaneous synthetic GH. This is very expensive.

B. TSH deficiency is a cause of primary hypothyroidism.

C. ACTH deficiency results in Addison's disease.

D. Gonadotropin deficiencies result in delayed or absent pubertal development.

E. GH excess is the cause of **acromegaly** (post-pubertal onset) and **gigantism** (early childhood onset).

1. Symptoms include headache, acral enlargement, vision deficits, and glucose intolerance.
2. It is usually due to a GH secreting adenoma.

F. Prolactinomas result in delayed or interrupted pubertal development and galactorrhea.

5.2.9 Disorders of the Posterior Pituitary Gland

A. Diabetes insipidus (DI) is due to lack of antidiuretic hormone (ADH) secretion from the pituitary or to renal insensitivity to ADH.

1. It can be an isolated deficiency or be seen in conjunction with anterior lobe defects.
2. Symptoms include polyuria and polydipsia.

3. Laboratory studies reveal a low urinary osmolality.
4. Diagnosis is made by performing a water deprivation test. After an initial fluid bolus, liquid is withheld and urine output, osmolality, and patient weight are carefully monitored. When serum osmolality rises to over 300 mosm/L in the absence of urinary concentration, desmopressin is administered and the child is allowed to drink. Rise in urine osmolality is indicative of ADH deficient DI.
5. Intranasal desmopressin is the treatment of choice for central DI.

B. **Syndrome of inappropriate secretion of antidiuretic hormone** (SIADH) results from excessive ADH release.
1. Hallmark of SIADH is fluid retention and hyponatremia.
2. It is commonly associated with central nervous system disease, trauma, or infection, as well as drug use such as desmopressin and chemotherapeutic agents.
3. Diagnosis is made by comparing serum (low) and urine (high) osmolarity.
4. Treatment is with fluid restriction.

5.2.10 Ambiguous Genitalia

A. **Male pseudohermaphrodism** is the incomplete masculinization of a genetically XY infant. Common causes include defects in testosterone synthesis, defects in androgenation (5α-reductase deficiency), and androgen resistance (testicular feminization).

B. **Female pseudohermaphrodism** is masculinization of the genetically XX infant. The most common etiology is CAH. Maternal androgen exposure in pregnancy can cause similar effect.

C. **Mixed gonadal dysgenesis** (45,X, 46,XY) is an example of true hermaphrodism.

D. Gender assignment should be made based on consideration of the possibility of normal adult sexual or reproductive capability as well as the ability to surgically correct the abnormalities of the genitalia.

5.2.11 Disorders of Puberty

A. **Delayed Puberty**
1. Delayed female puberty is defined as the absence of secondary sexual characteristics at age 14 years or menarche by age 16 years.
2. Male puberty is delayed if there is no evidence of change by 14 years old.
3. Etiologies
   a. Constitutional delay is associated with late puberty and a late growth spurt, but children ultimately fulfill their genetic potential.
   b. Other causes include primary ovarian failure (Turner's syndrome), hypogonadotropic hypogonadism, Klinefelter's syndrome, vanishing testes syndrome, and pregnancy.

B. **Precocious Puberty**
1. **Precocious puberty** is defined as the appearance of secondary sexual characteristics prior to age 8 years in females and age 9.5 years in males.
2. It may be caused by central nervous system disease, tumors, endogenous or exogenous hormone exposure, or be idiopathic.
3. **Premature thelarche** is isolated breast bud development usually occurring between 12 and 24 months of age. Treatment, other than removing the offending exogenous hormone if present, is not needed as the condition resolves spontaneously.
4. **Premature adrenarche** is the early appearance of pubic hair. This requires evaluation for disorders of androgen production.
5. **Isosexual Precocious Puberty**
   a. Gonadotropin-dependent is normal puberty beginning abnormally early. It is usually idiopathic or due to central nervous system disease. Patients tend to be tall for age, but have an advanced bone age and premature closure of the epiphysis, resulting in adult short stature. It can be treated with gonadotropin-releasing hormone (GnRH) antagonists.
   b. Gonadotropin independent precocious puberty is rare. It does not respond to GnRH antagonist. It has associations with McCune-Albright syndrome and familial male precocious puberty.

5.2.12 Disorders of Calcium Metabolism

A. Serum calcium and phosphorus are regulated by PTH and calcitonin, both acting on bone and kidney.

B. **Hyperparathyroidism**
1. **Primary hyperparathyroidism** results in hypercalcemia due to increased mobilization of calcium and phosphorus from the bone, with decreased tubular reabsorption of phosphorus, leading to hypophosphatasia.
   a. Hypercalcemia results in weakness, weight loss, fever, nausea, vomiting, anorexia, and constipation.
   b. Treatment is usually surgical excision of a portion of the parathyroid glands or an identified adenoma.
   c. This condition is not common in children.
2. **Secondary hyperparathyroidism** results in a normal calcium level, but decreased phosphorus.
   a. It is usually seen in conjunction with chronic renal or liver disease and decreased vitamin D intake.
   b. Initial hypocalcemia results in increased PTH, leading to the aforementioned finding of normal calcium and decreased phosphate.
   c. X-ray findings are those of rickets.
   d. Treatment is vitamin D supplementation.

C. **Hypoparathyroidism**

1. **Idiopathic hypoparathyroidism** is due to decreased PTH secretion with subsequent decreased calcium and increased phosphate. Symptoms include seizures, tetany, numbness to the face, and carpopedal spasm. Treatment is with vitamin D and calcium supplementation.
2. **Pseudohypoparathyroidism** is a condition of PTH unresponsiveness. PTH is high but the laboratory findings are that of hypoparathyroidism. Affected individuals have short stature and mental retardation, and are treated with Vitamin D.

D. Rickets

1. Rickets is a failure of bone mineralization, resulting in abnormal bending and twisting.
2. Bowing of the legs, thickening of the costochondral junctions (rachitic rosary), prominent wrists and knees, and craniotabes (thinning of skull plates) are characteristic findings.
3. **Nutritional rickets** is secondary to lack of vitamin D intake. It is treated by assuring adequate vitamin D intake.
4. **Vitamin D-dependent rickets** is an autosomal recessive disease with failure of conversion of $25(OH)D_3$ to $1,25(OH)_2D_3$. Successful treatment is sometimes achieved with vitamin D supplementation. Some patients, however, do not have resolution of symptoms with this therapy.
5. **Renal osteodystrophy (renal rickets)** is due to decreased 1α-hydroxylase activity in the kidneys with decreased conversion of $25(OH)D_3$ to $1,25(OH)_2D_3$.
6. Chronic liver disease leads to decreased intestinal absorption of vitamin D or decreased 25-hydroxylase activity in the liver with resultant vitamin D-dependent rickets. High enough doses of vitamin D to overcome malabsorption is effective therapy.
7. **X-linked hypophosphatemia** (vitamin D-resistant rickets) results in renal wasting of phosphate. Calcium levels are normal and phosphate is low. Alkaline phosphatase is elevated. Treatment is with vitamin D and oral phosphate.
8. **Rickets of prematurity** is due to loss of the benefit of bone mineralization that normally would occur in the third trimester of pregnancy. Treatment is with calcium and vitamin D.

5.2.13 Short Stature

A. Constitutional Growth Delay

1. This is a normal growth velocity occurring below the fifth percentile on standard growth curves.
2. It is usually associated with a delay in puberty.
3. There often is a family history of the same process in the parents.
4. Treatment is not needed as affected children will reach their genetic potential.
5. Bone age (BA) = height age (HA) < chronological age (CA).

B. Genetic Short Stature

1. Affected children have a normal growth velocity at less than the fifth percentile on standard curves.
2. Adult height is less likely to be in the normal range.
3. HA < BA = CA.

C. Growth Hormone (GH) Deficiency. Associated with a subnormal growth velocity where HA and BA<CA.

D. Primary Hypothyroidism

1. Like GH deficiency, growth velocity is < 5 cm/year.
2. BA<<CA.

E. Other causes of short stature include hypercortisolism, skeletal dysplasias, genetic syndromes, chronic disease, nutritional deficiencies, and psychosocial deprivation (functional GH deficiency).

5.3 METABOLIC DISEASE

5.3.1 Inborn Errors of Metabolism

A. The diseases of the "inborn errors of metabolism" are primarily caused by either deficiency of an enzyme or failure of enzymatic function, which leads to accumulation of a precursor and deficiency of the end product in a metabolic pathway.

B. Abnormalities result from either toxicity of the excessive precursor or harmful effects from the absent product.

C. Most of these diseases are inherited as autosomal recessive conditions.

D. Presentation is often of a clinically deteriorating neonate who had been previously normal.
   1. The clinical picture is similar to that of neonatal sepsis.
   2. Symptoms occur during the first week of life and include poor feeding, vomiting, tachypnea, central nervous system depression (lethargy, hypotonia), and often seizures.

E. Hypoglycemia, metabolic acidosis, hyperammonemia, ketonuria, and liver dysfunction are the usual laboratory findings.

F. Death, mental retardation, and failure to thrive are the sequelae if treatment available for a given disorder is not applied.

G. Diagnostic evaluation includes:
   1. Arterial blood gas for pH and pCO_2, glucose, free-flowing serum lactate, serum ammonia, liver functions, urinalysis for reducing substances, urine and serum metabolic screening including amino and organic acids, and specific enzyme assays from blood or fibroblasts.
   2. Differential based on serum ammonia:
      a. If ammonia level is high with a normal pH, think urea cycle defects.
      b. If ammonia is elevated in the presence of acidosis, think organic acidemias.
      c. If ammonia is normal, think aminoacidopathies.

H. Therapy consists of restriction of dietary protein, administration of intravenous glucose, and occasionally, supplementation of specific vitamins or cofactors.

I. Prognosis depends on the specific disorder.

5.3.2 Examples of Metabolic Diseases

A. Phenylketonuria (PKU)

1. Pathogenesis is a deficiency of phenylalanine hydroxylase that is normally responsible for the metabolism of phenylalanine to tyrosine, leading to a build up of phenylacetic acid and phenyllactic acid.
2. It is the most common disorder of amino acid metabolism.
3. If untreated, symptoms are seen in later childhood and include mental retardation, hypertonicity, tremors, and behavior disorders.
4. Treatment is dietary restriction of phenylalanine.
5. Pregnant women with PKU who do not follow dietary restrictions deliver infants with increased risk of mental retardation, congenital heart disease, and microcephaly.

B. Hereditary Fructose Intolerance (HFI)

1. HFI is due to the absence of hepatic fructose-1-phosphate aldolase.
2. Symptoms become apparent with introduction of fructose or sucrose to the diet and include hypoglycemia, nausea, hepatomegaly, and liver failure.
3. Treatment is elimination of dietary fructose.

C. Citrullinemia is a urea cycle disorder caused by deficient arginosuccinate synthetase, with affected patients having severe mental retardation or death in infancy.

D. Glycogen Storage Disease

1. These are a group of conditions caused by a deficiency of enzymes involved in glycogen synthesis or breakdown. The consequence is a build up of glycogen in the tissues.
2. Type I (von Gierke's disease) is hepatomegaly associated with deficient glucose-6-phosphatase.
3. Type II (Pompe's disease) is acidosis, hypoglycemia, and storage abnormalities affecting all tissues secondary to acid maltase deficiency. Death usually occurs in infancy.
4. Type III (Forbes' or Cori's disease) is a deficiency of amylo-1,6-glucosidase with resultant hepatomegaly, hypotonia, and hyperlipidemia.
5. Type IV (Andersen's disease) is a deficiency of amylo-1,4→1,6-transglucosidase with hepatomegaly, cirrhosis, and infant death.
6. Type V (McArdle's disease) is associated with muscle weakness and cramps with exercise. It is due to a deficiency of muscle phosphorylase.
7. Type VI (Hers' disease) is a deficiency of liver phosphorylase and is associated with hepatomegaly and hypoglycemia.
8. Type VII (Tarui's disease) presents with weakness and muscle cramping with exercise. It is due to a deficiency of phosphofructokinase.

57. Most genetic malformations are due to — B 5.1.1

A. mutant genes
B. multifactorial inheritance
C. deletions
D. translocations

58. An infant has prolonged jaundice, constipation, a large anterior fontanelle, and coarse facial features. He grows poorly and has obvious cognitive delay as he ages. What is your diagnosis — A 5.2.7

A. hypothyroidism
B. phenylketonuria
C. hyperthyroidism
D. congenital adrenal hypoplasia
E. congenital heart disease

59. A 3-week-old male presents to the emergency room with a history of vomiting. He appears dehydrated and quite ill, with poor capillary refill, cyanosis, and scrotal hyperpigmentation. He has a markedly elevated serum potassium and a metabolic acidosis. His disease occurs as — B 5.2.5

A. a sporadic mutation
B. an autosomal recessive disorder
C. an autosomal dominant disorder
D. an X-linked disorder

60. If an infant with congenital adrenal hyperplasia has hyponatremia, he is most likely to have a deficiency of what enzyme — C 5.2.5

A. 11β-hydroxylase
B. 17,20 lyase
C. 21-hydroxylase
D. glucose-6-phosphate dehydrogenase

61. A 16-year-old female presents with short stature and amenorrhea. On exam, you note a shield-shaped chest, absent secondary sexual characteristics, and a heart murmur. What is the chromosomal abnormality — E 5.1.3

A. 47,XXY
B. 46,XX
C. 46,XY
D. 47,XX
E. 45,X, 46,XX mosaicism

62. A child with Down's syndrome presents with anemia, bruising, fatigue, and neutropenia. The most likely diagnosis is — A 5.1.3

A. leukemia
B. viral syndrome
C. idiopathic thrombocytopenic purpura
D. congestive heart failure
E. hemophilia

63. A 16-year-old male presents with tall stature, small gonads, and behavior problems. His karyotype is most likely to reveal — D 5.1.3

A. 46,XY
B. 47,XY
C. 47,XXY, 46,XY
D. 47,XXY
E. 45,XO

64. Infants with which of the following abnormalities on chromosome analysis have a cat-like cry — B 5.1.3

A. 47,XX (13^+)
B. 46,XY ($5\ p^-$)
C. 46,XX, 45,XO
D. 47,XXY

65. All of the following conditions are associated with triplet repeat nucleotide sequences except — C 5.1.3

A. spinocerebellar ataxia
B. Huntington's disease
C. Prader-Willi syndrome
D. fragile X syndrome
E. myotonic dystrophy

66. The most common chromosomal abnormality in Down's syndrome is — C 5.1.3

A. a complete extra chromosome 18
B. a 14-21 translocation
C. a complete extra chromosome 21
D. an absent chromosome 13

67. Color blindness occurs with what type of inheritance pattern — C 5.1.3

A. autosomal dominant
B. autosomal recessive
C. X-linked
D. it is not an inherited trait

68. What level of pancreatic islet cell function is necessary to maintain normal glucose homeostasis — B 5.2.1

A. 5%
B. 10%
C. 15%
D. 20%
E. 50%

69. A child with known insulin-dependent diabetes mellitus presents with a dry mouth, Kussmaul's respiration, tachycardia, and abdominal pain. What is this child's primary acid-base defect — C 5.2.1

A. respiratory acidosis
B. respiratory alkalosis
C. metabolic acidosis
D. metabolic alkalosis

70. A child in diabetic ketoacidosis has a reported serum sodium of 129 mmol/L and a serum glucose of 550 mg/dL. The actual serum sodium (mmol/L) is closest to — A 5.2.1

A. 135
B. 132
C. 130
D. 127
E. 124

71. Waterhouse-Friderichsen syndrome is — B 5.2.5

A. acute adrenal insufficiency due to tumor
B. acute adrenal insufficiency due to sepsis
C. hypercortisolism due to neuroblastoma
D. hypercortisolism due to pheochromocytoma

72. What is the state of total body potassium in the child with diabetic ketoacidosis and a serum potassium of 5.0 mmol/L — B 5.2.1

A. high
B. low
C. normal
D. cannot tell from information provided

73. Which of the following is not a cause of hypoglycemia in an infant or child — E 5.2.3

A. maternal gestational diabetes
B. insulin administration
C. fasting
D. islet cell adenoma
E. cortisol excess

74. Which of the following deficiencies is not associated with ambiguous genitalia in female infants — D 5.2.5

A. 21-hydroxylase
B. 11β-hydroxylase
C. 3β-hydroxysteroid-dehydrogenase
D. 20,22-desmolase

75. Which of the following syndromes is associated with pituitary adenoma, pancreatic islet cell tumor, and hyperparathyroidism — A 5.2.6

A. multiple endocrine neoplasia (MEN) I
B. MEN II
C. MEN III
D. rickets

76. An infant has elevated levels of phenylacetic acid and phenyllactic acid on serum testing. What metabolic disease does he have — C 5.3.2

A. adrenal leukodystrophy
B. galactosemia
C. phenylketonuria
D. tuberous sclerosis

77. A 15-year-old presents with neck fullness, eyelid lag, rapid heart rate, tremor, and exophthalmos. What is the best therapy for her condition — A 5.2.7

A. propylthiouracil
B. levothyroxine
C. cortisone
D. observation

78. Prenatal α-fetoprotein is likely to be increased in each of the following except — A 5.1.2

A. trisomy 21
B. multiple gestation
C. neural tube defects
D. congenital nephrosis

79. Treatment for syndrome of inappropriate secretion of antidiuretic hormone is — D 5.2.9

A. administration of extra sodium containing fluids
B. desmopressin
C. diuretics
D. fluid restriction

80. What is the usual growth velocity in children with growth hormone deficiency — B 5.2.8

A. <1 cm per year
B. <5 cm per year
C. <10 cm per year
D. <15 cm per year

81. A child with meningitis has a serum sodium of 128 mmol/L and decreased urine output. What is your diagnosis — C 5.2.9

A. hyperthyroidism
B. diabetes insipidus
C. syndrome of inappropriate secretion of antidiuretic hormone
D. adrenal insufficiency

82. Thelarche refers to what pubertal change — D 5.2.11

A. testicular enlargement
B. axillary hair growth
C. menstruation
D. breast development
E. pubic hair growth

83. Premature thelarche may be due to all of the following except — B 5.2.11

A. normal variation
B. hypogonadism
C. exogenous estrogen
D. tumor
E. central nervous system trauma

84. A child has flared wrists, decreased bone mineralization, bowing of the legs, a normal calcium level, and decreased serum phosphorus. What is your diagnosis — B 5.2.12

A. primary hyperthyroidism
B. secondary hyperparathyroidism
C. hypoparathyroidism
D. pseudohyperparathyroidism

85. What is the recommended therapy for secondary hyperparathyroidism — C 5.2.12

A. oral calcium
B. renal dialysis
C. vitamin D supplementation
D. observation

86. A 1-week-old infant presents with vomiting, lethargy, and seizures. His serum ammonia level is elevated and his pH is normal. What is the most likely diagnosis — A 5.3.1

A. urea cycle defect
B. organic academia
C. sepsis
D. poisoning

6 IMMUNOLOGY

6.1 HOST DEFENSE

6.1.1 General Concepts

A. A host defense system helps ensure the homeostasis of the human organism by providing protection against infection, malignancy, and autoimmune diseases.
1. Some of the defense system is static, such as the skin barrier and mobile cilia.
2. Other defenses adapt to challenges presented to the organism as "foreign substances." The major components of the adaptive system of defense are the T lymphocytes, B lymphocytes, phagocytes and the complement system.

B. Host defense can be subdivided into nonspecific and specific components.
1. Nonspecific defense mechanisms include skin and mucosal barriers, complement system, phagocytic system, and normal intestinal flora (impeding bacterial or yeast overgrowth).
2. Specific defense mechanisms are antibody-mediated (humoral) immunity and cell-mediated immunity.
   - **a.** Antibody-mediated defense is directed primarily against bacterial and extracellular phases of viral infections.
   - **b.** Cell-mediated defense is directed against intracellular pathogens (fungi, viruses, parasites) and is responsible for the recognition and destruction of malignant cells and foreign tissue.

6.1.2 Humoral Immunity

A. B cells arise from undifferentiated stem cells that migrate to the bone marrow and enter the circulation to populate lymphoid follicles. In the follicles, they differentiate into plasma cells, which secrete immunoglobulin (Ig).

B. Immunoglobulin Classification and Function
1. **IgM** forms rapidly after antigenic stimulation. It accounts for 10% of the immunoglobulin pool and aids in opsonization and agglutination of antigen. Adult levels are produced by 1 year of age.
2. **IgG** comprises 70 to 75% of the immunoglobulin pool. It is the major antibody of rechallenge and persists after antigenic stimulation. Adult levels are produced by 5 to 7 years of age. It is capable of crossing the placenta in the latter half of the third trimester.
3. **IgA** is 15 to 20% of the Ig pool and is the secretory antibody in saliva, lacrimal fluid, colostrum, nasal secretions, bronchial secretions, and intestinal secretions. Adult levels are produced by 10 to 14 years of age.
4. **IgD** is less than 1% of the Ig pool. It serves as a receptor site on circulating B cells.
5. **IgE** accounts for a very small part of the Ig pool, although, allergic individuals often have elevated serum levels. It is found on the surface of mast cells and basophils. It is typically responsible for anaphylaxis (immediate hypersensitivity response).

6.1.3 Cell-Mediated Immunity

A. Stem cells migrate to the thymus and develop under the influence of local humoral factors to become T cells.
1. **T cells** release soluble mediators (**lymphokines**) in response to appropriate antigenic challenge which in turn, recruit macrophages, granulocytes and other immunocompetent cells.
2. **Helper T cells** have the CD4 surface antigen marker and interact with B cells, helping them to divide, differentiate, and make antibody. They also interact with macrophages, helping them to destroy intracellular pathogens.
3. **Cytotoxic T cells** have the CD8 surface antigen. They recognize antigen presented on other cells' membranes by the major histocompatibility complex (MHC) and lyse what is not considered "self."

6.1.4 Auxiliary Cells of Immune Function

A. **Phagocytes** migrate toward a chemical stimulus initiated by an inflammatory response, ingest, and then destroy engulfed microorganisms.

B. **Mast cells** and **basophils** are mediators of the immediate hypersensitivity response.
1. They have receptors with a high affinity to IgE, but can be activated by non-IgE mechanisms as well.
2. Upon activation, they secrete mediators of an inflammatory response within seconds, the most prominent being histamine, leading to the allergic response.

C. **Natural killer cells** recognize surface changes that occur on the surface of tumor cells and virally infected cells, without aid of the MHC.

D. **Eosinophils** damage extracellular parasites by releasing the contents of their intracellular granules in close proximity to the antigen.

E. Platelets can release inflammatory mediators when activated by antigen-antibody complexes or when forming a thrombus.

6.1.5 Complement System

A. Components of the complement system are involved in the inflammatory response in both effector and regulatory functions.

B. There are two pathways of complement activation: the classic and the alternative pathway. Either leads to activation of a common final pathway which results in the formation of a membrane attack complex. The process is modulated by regulatory proteins.
1. The classic pathway is initiated by IgG or IgM antigen-antibody complexes.
2. The alternative pathway does not require antibody

for its activation. Activation occurs only as a result of loss of inhibition mediated by regulatory proteins.

3. Bacteria rich in sialic acid (group B *Streptococcus, Neisseria* and *Escherichia coli*) are able to resist alternative pathway activation and therefore, are more pathogenic in individuals who lack sufficient antibody activators of the classic pathway, such as neonates.

6.1.6 Diagnostic Modalities

A. Perform a complete history with emphasis on previous growth deficiency, chronic, recurrent or opportunistic infections, skin rashes, continual infections (without intervals of good health), and infections with microbial agents of normally low pathogenicity.

B. On physical examination pay close attention to growth parameters, general appearance, energy level, (pale, apathetic, irritable), skin rashes (eczema, abscesses), mucous membranes (*Candida*), lymphatic tissue, liver and spleen size, and the presence of neurologic findings such as ataxia or developmental delay.

C. Diagnostic Evaluation

1. Perform general testing of complete blood count with manual differential of cell types, x-rays and bone scans to identify infections, cultures, and erythrocyte sedimentation rate.
2. Tests of antibody-mediated (humoral B cell) immunity can be performed and include quantitative Ig levels of IgG, IgM, IgA, IgE, isohemagglutinin titer (anti-A, anti-B) to measure IgM function, and the patient's antibody response to immunization with diphtheria, tetanus toxoid and measles-mumps-rubella vaccine.
3. Tests of cell-mediated (T cell) immunity include absolute lymphocyte count and delayed hypersensitivity skin testing to common antigens (*Candida*, tetanus toxoid, mumps).
4. Absolute neutrophil count and nitroblue tetrazolium (NBT) dye test to measure neutrophil metabolic function are tests of phagocytosis-mediated immunity.
5. Test total hemolytic complement (CH50) to measure complement activity and both C3 and C4 levels to measure important pathway components.

D. Advanced immunologic tests such as B cell quantitation, T cell quantitation, mixed lymphocyte cultures, mitogen stimulation, enzyme assays, and individual complement pathway component testing can be performed based upon suspected diagnosis.

6.2 MANIFESTATIONS OF IMMUNE SYSTEM DEFECTS

6.2.1 Clinical Characteristics of B Cell Defects

A. History is significant for recurrent pyogenic infections with extracellular encapsulated organisms (*Streptococcus pneumoniae, Haemophilus influenzae, Neisseria meningitidis*). Also noted are recurrent episodes of otitis media, conjunctivitis, sinusitis, pneumonia, and bronchiectasis, especially without risk factors (daycare or passive smoke exposure).

B. Patients may have chronic or recurrent episodes of diarrhea, especially due to *Giardia lamblia* infection.

C. Decreased serum levels of Igs are identified by specific testing.

D. Growth is usually normal.

E. An increased rate of viral and fungal infections are rare (except for enterovirus encephalitis and poliomyelitis).

F. Prognosis is for survival to adulthood or at least for survival several years after onset.

6.2.2 Clinical Characteristics of T Cell Defects

A. Patients have a history of recurrent infections with opportunistic or less virulent organisms (viruses, fungi, protozoa, mycobacteria).

B. Malabsorption, diarrhea, growth retardation, and failure to thrive are common.

C. Anergy is present on challenge testing.

D. Affected individuals may develop graft-versus-host reaction if given non-irradiated blood.

E. Live virus vaccinations or bacille Calmette-Guérin (BCG) vaccinations can be fatal.

F. There is a high incidence of malignancy.

G. Survival beyond infancy or childhood is rare, but is improving with better treatments.

6.2.3 Clinical Characteristics of Phagocytic Defects

A. Recurrent skin infections with bacteria and fungi (*Staphylococcus, Pseudomonas, Escherichia coli,* and *Aspergillus*) are common.

B. Abscesses of lymph nodes, subcutaneous tissue, liver, and lung are frequent. The pulmonary infections contribute to chronic lung disease seen in these patients.

C. Bone and joint infections also occur often.

6.2.4 Clinical Characteristics of Complement Defects

A. Recurrent bacterial infections with extracellular pyogenic organisms (*Streptococcus pneumoniae, Haemophilus influenzae*) are seen.

B. Recurrent or severe skin and respiratory tract infections occur.

C. Patients have an unusual susceptibility to recurrent *Neisseria* infections (gonococcus and meningococcus).

D. Individuals have an increased incidence of autoimmune disease (systemic lupus erythematosus, rheumatoid arthritis, sarcoidosis).

6.3 DISEASE PROFILES

6.3.1 Selected Primary Immunodeficiency Disorders (Table 6.3.1).

6.3.2 Pediatric Acquired Immunodeficiency Syndrome

A. Etiology is infection with the human immunodeficiency virus human immunodeficiency virus (HIV) type 1.

B. Affected patients demonstrate depletion of CD4 cells, anergy, poor antibody response to *de novo* antigens, and hypergammaglobulinemia.

C. HIV can be contracted through vertical transmission (transplacental, perinatal, breast feeding), blood inoculation, sexual abuse, sexual activity, injectable drug use, or any condition that allows exposure to HIV-positive body fluids.

D. Symptoms that suggests a child is at risk are recurrent infections, poor growth, and infection with opportunistic organisms.

E. Physical findings include hepatosplenomegaly, lymphadenopathy, growth failure, candidiasis, and diarrhea.

F. Laboratory analysis reveals anti-HIV antibodies or the presence of viral copies by polymerase chain reaction (PCR). Remember, infants may have persistent maternal IgG anti-HIV for up to 15 months.

Table 6.3.1 Selected primary immunodefiency disorders

DISORDER	CLINICAL MANIFESTATIONS	INHERITANCE
B Cell (antibody-mediated)		
X-linked (Bruton) agammaglobulinemia	Recurrent pyogenic infections of the central nervous system, sinuses, middle ear, lungs, skin	Xq22
Dysgammaglobulinemia IgA deficiency IgM deficiency IgG subclass of deficiency	Recurrent infections of sinuses, lungs, gastrointestinal disease	Variable Autosomal recessive Gene deletion
Common variable immunodeficiency	Infections of sinuses, middle ear, lungs, giardiasis, malabsorption, autoimmune disease	Autosomal recessive, Autosomal dominant
Transcobalamin II deficiency	Recurrent infections, megaloblastic anemia, intestinal villous atrophy; defective granulocytic bactericidal activity	Autosomal dominant
T Cell (cell-mediated)		
Wiskott-Aldrich syndrome	Eczema, thrombocytopenia, recurrent infections, malignancy	X-linked
DiGeorge's syndrome	Hypoparathyroidism, facial abnormalities, cardiac anomalies	90% have 22q11 deletion
Ataxia-telangiectasia	Occulocutaneous telangiectasia, progressive cerebellar ataxia, bronchiectasis, malignancy	Autosomal recessive
Severe combined immunodeficiency	Recurrent infections, chronic diarrhea, failure to thrive	X-linked, Autosomal recessive
Complement		
Hereditary angioedema (C1 inhibitor deficiency)	Recurrent facial, laryngeal, gastrointestinal or limb edema	Autosomal dominant
Neutrophil		
Hyper IgE (Job) syndrome	Recurrent staphylococcal skin abscesses, chronic eczema, otitis media, severe periodontal disease	Unknown
Chronic granulomatous disease	supportive lymphadenitis, hepatosplenomegaly, pneumonitis, osteomyelitis	X-linked, Autosomal

G. Differential diagnosis is severe combined immunodeficiency (SCID) and hypogammaglobulinemia.

H. Potential complications are infections with encapsulated organisms, Gram-negative bacteria, opportunistic organisms, and continued poor growth, leading eventually to death.

I. Therapy is treatment of specific infections, infection prophylaxis and antiretroviral therapy.

6.3.3 Secondary Immunodeficiency Disorders

A. Many diseases interfere temporarily or permanently with the function of the normal immune system.

B. The two most common significant diseases resulting in immunodeficiency are HIV (section 6.3.2) and protein-calorie malnutrition.

C. Examples of Secondary Immunodeficiency

1. Premature and newborn infants have an immature immune system for up to several months after birth.
2. Infections can result in immunosuppression by direct effect on individual immune cell number and function, or by overall suppression of bone marrow function. This can be seen with bacterial (tuberculosis, sepsis), viral (HIV, cytomegalovirus, measles, rubella, hepatitis, Epstein-Barr virus), fungal, and parasitic (malaria) infections.
3. Chronic disease such as sickle-cell disease (functional splenectomy) and cystic fibrosis (malnutrition, impairment of nonspecific host defenses) leads to decreased immune response to pathogens.
4. Neoplastic disease (leukemia, Hodgkin's disease, nonlymphoid cancer) destroys and replaces functional immune tissue.
5. Surgery and trauma result in consumption or loss of immune mediators (burns, stress) or mechanical loss of immune tissue (splenectomy).
6. Autoimmune disease (systemic lupus erythematosus, rheumatoid arthritis, acute graft-versus-host disease) results in disordered function of the immune system. Treatments which usually involve immunosuppressive drugs increase the risk of infection.
7. Other miscellaneous causes of altered immune function or decreased immune system components include protein-losing states (protein-losing enteropathy, nephrotic syndrome), immunosuppressive treatments (chemotherapy, radiation, corticosteroids), heredity, and metabolic disease.

6.3.4 Hypersensitivity Reactions

A. Mechanisms which provide host defense can also cause tissue damage if the reaction is exaggerated.

B. Four major types of reaction are recognized:

1. Type I is the anaphylactic, atopic, or reaginic reaction mediated by IgE triggered release of histamine and other substances (hay fever, extrinsic asthma, anaphylactic shock).
2. Type II is an antibody-mediated cytotoxic reaction. IgG or IgM binds to cell-carried antigens, resulting in lysis (autoimmune hemolytic anemia).
3. Type III is associated with tissue deposition of immune-complexes. Complement activation is involved (autoimmune diseases, serum sickness, Arthus reactions).
4. Type IV occurs when sensitized T cells bind to cellular antigens and result in lysis (graft rejection, acute graft-versus-host disease, contact dermatitis).

6.3.5 Autoimmune Diseases

A. Autoimmune diseases arise in situations where the host defense mechanisms recognize the individuals own cell antigens as foreign.

B. The most common mediators of autoimmune diseases are misdirected type I and type III hypersensitivity reactions.

C. Some of the conditions that occur when the system goes awry are systemic lupus erythematosus, rheumatoid arthritis, rheumatic fever, serum sickness, mucocutaneous lymph node syndrome (Kawasaki disease), Henoch-Schönlein purpura, atopic dermatitis, and Lyme disease.

D. Diagnosis and treatment are dependent on the specific suspected etiology.

87. Which of the following are nonspecific host defenses — B 6.1.1

A. antibodies
B. oral mucosa
C. T cells
D. B cells
E. natural killer cells

88. Which immunoglobulin (Ig) is the major antibody that persists after an antigenic challenge — A 6.1.2

A. IgG
B. IgM
C. IgD
D. IgE
E. IgA

89. What is the function of a helper T cell — D 6.1.3

A. precursor for other T-cell subtypes
B. kill foreign cells
C. recruit macrophages
D. aid in B-cell antibody production

90. A 3-year-old has a history of recurrent infections with pneumococcus and *Haemophilus influenzae,* and experienced severe enteroviral sepsis at 1 year of age. He has bronchiectasis. He is growing normally. He has a deficiency in which type of immunity — B 6.2.1

A. T cell
B. B cell
C. complement
D. he is not immune deficient

91. Which genetic syndrome is associated with seizures, hypoparathyroidism, cardiac disease, and recurrent infections — C 6.3.1

A. Wiskott-Aldrich syndrome
B. ataxia-telangiectasia
C. DiGeorge's syndrome
D. severe combined immunodeficiency

92. An 8-month-old child is in foster care. His family history is unknown. His medical history includes 2 prior hospitalizations for pneumonia, 3 episodes of candidiasis, growth failure, and intermittent diarrhea. His evaluation should include — D 6.3.2

A. immunoglobulin G anti-human immunodeficiency virus
B. immunoglobulin A anti-human immunodeficiency virus
C. human immunodeficiency virus polymerase chain reaction
D. A and C
E. B and C

93. Anaphylaxis is mediated by which of the following immunoglobulin (Ig) types — C 6.3.4

A. IgG
B. IgA
C. IgE
D. IgD
E. IgM

94. Which immunoglobulin (Ig) is present in the highest concentration in the serum — A 6.1.2

A. IgG
B. IgA
C. IgM
D. IgD
E. IgE

7 INFECTIOUS DISEASE

7.1 GENERAL CONCEPTS

7.1.1 Age Related Considerations

A. Infants under 2 to 3 months of age are not able to isolate and localize infections very effectively. Also, they may not at that age show signs of infection other than temperature changes, either fever or hypothermia. Therefore, infants under 2 months of age with a rectal temperature over 38.0° C or who are hypothermic should have a "sepsis work-up" (cultures of blood, urine, and cerebrospinal fluid (CSF), at a minimum).

B. Even if their temperature is less than 38.0° C, infants under 2 months of age who are found to have an infection presumably, due to a bacterial cause (pneumonia, otitis media, urinary tract infection), should be assumed to be incapable of localizing the infection and started on intravenous antibiotics after a sepsis work-up is completed.

C. Placentally-transferred maternal immunity lasts a few months.

D. Children in daycare get more upper respiratory tract infections ("common colds") for their age than those exposed to fewer contacts. It is unknown to what extent these children are protected from upper respiratory tract infections in later school years because of an already acquired immunity to certain viral agents.

7.1.2 Temperature Regulation and Fever

A. A child's temperature is normally lower in the early morning than late in the afternoon after they have been active. The maximal daily temperature of children usually occurs between 5:00 and 7:00 PM.

B. Excessive clothing can interfere with the child's ability to dissipate normal body heat and result in a raised body temperature.

C. A normal homeostatic mechanism establishes the temperature threshold in children at around 41.1° C (106° F).

D. Leukocytes have greater phagocytic activity at 38° to 40° C than at lower temperatures.

E. A decrease in temperature after administration of antipyretics does not distinguish between bacterial and viral infections.

F. Because of its association with Reye's syndrome in children and adolescents, aspirin should not be used to treat fever in these groups.

G. There are literally hundreds of diseases, not all infectious, which have fever as one of their components. Since there are so many causes of fever, the finding of fever alone does not narrow the list of diagnostic possibilities much.

H. A fever without obvious cause does not necessarily mean the child has a viral infection.

7.2 DIAGNOSIS

7.2.1 Physical Examination (Table 7.2.1)

7.2.2 Laboratory Studies

A. **Gram staining** is useful for classifying bacteria, thus narrowing the list of diagnostic possibilities.

B. **Cultures**

1. Bacteria and Fungi. Selective media is used to classify the bacteria or fungus as to type and subtype. This information can then be used to guide selection of a therapeutic agent.
2. Viral Cultures. Usually done in tissue culture which can take significantly longer than that available for bacteria and fungi.

C. **Immunologic Techniques**

1. **Immunofluorescence**. Fluorescent antibodies (FA) are specific antisera that are used to identify bacteria by fluorescence which results when added to sera containing the pathogen.
2. **Agglutination Tests**. A substance, usually latex, is coated with antibodies that will agglutinate when added to sera containing their antigen. It is more sensitive than countercurrent immunoelectrophoresis (CCIE).
3. **CCIE**. Able to detect antigens in body fluids, including cerebral spinal fluid and urine. It can identify antigens of *Haemophilus influenzae* type b, *Streptococcus pneumoniae*, and some types of *Neisseria meningitidis*.
4. **Enzyme-Linked Immunosorbent Assay** (ELISA). Used to detect viral antibodies. It is now available for detecting most viruses.
5. **Polymerase Chain Reaction** (PCR). Uses deoxyribonucleic acid and ribonucleic acid probes to identify pathogen nucleic acid in clinical specimens.

D. **Sepsis Work-Up**. A sepsis work-up is done when a significant infection is feared and a source or the extent of infection is not evident. The following tests are performed:

1. **Blood Cultures**. A minimum of one blood culture is obtained.
2. **Lumbar Puncture**. Cerebral spinal fluid (CSF) is sent for protein, glucose, culture and sensitivity, CCIE, cell count, and other studies based on clinical suspicion.
3. **Chest x-ray** is obtained to rule out pneumonia, as well as other chest pathology.
4. **Chem 7** (sodium, potassium, chloride, carbon dioxide, glucose, blood urea nitrogen, creatinine).
   a. The glucose is needed for comparison with the CSF glucose and blood urea nitrogen and creatinine to assess hydration status and guide dosing of potentially nephrotoxic drugs.
   b. Electrolytes provide guidance in fluid therapy and assess the potential of inappropriate antidi-

uretic hormone (ADH) secretion found in some cases of meningitis (especially *Haemophilus influenzae*).

5. **Urine** is collected for culture and sensitivity as well as routine studies. It should be obtained by suprapubic tap or by bladder catheterization in children whom a mid-stream clean catch urine cannot be obtained.
6. **White Blood Cell** (WBC). Elevated WBC counts can be supportive of, but are not diagnostic of a bacterial infection.
   a. Typically, the WBC count is elevated in bacterial infections and normal or low in viral infections. However, early viral infections may have an elevated WBC count and overwhelming bacterial infections may cause a decreased number of WBCs.
   b. Other conditions, such as leukemia, can obscure the interpretation of the WBC count. (CAUTION: An automated blood cell counter cannot differentiate between blast cells and lymphocytes and will report them as lymphocytes or monocytes.)

7.2.3 Infectious Diseases Grouped by Patient Categories (Table 7.2.3)

7.2.4 Diseases Identified by Typical Childhood Exanthems (Table 7.2.4)

7.3 DISEASE PROFILES

7.3.1 Occult Bacteremia

A. Occult bacteremia is the presence of bacteria in the bloodstream without clinical manifestations other than fever.

B. *Streptococcus pneumoniae* (70 to 80%), *Haemophilus influenzae* type b, *Neisseria meningitidis*, group A streptococcus, and *Staphylococcus aureus* are the most common bacterial etiologies.

C. Risk Factors
   1. Children ages 3 months to 3 years have the highest incidence of occult bacteremia (approximately 4%).
   2. Incidence increases when the temperature exceed-

Table 7.2.1 Physical examination

REGION	FOCUS	SIGNIFICANT ABNORMALITIES
General Appearance	Playfulness Interactiveness Alertness Consolability Irritability with movement Color Hydration	Disinterest in activities or play Withdrawn demeanor Unaware of those in room Unresponsive to comforting Movement of inflamed tissue, including the meninges, causes pain Pallor or cyanosis Sunken eyes or fontanelle, dry mucous membranes
Head, Eyes, Ear, Nose, and Throat (HEENT)	Fontanelle Nuchal rigidity Rhinorrhea Tympanic membranes Drooling	Bulging or depressed Brudzenski and Kernig signs Purulent discharge may be due to sinusitis Erythema, lack of mobility Pharyngitis, gingivostomatitis, retropharyngeal abscess, and epiglottitis
Heart	Murmurs Friction rubs Distant heart sounds	Rheumatic fever, endocarditis Suspect pericarditis Suspect pericardial effusion
Lungs	Persistant cough, tachypnea, expiratory grunting, retractions, flaring of nasal alae	Suspect pneumonia
Abdomen	Localized tenderness	Appendicitis, hepatitis, pyelonephritis
Extremities	Joint swelling, pain Bone pain	Septic joint, arthritis Osteomyelitis, leukemia, sickle cell disease
Integument	Petechial rashes, cellulitis	Meningococcemia, Rocky Mountain spotted fever, leukemia

ing 39° C, with risk proportional to the degree of fever. These febrile children are usually irritable as well.

3. WBC count >15,000 cells/mm^3, increased absolute granulocyte count, increased erythrocyte sedimentation rate (ESR) or increased C-reactive protein are indicators of possible occult bacteremia, although no combination of laboratory tests are 100% accurate in predicting this condition in any given child.

D. Blood culture should be obtained in any child with suspected occult bacteremia.

E. Therapeutic Plan
1. If the organism is not *Streptococcus pneumoniae*, treat as sepsis. Complete the sepsis work-up, if not already done, and begin antibiotics appropriate for the patients age.
2. If the organism is *Streptococcus pneumoniae,* and the child is afebrile and appears well when culture results become known, repeat the culture observe. If the child is still febrile, complete the sepsis work-up, repeat the blood culture, and decide on inpatient or outpatient treatment based upon the age and condition of the child.

F. With appropriate treatment, spontaneous resolution of the fever should occur in 24 to 48 hours with *Streptococcus pneumoniae* and sepsis with other organisms.

7.3.2 Sepsis

A. Sepsis is life-threatening invasion of the bloodstream usually by bacteria.

B. The most common causative agents are *Haemophilus influenzae*, *Neisseria meningitidis*, and *Streptococcus pneumoniae.*

C. Predisposing conditions are compromised host defense, immaturity, or infection with a particularly virulent strain of organism.

D. Symptoms can include high fever, respiratory distress, shock, altered mental status, local pain (if invasive), and petechial or purpuric rashes.

E. Laboratory analysis may reveal either WBC pleocytosis or neutropenia, an increase in the immature forms of WBCs, and a positive blood culture, with or without other positive body fluid cultures.

F. Focal infections of the central nervous system, bone, or other organ tissues are potential complications.

G. Treatment is age and problem specific.
1. In infants <2 months old, initial coverage includes ampicillin and either gentamicin or cefotaxime.
2. In infants and children >2 months old, initial therapy is with ceftriaxone or cefotaxime.
3. If meningitis is present and the causative agent is identified as potentially being pneumococcus, empiric coverage should also include vancomycin until susceptibility patterns of the bacterial pathogen are known. Such treatment is necessary due to the high incidence of multiple drug resistance in these organisms.

7.3.3 Meningitis

A. Meningitis is inflammation of the meninges surrounding the brain.

B. It can be caused by bacteria, fungi, atypical bacteria, and viruses. When a specific etiologic agent cannot be identified, the term aseptic meningitis is applied.

C. Signs and symptoms include severe headache, altered sensorium, seizures, vomiting, meningeal signs (nuchal rigidity, Kernig's or Brudzinski's signs), and bulging fontanelle (if the anterior fontanelle is still palpable).
1. **Kernig's sign** is performed by flexing the hip to 90° and extending the leg at the knee. If meningeal irritation is present, pain is produced upon leg extension.
2. **Brudzinski's sign** is involuntary flexion of the knees and hips during passive flexion of the neck while supine.

D. **Bacterial meningitis**
1. Usually arises from hematogenous spread of pathogens.
2. Neonates are typically infected with organisms that reflect maternal flora (group B streptococcus, *Listeria monocytogenes,* and enteric bacteria).
3. Children between 2 and 12 years of age most commonly become infected with pneumococcus and *Neisseria meningitides.*
   a. Serogroup B meningococcus is the usual agent in sporadic cases, with A and C comprising the agents in epidemic meningococcal meningitis.
   b. Previously, *Haemophilus influenzae* type B was the most prevalent etiology of bacterial meningitis in this age group. Universal vaccination has lead to a dramatic decline in its incidence.
4. The median age for bacterial meningitis is now 25 years versus 15 months in 1986. This is largely due to the development and widespread use of vaccines, beginning in infancy, against common pathogens.
5. CSF pleocytosis, increase in CSF protein, decrease in CSF glucose, and positive CSF fluid cultures or antigen tests are seen in meningitis. Gram stain may be positive as well.
6. Complications can include shock, disseminated intravascular coagulation (DIC), subdural effusion, cerebral edema, seizures, syndrome of inappropriate antidiuretic hormone (SIADH), and permanent neurologic sequelae.
7. Antibiotic choices for treatment are the same as for sepsis. Acyclovir is used if herpes simplex virus (HSV) is suspected.

E. **Aseptic meningitis** is nonbacterial inflammation of the meninges.

1. Numerous etiologies exist: enteroviruses (85% of cases), coxsackie virus, echoviruses, arboviruses (St. Louis encephalitis virus, California encephalitis virus), human immunodeficiency virus (HIV), varicella, Ebstein-Barr virus (EBV), measles, rubella, rabies, influenza, parainfluenza, cytomegalovirus (CMV), mumps, *Mycoplasma, Chlamydia,* fungi, protozoa and other parasites, and postinfectious reactions. Less common pathogens are leptospirosis, syphilis, Lyme disease, cat-scratch disease, nocardiosis, Rocky Mountain spotted fever (RMSF), vasculitis, intracranial hemorrhage, reactions to nonsteroidal antiinflammatory drugs, and heavy metal poisoning.
2. Headache, irritability, fever, nausea, vomiting, and retrobulbar pain are reported symptoms, with nuchal rigidity, exanthems, and signs of underlying disease present on exam.
3. Laboratory findings are elevated CSF WBCs (often predominately polymorphonuclear cells early, lymphocytes and mononuclear cells later), normal or slightly elevated CSF protein, normal CSF glucose in viral causes, and a negative CSF Gram stain.
4. Care is supportive in the presence of viral etiologies. Often, children seem to have improvement in the severity of headache after the diagnostic lumbar puncture. If HSV is suspected, initiate treatment with intravascular acyclovir.
5. The disease is usually self-limiting when caused by viral infection.

7.3.4 Other Central Nervous System Infections

A. Encephalitis

1. **Encephalitis** is an acute inflammation of brain parenchyma.
2. Common causative agents are HSV, St. Louis encephalitis virus, California encephalitis virus, eastern equine encephalitis virus, western equine encephalitis virus, coxsackie virus, echoviruses, or postinfectious encephalitis following measles, mumps, varicella, rubella, *Mycoplasma pneumoniae,* amebas (*Naegleria, Acanthamoeba*), and *Toxoplasma gondii.*

Table 7.2.3 Likely infectious diseases etiologies for febrile patients catagorized by group

PATIENT GROUP	AT RISK FOR
Previously Normal	
Neonate <1 month of age	Group B streptococcus, *Escherichia coli*, *Listeria monocytogenes*, herpes simplex, enterococcus
Infant 1 to 3 months of age	Group B streptococcus, *Escherichia coli, Listeria monocytogenes,* respiratory syncytial virus, enterovirus, *Haemophilus influenzae, Neisseria meningitis*
Temperature >41° C	Meningitis, bacteremia, pneumonia, heat stroke, hemorrhagic shock-encephalopathy syndrome
Petechial rash with fever	Meningococcus, *Hemophilus influenzae* type b, pneumococcus, Rocky Mountain spotted fever
Immunocompromised	
Sickle cell anemia	Pneumococcal sepsis, meningitis, *Salmonella*
Asplenia	Encapsulated bacteria (esp. pneumococcus), *Salmonella*
Agammaglobulinemia	Bacteremia, sinopulmonary infection
Acquired immunodeficiency syndrome	Pneumococcus, *Haemophilus influenzae* type b, *Salmonella*
Immunosuppressive drugs	*Pseudomonas aeruginosa, Staphylococcus aureus, Candida, Staphylococcus epidermidis*
Left-to-right shunt heart lesions	endocarditis
Central venous lines	*Staphylococcus aureus, Staphylococcus epidermidis, Corynebacterium, Candida*

3. Symptoms are similar to aseptic meningitis, but with more severe central nervous system manifestations (confusion, delirium, hallucinations, memory loss, combativeness, seizures, coma).
4. Physical exam reveals focal neurologic signs, ataxia, and signs of increased intracranial pressure.
5. Laboratory findings include increased CSF red blood cells with HSV, increased CSF WBCs (usually 10 to 500 cells/mm^3), increased CSF protein, and a normal CSF glucose.
6. Diagnostic plan is geared toward identification of the etiologic agent and includes culture, PCR, antigen testing, serology, magnetic resonance imaging (MRI), and potentially, brain biopsy.
7. Treatment
   a. Acyclovir is indicated for HSV and complicated herpes zoster.
   b. Supportive care for increased intracranial pressure.
   c. Other pharmacologic agents may be needed based upon the diagnosis (amphotericin B in fungal or amebic infection).
8. Prognosis varies with etiology. Examples include:
   a. St. Louis, California and Western equine encephalitis have a good prognosis with likely full neurologic recovery.
   b. Eastern equine and HSV encephalitis have a 60% death rate and high incidence of serious neurologic sequelae in survivors.
   c. *Acanthamoeba* and *Naegleria* infections are almost universally fatal.

B. Brain Abscess

1. This is a common central nervous system infection in 4 to 8 year olds.
2. The condition arises from embolization in those with congenital heart disease or local spread from meningitis, otitis media, sinusitis, or mastoiditis.
3. The agents are pneumococcus, *Staphylococcus aureus,* anaerobes, and Gram-negative bacteria.
4. Early symptoms (lethargy and low grade fever) are

Table 7.2.4 Diseases identified by typical childhood exanthems

DISEASE	INCUBATION PERIOD	TYPICAL DISTRIBUTION	CLINICAL FEATURES
Maculopapular Lesions			
Measles (Rubeola)	10-14 days	Begins at hairline and descends downward; Generalized by 3rd day; Confluent on face, neck, upper trunk	3 day prodrome with 3 C's: Cough, Conjunctivitis, Coryza: Koplik's spots 2 days before rash; Desquamates after 7-10 days
Rubella (German Measles; Three-Day Measles)	14-21 days	Begins on face, progresses rapidly downward; Generalized by second day; Fades in order of appearance	Postauricular and suboccipital lymphadenopathy; Arthritis common in women
Roseola (Exanthema Subitum)	10-14 days	Appears after defrevescence of fever; Initially on chest, then face, extremities; fades quickly	3-4 day prodrome of high fever in otherwise well appearing 1 to 4 year old child
Erythema Enfectiosum (Fifth Disease; Parvovirus B19)	7-14 days	Red flushed cheeks with circumoral pallor (slapped cheek); Followed by reticular, lacy rash on extremities; May recur on exposure to trauma, sunlight, heat	Patients with diseases that shorten red blood cell life span may have aplastic crisis
Enterovirus (esp. Echovirus Type 9)	few days	Rubella-like lesions; Nonpuritic; May be petechial; Lasts 3-5 days	Fever, malaise, sore throat, rhinorrhea, vomiting, diarrhea, herpangina; Illness may mimic meningococcemia
Scarlet Fever (Group A Streptococci)	2-4 days	Sandpaper texture; Appears 1st on flexor surfaces, then generalized; Most intense on neck, shoulders, axilla, inguinal, popliteal skin folds; Circumoral pallor, Lasts 7 days then desquamates	Pharyngitis, tonsillitis, strawberry tongue, palatal petechiae

(continued)

nonspecific. Later, the child develops vomiting, headache, seizures, focal neurologic deficits, coma, shock, and ultimately, death.

5. The WBC count is normal to elevated and the blood culture is positive in 10% of patients. CSF studies reveal normal to minimally increased WBC and protein, and a slightly low glucose. (Do not do a lumbar puncture if an abscess is suspected based on initial presentation).
6. Diagnosis is usually made by neuroimaging.
7. Treatment is generally with parenteral antibiotics alone based on the suspected pathogen. Aspiration or excision are performed only if gas is present on imaging studies, the lesion is multiloculated, mass effect is evident, or the lesion is fungal.
8. Mortality is 5 to 10%, worse if the lesions are multiple. Neurologic sequelae are common in survivors (hemiparesis, seizures, hydrocephalus, learning disability, behavior problems).

7.3.5 Head, Eyes, Ears, Nose, and Throat (HEENT) Infections

A. Periorbital (Preseptal) Cellulitis

1. This is an inflammatory process occurring in the structures superficial to the orbital septum.
2. A bacterial pathogen is identified in only 30% of cases. The infecting organism is generally related to the route of infection.
   a. Trauma, such as insect bite, leads to infection with *Staphylococcus aureus* or *Streptococcus pyogenes.*
   b. *Haemophilus influenzae* type b and *Streptococcus pneumoniae* arise from local extension of infection from a sinusitis.
   c. *Haemophilus influenzae* type b and *Streptococcus pneumoniae* also cause disease by seeding

Table 7.2.4 Diseases identified by typical childhood exanthems (continued)

DISEASE	INCUBATION PERIOD	TYPICAL DISTRIBUTION	CLINICAL FEATURES
Vesicular/pustular Lesions			
Varicella (Chickenpox)	10-21 days	Discrete puritic macules which progress to vesicles, umbilicated pustules and then crusted lesions; All stages are present at the same time; Can involve mucous membranes	Avoid asprin; Contagious until all lesions are crusted over
Herpes Zoster (shingles)		Erythema, followed by red papules, then vesicles in 12-24 hours, then pustules in 72 hours, then crusts in 10-12 days; Unilateral peripheral dermatome distribution; does not cross midline	History of varicella; Pre-eruptive pain common
Hand, Foot, and Mouth Syndrome (Coxsackievirus A16)	4-6 days	Palmar and plantar pustules have typical elliptical football-shaped appearance	Fever, myalgia, malaise, herpangina, rhinorrhea, vomiting, diarrhea
Disseminated Gonococcemia		Erythema or hemorrhagic papules that evolve into pustules or vesicles with an erythematous halo	Affects primarily young women; Fever and migratory polyarthralgias are common
Impetigo (Group A Streptococcus; Bullous lesions are caused by Staphylococci)		Honey-colored crusted lesions with a predilection for the face and exposed areas; Bullous lesions are round bullae which rupture quickly	Poststrptococcal glomerulonephritis is a potential complication; Bullous impetigo may be mistaken for cigarette burns
Insect Bites		Local reactions may resemble infectious exanthems or may be secondarily infected	

of the preseptal tissue during bacteremia.

3. The child presents with acute swelling, redness, and pain of the eyelids and periorbital tissues. Proptosis is absent, as is pain with eye movement, helping to distinguish periorbital cellulitis from orbital cellulitis or abscess.
4. Orbital cellulitis may be a complication.
5. It is sometimes difficult to distinguish periorbital cellulitis from local trauma, noninfectious periorbital edema, and local allergic reactions.
6. Oral or parenteral antibiotics are prescribed to cover likely etiologic agents. Careful monitoring to detect progression to orbital cellulitis is essential.
7. Recovery generally occurs without sequelae.

B. Orbital Cellulitis

1. Orbital cellulitis is an inflammatory process deep to the orbital septum.
2. The etiologic agents are the same as seen in periorbital cellulitis.
3. Affected patients have pain with movement of the eyes and fever.
4. Exam is very similar to periorbital cellulitis except for the presence of proptosis and chemosis.
5. Leukocytosis is present on complete blood cell count, and blood culture may be positive.
6. Complications can be severe and include cavernous sinus thrombosis, meningitis, and epidural, subdural or brain abscess.
7. Sepsis work-up should be strongly considered.
8. Therapy should incorporate intravenous antibiotics and an ophthalmology consult.

C. Buccal Cellulitis

1. Except for the location, the implications of this entity parallel those of periorbital cellulitis.
2. Prior to widespread availability of *Haemophilus influenzae* vaccine, this agent was the most common cause of buccal cellulitis. A full sepsis work-up was indicated due to the significant association with meningitis. The same was true for preseptal cellulitis.

D. Candidal Gingivostomatitis (Thrush)

1. Thrush is the formation of adherent white plaques on the buccal mucosa, palate, and tongue, caused by candida species, usually *Candida albicans.*
2. Thrush is common in infants. When it occurs after infancy, consider immune deficiency.
3. Infants exhibit poor feeding and fussiness. Older children and adults may complain of mouth or throat irritation.
4. Treatment is with nystatin oral suspension or oral fluconazole in resistant cases.

E. Herpetic Gingivostomatitis

1. Herpetic gingivostomatitis is a vesiculoulcerative condition affecting the mouth.
2. The etiologic agents are HSV, usually type I, and type II.
3. Primary infection involves the mouth and gums, and can be extensive and severe. Recurrent infection tends to be localized to the lips.
4. After the primary infection, the virus lies dormant in nerve tissue until reactivation occurs.
5. Recurrence is precipitated by stress, either physical or emotional.
6. Chronologic Sequence of Manifestations
   a. The incubation period is 3 to 9 days.
   b. Once the lesions erupt, improvement occurs after 3 to 10 days, with resolution in 2 weeks.
7. Dehydration requiring intravenous fluid rehydration may occur, especially in primary HSV gingivostomatitis.
8. Treatment is primarily supportive. Cold foods and liquids, oral painting with a mixture of Maalox® and diphenhydramine, and analgesics are employed for pain control. Oral acyclovir may shorten the duration of illness if administered within the first day or two of illness.
9. Complications include herpetic whitlow, keratoconjunctivitis, and skin infection secondary to autoinoculation.

F. Acute Necrotizing Ulcerative Gingivitis (ANUG)

1. Alternate terminology is Vincent's stomatitis or trench mouth.
2. Fusiform bacilli and spirochetes invade areas of interdental papillae eroded by plaque.
3. Severe dental plaque predisposes to the condition.
4. Physical findings include fever, malodorous breath, and gingival pain.
5. Treatment is with penicillin.

G. Coxsackievirus Infections

1. **Herpangina** is the formation of yellow ulcers on an erythematous base, usually located on the soft palate and tonsillar pillars. It is associated with sudden onset of fever. It is caused by group A coxsackieviruses.
2. **Hand, foot, and mouth disease** presents with fever, malaise, oral mucosal ulcers, and erythematous papules on the hands, feet, and diaper area. It is caused by coxsackie A16. It has a summer and fall seasonal pattern.
3. **Pleurodynia** is sudden onset of fever and pain in the upper abdomen and chest caused by Coxsackieviruses B1, B2, B3 and B5, and echoviruses. The pain is paroxysmal and knife-like. The illness usually resolves in days to a few weeks without sequelae.
4. Group B coxsackieviruses have been associated with myocarditis and pericarditis.
5. Coxsackie infection is second only to mumps as the etiologic agent in orchitis.

H. Sinusitis

1. Etiologic agents are *Staphylococcus pneumoniae*, unencapsulated strains of *Haemophilus influenzae*, and *Bacteroides catarrhalis*.
2. Allergic rhinitis, viral upper respiratory tract infections, swimming, structural anomalies, dysmotile cilia disorders, cystic fibrosis, and trauma predispose to acute and chronic sinusitis.
3. Sinus Development
   a. Maxillary and ethmoid sinuses are present in utero, although further development (enlargement and aeration) occurs after birth.
   b. The frontal and sphenoid sinuses begin to develop around 2 years of age, but are not visible by radiology until age 6 years or later.
4. Fever, headache, chronic nasal discharge (if terribly malodorous, look for a foreign object), persistent cough, and sometimes facial pain are symptoms reported by children. These symptoms are confirmed by exam. Additionally, the examiner may note halitosis.
5. Diagnosis is primarily by history and exam, since x-ray findings are unreliable, especially under age 3 years. If x-rays are performed, they may show air fluid levels or opacity. (Be careful when interpreting these films, as a crying child may also demonstrate air fluid levels in the absence of sinusitis).
6. Potential complications include orbital cellulitis, meningitis, brain abscess, and cavernous sinus thrombosis.
7. Treatment is primarily with amoxicillin, amoxicillin-clavulanate, and second and third generation cephalosporins.

I. Acute Otitis Media (AOM)

1. AOM is a suppurative infection of the middle ear space caused by *Streptococcus pneumoniae*, unencapsulated *Haemophilus influenzae*, *Bacteroides catarrhalis*, group A streptococcus, and *Staphylococcus aureus*.
2. The pathophysiology of the condition is eustachian tube dysfunction, leading to adsorption of air from middle ear, leaving a vacuum with subsequent accumulation of fluid that acts as a growth medium for bacteria migrating from the nasopharynx.
3. The primary symptoms are ear pain, with or without fever, hearing impairment, vomiting, as well as symptoms associated with predisposing infections such as an upper respiratory tract infection.
4. An erythematous, bulging, nonmobile tympanic membrane is noted on exam.
5. Potential complications include hearing deficit with subsequent impaired language acquisition.
6. The incidence of otitis media is increased in children who use pacifiers, drink from bottles, attend daycare, or are exposed to passive smoke.
7. The drug of choice for treatment is amoxicillin given in doses of 80 mg/kg/day in children at risk for infection with multidrug resistant bacteria (daycare, recurrent infection, recent antibiotic therapy).

J. Streptococcal Pharyngitis

1. This is inflammation of the oropharyngeal structures caused by group A β-hemolytic streptococcus (GABHS).
2. Presenting symptoms can include fever, sore throat, headache, abdominal pain, nausea, and vomiting, with or without a scarlatiniform rash.
3. Examination alone cannot distinguish GABHS infection from other bacterial and viral causes of pharyngitis, but may be significant for fever, exudative tonsillar hypertrophy, petechiae on the soft palate, tender anterior cervical nodes, and a fine, erythematous, sandpaper rash. Other associated findings may include desquamation and swelling of the fingers and toes, and in females, vulvovaginitis.
4. Diagnosis is by positive rapid streptococcus screen or a positive culture for the organism. A negative rapid streptococcus screen should always be followed up with a culture for confirmation.
5. Complications include otitis media, acute sinusitis, peritonsillar abscess, cervical lymphadenitis, acute rheumatic fever, and acute glomerulonephritis.
6. Viral pharyngitis, *Corynebacterium diphtheriae*, *Mycobacteria pneumoniae*, infectious mononucleosis, *Neisseria gonorrhoeae*, *Arcanobacterium haemolyticum,* and opportunistic infections in leukemia should be considered in the differential diagnosis.
7. Penicillin is the drug of choice for treatment.

K. Infectious Mononucleosis Syndromes

1. The most common causative agents are EBV and CMV.
2. Symptoms include malaise, headache, fever, sore throat, fatigue, abdominal pain, decreased appetite, and weight loss.
3. On physical exam, pharyngitis, tender anterior and posterior cervical nodes, splenomegaly, and maculopapular rash may be noted. The rash is very likely to develop if the child is treated with ampicillin for concurrent GABHS pharyngitis.
4. Laboratory findings reveal positive monospot test (heterophile antibody) in EBV, antibodies to EBV (titers more sensitive in patients <5 years), and antibodies to CMV if it is the causative agent.
5. Providers should be aware of potential complications of splenic rupture, hepatitis, airway obstruction, aseptic meningitis, and Guillain-Barré syndrome.
6. Patients should avoid contact sports until the spleen is normal.

L. Acute Epiglottitis

1. Epiglottitis is defined as inflammation and edema,

usually infectious, of the epiglottis and surrounding tissues.

2. Previously, it was primarily attributed to *Haemophilus influenzae* type b.
3. Symptoms are rapid in onset and include, high fever, sore throat, and respiratory distress. They may be acutely life threatening.
4. On physical exam, respiratory distress with stridor, drooling, and air hunger (sitting forward with mouth open) are evident. A cherry red epiglottis is seen on direct visualization in the operating room.
5. Lateral neck x-rays, if obtained, show the classic "**Thumbprint Sign.**"
   a. Remember, epiglottitis is not meant to be an x-ray diagnosis. If the child is suspected to have epiglottitis, direct, controlled visualization of the structure by individuals skilled in intubation is the diagnostic modality of choice.
   b. NEVER send a child with suspected epiglottitis to radiology without skilled medical supervision.
6. The feared complication is complete airway obstruction.
7. Management is to maintain the child in a position of comfort, avoiding activities that cause agitation. Transport the child to the operating room as soon as possible for examination and definitive airway support.
8. Treat the child with endotracheal intubation, ventilatory support, and intravenous antibiotics to cover beta-lactamase producing organisms until airway edema resolves.
9. Prognosis for recovery is good if airway control is maintained and antibiotics are effective.

M. Acute Laryngotracheobronchitis (Croup)

1. Croup is a condition of laryngeal edema caused by any of a number of respiratory viruses. Parainfluenza is the most common causative agent.
2. The child with croup usually has symptoms of an upper respiratory tract infection and awakens in the early morning hours with a barking cough, vocal hoarseness, respiratory distress, and stridor, with or without fever.
3. An anteroposterior soft tissue neck x-ray may reveal subglottic narrowing (**Steeple sign**).
4. Symptoms progress over several days. The episodes of croup are usually worse on the second and third nights of the illness.
5. Treatment
   a. Home care includes humidification (cool mist humidifier or steamy shower). Oral dexamethasone or prednisone may also be prescribed.
   b. Clinic or hospital care includes dexamethasone, nebulized saline, and nebulized racemic epinephrine. Contrary to previous practice, the use of nebulized racemic epinephrine in the acute management of croup does not always necessitate inpatient hospitalization.

7.3.6 Lung Infections

A. Bronchiolitis

1. Bronchiolitis is an infectious edema of bronchiolar mucosa usually caused by respiratory syncytial virus (50%), parainfluenza virus, or adenovirus.
2. Children with these infections can present with cough, wheezing, tachypnea, respiratory distress or failure, nasal congestion, difficulty feeding, and dehydration.
3. The natural course of the condition is to initially resemble a mild upper respiratory tract infection, before progressing, over a week, to respiratory distress. Symptom resolution is slow and occurs over several weeks. Infants, especially those born premature, are more likely to have severe disease.
4. Diagnosis can be made by rapid viral antigen assays and fluorescent antibody testing.
5. The dire complications are respiratory failure, apnea, and cardiorespiratory arrest.
6. Asthma, pertussis, congestive heart failure, pneumonia, and foreign body aspiration are in the differential diagnosis.
7. The incidence of disease can be diminished by prophylaxis, with monthly injections of specific antibody against several strains of respiratory syncytial virus.
8. Treatment
   a. Supportive care with oxygen and intravenous fluids is provided if needed.
   b. Bronchodilators, steroids, and Ribavirin are unlikely to be of benefit.
9. Children hospitalized with bronchiolitis in infancy have a higher incidence of asthma later in childhood.

B. Pneumonia is infection of lung parenchyma caused by bacterial, viral, fungal, or rickettsial agents.

1. **Bacterial Pneumonia**
   a. The most common bacterial etiology is *Streptococcus pneumoniae. Haemophilus influenzae*, GABHS, and *Staphylococcus aureus, Mycoplasma pneumoniae* are also likely causes.
   b. Symptoms include abrupt fever, shaking chills, cough, and chest pain.
   c. Crackles, decreased breath sounds, and signs of respiratory distress may be present on exam. Tachypnea is the most sensitive indicator of pneumonia in children.
   d. Consolidation is evident on chest x-ray and complete blood cell count shows a leukocytosis. Blood cultures may be positive.
   e. Treatment is age dependent: Infants less than 2 months old are treated with ampicillin and

cefotaxime or gentamicin; between 2 months and 8 years with amoxicillin, amoxicillin-clavulanate, or macrolides (if atypical bacteria are suspected); and in children >8 years old, treatment should be geared to the suspected etiologic agent, either mycoplasma or pneumococcus.

2. **Viral Pneumonia**
   a. Respiratory syncytial virus is the most common agent, but other viruses are associated as well.
   b. Treatment is primarily symptomatic and supportive.
3. **Mycoplasma Pneumonia**
   a. This is also known as atypical pneumonia or "walking" pneumonia.
   b. It is caused by *Mycoplasma pneumoniae.*
   c. It is most common between the ages of 5 and 15 years and in individuals who live in dormitory settings.
   d. Symptoms are sore throat, non productive cough, fever, headache, and malaise. Few findings may be present on exam.
   e. Diagnostic evaluation may reveal elevated titers of cold agglutinating antibodies and infiltrate on chest x-ray.
   f. Treatment is with macrolide antibiotics (erythromycin, azithromycin, clarithromycin).
4. ***Pneumocystis Carinii* Pneumonia**
   a. This condition is seen in immunocompromised patients.
   b. Patients present with severe respiratory distress.
   c. Tracheal washings are positive for the organism.
   d. Patients at risk (human immunodeficiency virus-positive, immune deficient, chemotherapy) should receive trimethoprim-sulfamethoxazole prophylaxis 3 days per week.

7.3.7 Cardiac Infections

A. **Endocarditis**
1. This is a condition where infectious vegetations are found on heart valves.
2. The etiologic agents are β-hemolytic streptococcus, *Staphylococcus aureus*, and *Staphylococcus epidermidis.*
3. Central venous lines, injectable drug use, valvular heart lesions, and cardiac shunts with high turbulence are predisposing risk factors.
4. Symptoms include fatigue, fever, and malaise.
5. Roth's spots, Janeway lesions and Osler's nodes are rare physical findings. Changing murmurs and splinter hemorrhages are more common.
6. Laboratory studies reveal positive blood cultures. Vegetations are seen on echocardiogram.
7. Potential Complications include emboli, mycotic aneurysms, and CHF.
8. Treatment is long-term IV antibiotics (at least 4 weeks).

B. **Myocarditis** is inflammation of the cardiac muscle with associated myocardial dysfunction.
1. Myocarditis is caused by enteroviruses (coxsackie B, echovirus).
2. Symptoms include fever and symptoms of congestive heart failure.
3. Findings on clinical and technical evaluation include dysrhythmias, signs of congestive heart failure, and an abnormal electrocardiogram (EKG).
   a. EKG: ST segment depression, T wave inversion.
   b. Chest x-ray: cardiomegaly, pulmonary vascular congestion, edema.
4. Coxsackie myocarditis is extremely sensitive to digitalis. Regular digitalizing doses can be highly toxic.
5. Treatment is primarily supportive.
6. Spontaneous resolution occurs in 10 to 20%.

C. **Pericarditis** is inflammation, with fluid accumulation in the pericardial sac.
1. Etiologic agents are bacteria, viruses, fungi and tuberculosis.
2. Symptoms include left shoulder pain and back pain relieved by sitting forward, fever, cough, and dyspnea.
3. Physical Findings are a pericardial friction rub and distant heart sounds.
4. Special Testing
   a. Echocardiography: pericardial fluid.
   b. Chest x-ray: enlarged heart with normal pulmonary vascularity.
   c. EKG: ST segment elevation.
5. Cardiac tamponade is a life-threatening condition.
6. Treatment is by pericardial drainage and antibiotics if bacterial etiology is suspected.

7.3.8 Gastrointestinal System Infections

A. **Hepatitis A** is inflammation of the liver caused by hepatitis A virus, a ribonucleic acid virus. It is also known as **infectious hepatitis.**
1. Transmission is by the fecal-oral route.
2. Symptoms may be mistaken for a "common cold" or gastroenteritis in children, as they often do not become jaundiced. Some commonly reported symptoms include right upper quadrant pain, anorexia, nausea, vomiting, and diarrhea.
3. Jaundice, hepatomegaly, and right upper quadrant tenderness can be present on exam.
4. Laboratory findings include elevated liver transaminases, elevated direct and indirect bilirubin, and positive immunoglobulin M anti-hepatitis A virus antibody.
5. Chronologic Sequence of Manifestations
   a. The incubation period is 2 to 6 weeks. The pro-

dromal phase may not be noticed in children.

b. gastrointestinal symptoms, dark urine, and jaundice subsides after 1 to 2 weeks.

6. Children may rarely develop fulminant hepatitis.
7. Infectious mononucleosis, leptospirosis, CMV, Wilson's disease, and other forms of viral hepatitis are considered in the differential diagnosis.
8. Treatment is supportive care.
9. Prognosis is good with complete recovery being the norm.
10. Prevention is accomplished by immunoglobulin G administration to household contacts of the index case within 2 weeks of exposure. Also, disease can be prevented by administration of hepatitis A virus vaccine to susceptible individuals.

B. **Hepatitis B** (serum hepatitis) is caused by hepatitis B virus, a deoxyribonucleic acid virus, with blood borne transmission.

1. Symptoms include fever, arthralgia, right upper quadrant pain, anorexia, nausea, vomiting, and diarrhea.
2. Jaundice, hepatomegaly, and right upper quadrant tenderness are found on exam.
3. Laboratory studies reveal elevated liver transaminases and elevated direct and indirect bilirubin. Antigen and antibody tests allow determination of disease state.
   a. Elevated hepatitis B surface antigen (HBsAg) indicates acute disease.
   b. Antibodies against the hepatitis B surface antigen (HBsAb) indicates immunity.
   c. Presence of hepatitis B e antigen (HBeAg) indicates infectivity.
4. Chronologic Sequence of Manifestations
   a. Incubation period is 2 to 6 months.
   b. Gastrointestinal symptoms, dark urine, and jaundice subsides after 1 to 2 weeks.
   c. The disease may remit or become chronic.
5. Potential complications include fulminant hepatitis, carrier state, or chronic active hepatitis which predisposes to hepatocellular carcinoma.
6. Infectious mononucleosis, leptospirosis, CMV, Wilson's disease, and other viral hepatitis syndromes are in the differential diagnosis.
7. Therapy includes supportive measures.
8. Prevention is available with hepatitis B virus vaccine.

7.3.9 Urinary Tract Infections (UTI)

A. **Cystitis** is infection of the bladder, usually caused by enteric bacteria.

1. Female gender and urologic anatomic abnormalities are risk factors.
2. Symptoms are dysuria, urgency, and frequency.
3. Definitive diagnosis is by positive urine culture.
4. Pyelonephritis is a recognized complication.
5. Treatment is with oral antibiotics.

B. **Pyelonephritis** is inflammation and infection in the kidneys.

1. Symptoms include gastrointestinal symptoms, fever, chills, and flank pain.
2. Costovertebral angle tenderness is usually noted on exam.
3. Hypertension and renal insufficiency may complicate the condition.
4. If the child is very young or toxic in appearance, hospitalization for intravenous fluid and parenteral antibiotics is indicated, otherwise, outpatient therapy with oral antibiotics may be acceptable.
5. All males and most females (especially under age 5) should undergo radiologic evaluation of their urinary tract to rule out vesicoureteral reflux.
   a. Nuclear cystogram is more sensitive than voiding cystourethrography (VCUG) for reflux, but does not define anatomy well. It is acceptable for use in females undergoing evaluation for reflux.
   b. Since boys are at risk for posterior urethral valves, their initial evaluation after a UTI should include a VCUG. It identifies vesicoureteral reflux disease as well as defining lower urinary tract anatomy.

7.3.10 Bone and Joint Infections

A. **Septic Arthritis** is the invasion of the joint space by bacteria.

1. Etiology
   a. *Staphylococcus aureus* is the most common cause and is often preceded by trauma.
   b. *Haemophilus influenzae* type b, is often associated with infection elsewhere (meningitis, otitis media).
   c. *Kingella kingae* is becoming a more prevalent causative agent in toddlers.
   d. Streptococci (group A and B, anaerobic, *Streptococcus viridans*) can cause disease in otherwise healthy children.
   e. *Streptococcus pneumoniae*, and *Neisseria gonorrhoeae* occurs primarily in the hands, wrists, knees, and ankles.
   f. Gram-negative enteric bacteria are found in neonates and immunosuppressed patients.
   g. *Pseudomonas* species are seen in immunosuppressed patients, neonates, and puncture wounds (especially punctures into the foot through athletic shoes).
2. Patients may have fever, irritability, joint pain, and may appear toxic. They may also have effusion, swelling, and limitation of motion about the affected joint.
3. Laboratory Findings
   a. The ESR is elevated as is the WBC count.

b. Blood cultures are positive 50% of the time.
c. Joint aspirate shows the WBC count > 50,000 cells/mm^3, Glucose < 50% of blood glucose, and poor mucin clot formation.
d. X-ray may demonstrate bone demineralization (late finding) and joint distention.
e. Technetium bone scan is positive within 24 hours and may be able to differentiate between arthritis and osteomyelitis.
f. Gallium scan is positive within 24 to 48 hours and becomes normal with effective treatment.

4. Complications. Destruction of cartilage and the growth plate.
5. Differential Diagnosis. See section 7.3.10.
6. Treatment
   a. Parenteral antibiotic therapy with oxacillin, nafcillin, or ceftriaxone is required, depending upon the susceptibility patterns of the pathogen.
   b. Surgical drainage is often required.

B. **Osteomyelitis** is infection of the bone, with a predilection for the metaphysis of long bones.
1. Etiology is similar to septic arthritis plus *Mycobacterium* and, in immunocompromised patients, fungal agents. Patients with sickle cell disease have a high incidence of *Salmonella* infection, although *Staphylococcus aureus* is still the most common agent in this group.
2. Risk factors are trauma, systemic bacterial infection, immunocompromised status, sickle cell disease, and drug abuse.
3. Symptoms include fever and local pain. Infants may have little systemic toxicity.
4. On exam, findings can be local warmth, swelling, tenderness, limp, and restricted movement.
5. Laboratory Findings
   a. WBC and ESR may be elevated.
   b. Blood culture is positive in > 50% of patients.
   c. X-ray shows soft tissue swelling in 3 to 4 days and bone changes in 7 to 10 days (periosteal elevation, lytic changes, sclerosis).
   d. Technetium bone scan demonstrates disease within 24 hours.
6. Complications include chronic osteomyelitis, septic joint, and growth plate damage.
7. Differential diagnosis is septic arthritis, cellulitis, fracture, and Ewing's sarcoma.
8. Therapy is parenteral antibiotics determined by culture susceptibility patterns (initial coverage to include *Staphylococcus aureus*).

7.3.11 Disseminated Infections

A. **Rocky Mountain spotted fever** (RMSF) is a tick-borne vasculitic infection caused by *Rickettsia rickettsii.*
1. Symptoms include fever, chills, headache, irritability, confusion, delirium, myalgia, photophobia, and rash.
2. Physical exam reveals conjunctivitis, profuse nonpitting edema, and rash (rose-colored macules beginning on the wrists, hands, ankles and feet, involving palms and soles, then becoming petechial and purpuric lesions over the entire body).
3. Laboratory Findings include hyponatremia, thrombocytopenia, and positive immunofluorescence antibody.
4. Chronologic Sequence of Manifestations
   a. Abrupt onset of symptoms after a 2 to 8 day incubation period.
   b. Symptoms improve rapidly with antibiotic treatment in mild cases.
5. Complications may include neurologic deficits, coma, renal failure, DIC, gangrene of distal extremities, shock, and death.
6. RMSF must be distinguished from meningococcemia.
7. Treatment is with doxycycline.

B. **Meningococcemia** is a fulminant, multisystem disease caused by *Neisseria meningitides.*
1. Symptoms may be very mild initially and rapidly progress to overwhelming sepsis. They are fever, headache, malaise, arthralgias, and vomiting.
2. Exam reveals a pink maculopapular rash, generalized petechiae, including palms and soles, or purpura and ecchymosis (expect high mortality).
3. Scraping of purpuric lesions may show Gram-negative diplococci and may grow the organism.
4. Onset is insidious or fulminant. The patient may progress to death within12 hours or less of symptom onset.
5. Complications include meningitis, pericarditis, DIC, Waterhouse-Friderichsen syndrome, cardiovascular collapse, and death.
6. Differential diagnosis is RMSF, *Haemophilus influenzae* (rarely), leukemia, idiopathic thrombocytopenic purpura, infectious mononucleosis, measles, Henoch-Schönlein purpura, and viral infections.
7. Treatment
   a. The organism is susceptible to intravenous penicillin. Ceftriaxone and cefotaxime are acceptable alternatives.
   b. Close contacts should receive prophylactic treatment with rifampin, ceftriaxone, or ciprofloxacin.

7.3.12 TORCHS Infections

A. This is an acronym used to identify a group of congenitally acquired infectious agents.
1. **T**: Toxoplasmosis
2. **O**: Other infections
3. **R**: Rubella
4. **C**: Cytomegalovirus
5. **H**: HSV
6. **S**: Syphilis

B. The clinical features of these illnesses overlap to a significant degree and include prematurity, intrauterine growth retardation, non-immune hydrops, skin rash, congenital malformation, chorioretinitis, neutropenia, thrombocytopenia, hepatitis, myocarditis, pneumonia, microcephaly, macrocephaly, hydrocephalus, and intracranial calcifications.

C. Some affected infants are asymptomatic until after nursery discharge.

D. "TORCH titers" are unreliable for diagnosis. Specific testing needs to be geared toward the suspected diagnosis, based on maternal history, and infant physical findings and symptomatology.

95. In normal children, homeostatic mechanisms establish maximum temperature threshold during febrile illnesses at what level — C 7.1.1

- **A.** 104° F
- **B.** 105° F
- **C.** 106° F
- **D.** 107° F
- **E.** 108° F

96. The afebrile infant with tachypnea is more likely to have which of the following infections — B 7.1.1 7.2.1

- **A.** otitis media
- **B.** pneumonia
- **C.** tonsillitis
- **D.** chicken pox
- **E.** conjunctivitis

97. Which of the following infections is more common in infants compared to older children — D 7.2.3

- **A.** salmonella enteritis
- **B.** meningococcemia
- **C.** Rocky Mountain spotted fever
- **D.** group B streptococcus
- **E.** pneumococcus

98. A 5-year-old presents with low-grade fever, bright red cheeks, and a lacy rash on his extremities. What is the diagnosis — A 7.2.4

- **A.** erythema infectiosum
- **B.** erythema toxicum
- **C.** rubella
- **D.** rubeola
- **E.** roseola

99. A 2-year-old presents with low-grade fever, red papules on the hands and feet, and shallow ulcers on the tongue. What is the etiologic agent — C 7.2.4

- **A.** *Neisseria*
- **B.** group A β-hemolytic streptococcus
- **C.** coxsackie A16
- **D.** parvovirus B19
- **E.** human herpesvirus 6

100. A child has a red sandpaper rash with Pastia's lines and circumoral pallor. He has had fever, headache, sore throat, and stomachache. What is the drug of choice for his condition — B 7.3.5

- **A.** no treatment
- **B.** penicillin
- **C.** sulfasoxazole
- **D.** diphenhydramine
- **E.** prednisone

101. A 4-year-old child with congenital heart disease presents with vomiting, headache, seizures, and fever. A computed tomography scan of the brain is performed that reveals a probable brain abscess. What is next step in evaluation or treatment — C 7.3.4

- **A.** perform an lumbar puncture to identify the organism
- **B.** administer corticosteroids
- **C.** administer parenteral antibiotics
- **D.** consult a neurosurgeon to aspirate the lesion

102. A 2-year-old male develops a sudden fever which rises to 106° F and persists for 3 days. The temperature then abruptly drops to normal and a generalized skin rash appears which lasts for only 18 hours. The most likely diagnosis in this case is — D 7.2.4

A. measles (rubeola)
B. chickenpox (varicella)
C. Rocky Mountain spotted fever
D. roseola infantum (exanthem subitum)
E. German measles (rubella)

103. The incidence of occult bacteremia is highest in what age group — C 7.3.1

A. 0 to 3 months
B. 3 to 6 months
C. 3 months to 3 years
D. 3 to 6 years

104. A 2-year-old child with fever has a blood culture performed. Two days later, the culture grows pneumococcus. On contacting the parents, you discover that the child is afebrile and acting well. Appropriate management at this point is to — C 7.3.1

A. admit to the hospital for intravenous antibiotics
B. perform a sepsis work-up
C. repeat the culture and observe
D. evaluate for immune deficiency

105. Why do children <2 months of age need treatment with ampicillin, in conjunction with gentamicin or a third generation cephalosporin, for sepsis — B 7.3.2

A. ampicillin is added to cover group B streptococcus
B. ampicillin is added to cover enterococcus
C. infants immune systems are immature, so they need extra antibiotic coverage
D. ampicillin is necessary for coverage of chlamydia
E. ampicillin is necessary as adjunctive coverage for Gram-negative enterics

106. What organism is the cause of the majority of aseptic meningitis — E 7.3.3

A. group A β-hemolytic streptococcus
B. pneumococcus
C. herpes simplex virus
D. echovirus
E. enterovirus

107. The approach to the child with suspected epiglottitis includes all of the following except — A 7.3.5

A. use a tongue depressor to get a good look at the epiglottis
B. keep the child in a position of comfort
C. have the parent hold blow by oxygen on the child's face in the least anxiety provoking method possible
D. call an otolaryngologist
E. transport the child with the parent to the nearest hospital via ambulance

108. An 8-year-old boy became febrile and anorectic four days ago, five days after his return from a summer camping trip. Yesterday, a red macular rash appeared on his ankles and wrists. The rash rapidly spread to the entire body, including scalp, palms and soles. There are now many petechiae and the child complains of headache, malaise, and myalgia. The most likely diagnosis is — A 7.3.11

A. Rocky Mountain spotted fever
B. anaphylactoid (Henoch-Schönlein) purpura
C. meningococcemia
D. Lyme disease
E. Kawasaki disease (mucocutaneous lymph node syndrome)

109. Physical examination findings in preseptal cellulitis may include all of the following except A 7.3.5

A. proptosis
B. skin redness
C. periorbital edema
D. evidence of a insect bite on the eyelid
E. pain in the eyelids

110. A 2-year-old child presents with a history of low-grade fever and mouth pain. On exam you note swollen gums, shallow ulcers on a red base throughout the mouth, and signs of dehydration. What is the etiology of her condition B 7.3.5

A. parvovirus B19
B. herpes simplex virus
C. coxsackievirus
D. Epstein-Barr virus
E. varicella virus

111. A 2-year-old child presents following recent treatment for sinusitis due to persistent nasal discharge. You note copious, foul smelling, discolored mucous draining from the right nostril. What do you suspect D 7.3.5

A. recurrence of sinusitis
B. chronic sinusitis
C. allergic rhinitis
D. intranasal foreign body
E. noncompliance with therapy

112. A 13-year-old female presents with a 1 week history of sore throat, headache, fever, nausea, and anorexia. She was started on ampicillin 3 days ago for presumed group A β-hemolytic streptococcus throat. She now has a diffuse maculopapular, pruritic, red rash. What is her likely diagnosis E 7.3.5

A. scarlet fever
B. toxic shock syndrome
C. group A β-hemolytic streptococcus
D. parvovirus B19
E. Epstein-Barr virus

113. Which of the causes of encephalitis has the highest mortality rate E 7.3.4

A. St. Louis encephalitis
B. western equine encephalitis
C. eastern equine encephalitis
D. herpes simplex virus
E. *Naegleria*

114. What is the most common cause of bronchiolitis C 7.3.6

A. adenovirus
B. parainfluenza virus
C. respiratory syncytial virus
D. herpes simplex virus
E. influenza virus

115. The mainstay of treatment for respiratory syncytial virus is B 7.3.6

A. ribavirin
B. supportive care
C. acyclovir
D. monoclonal antibody therapy
E. steroids

116. The most common bacterial etiology of pneumonia is D 7.3.6

A. *Haemophilus influenzae*
B. *Staphylococcus aureus*
C. *Moraxella catarrhalis*
D. pneumococcus
E. group A β-hemolytic streptococcus

117. A 14-year-old presents with cough, fever, and wheezing. Chest x-ray shows patchy infiltrates and blood work is positive for cold agglutinating antibodies. Of the following choices, which is the best treatment for this child's illness D 7.3.6

A. penicillin
B. amoxicillin-clavulanate
C. sulfamethoxazole and trimethoprim
D. erythromycin
E. cefuroxime

118. A 15-year-old with systemic lupus erythematosus presents with left shoulder and back pain, relieved by sitting forward, cough, and dyspnea. He has evidence of jugular venous distension. Treatment is C 7.3.7

A. observation
B. chest tube placement
C. pericardiocentesis
D. antibiotics alone
E. steroids alone

119. A 2-year-old daycare attendee has upper respiratory infection symptoms, diarrhea, abdominal pain, and increased aspartate aminotransferase (AST) and alanine aminotransferase (ALT). On exam you note the absence of jaundice and right upper quadrant tenderness. What is the most likely diagnosis A 7.3.8

A. hepatitis A
B. hepatitis B
C. hepatitis C
D. Epstein-Barr virus
E. giardiasis

120. A 6-month-old female has pyelonephritis, fever, and vomiting. Management should include all of the following except D 7.3.9

A. hospitalization for parenteral antibiotics
B. nuclear cystogram
C. a repeat urine culture while on antibiotics
D. outpatient care with oral antibiotics

121. A 15-year-old stepped on a nail while wearing tennis shoes 2 weeks ago. He now has a 3 day history of heel pain, swelling, erythema, fever, and inability to walk. A diagnosis of osteomyelitis is made. Of the following organisms, which is the most likely cause of his infection A 7.3.10

A. *Pseudomonas aeruginosa*
B. group A β-hemolytic streptococcus
C. *Salmonella*
D. *Kingella kingae*
E. *Escherichia coli*

8 RHEUMATOLOGY

8.1 GENERAL CONCEPTS

8.1.1 Definitions

A. **Self-tolerance** is the ability of the immune system to avoid initiating an immune response against self-antigen.

B. **Autoimmunity** is the loss of self-tolerance resulting in an immune assault on self antigens by B or T cell lymphocytes.

8.1.2 Basis of Disease

A. Naturally occurring autoimmune disease tends to be specific for organs or tissues as opposed to the response seen in graft-versus-host disease where the immune dysfunction is seen because of differences in major histocompatibility complex (MHC) antigens.

B. Although no Mendelian inheritance pattern has been identified, autoimmunity and rheumatic disease appears to have a genetic basis. Environmental factors also exert influence.

C. Treatment of autoimmune disease is based on the ability to modify the course of the illness by influencing or interrupting the steps of the immunologic cascade.
   1. Corticosteroids are the most widely used agent in this process.
   2. Intravenous immunoglobulin (IVIG), chemotherapeutic agents such as methotrexate and cyclosporin, and nonsteroidal anti-inflammatory drugs are also frequently utilized.

8.1.3 Immunologic Indicators of Autoimmune Disease

A. **Acute Phase Reactants**
   1. These are substances that present during periods of disease activity.
   2. They are not specific for any given disease process but are elevated in any condition that causes inflammation.
   3. Examples include the erythrocyte sedimentation rate (ESR), C-reactive protein, platelet count, and immunoglobulins.

B. Complement levels can be increased or diminished in autoimmunity.

C. **Autoantibodies** ("anti-self" antibodies) such as antinuclear antibodies (ANA), with few exceptions, are not diagnostic or specific for any one disease.
   1. They may be seen in juvenile rheumatoid arthritis (JRA), systemic lupus erythematosus (SLE), chronic active hepatitis, antiepileptic drug use, birth control pill use, infectious mononucleosis, malignancy, and with aging.
   2. The highest titers are found in SLE and mixed connective tissue disease.
   3. Common associations include anti-double stranded deoxyribonucleic acid in SLE, and both anti-rho and anti-la in neonatal lupus.

D. LE cells are white blood cells that have phagocytized other white blood cell nuclei. This test is not performed much anymore, but was utilized in the past to diagnose SLE.

E. Antineutrophil cytoplasmic antibody (ANCA) and perinuclear antineutrophil cytoplasmic antibody (pANCA) are seen in numerous autoimmune diseases including Kawasaki disease, Wegener's granulomatosus, Henoch-Schönlein purpura, glomerulonephritis, and inflammatory bowel disease.

F. **Histocompatibility antigens** are antigens of the MHC expressed on cell surfaces to identify the cell as "self." Several classes of histocompatibility antigens, called human leukocyte antigens (HLA), have been associated with the occurrence of certain diseases.
   1. HLA-B27 – spondyloarthropathy.
   2. HLA-B8, -DR2, -DR3 – SLE.
   3. HLA-B8, -DR3 – childhood dermatomyositis, Grave's disease, celiac sprue, insulin-dependent diabetes mellitus, and Addison's disease.
   4. HLA-DR4 – insulin-dependent diabetes mellitus.

G. Antiphospholipid antibody, lupus anticoagulants, and anticardiolipin are associated with autoimmune thrombotic disorders.
   1. These substances may be present in up to 40% of people with SLE.
   2. Primary antiphospholipid syndrome causes thrombocytopenia, thrombosis, recurrent abortion, and stroke. It is caused by antiphospholipid antibody.

8.2 DISEASE PROFILES

8.2.1 Juvenile Rheumatoid Arthritis (JRA)

A. JRA is a chronic synovitis associated with extraarticular signs and symptoms.
   1. Patients present with joint effusion, redness, swelling, joint pain, stiffness, and loss of range of motion.
   2. The articular cartilage is eroded and eventually destroyed, yet many children do not experience permanent joint injury.
   3. Those with JRA experience "gelling," which is stiffness upon awakening or after other periods of inactivity, as opposed to osteoarthritis where the joint symptoms are more prominent with activity.
   4. Long-term disability is more common in children with hip disease.
   5. Any affected body part in JRA may experience increased or decreased growth velocity.
   6. Rheumatoid factor (RF)is a group of antibodies that react to the Fc portion of immunoglobulin G that is present in some forms of JRA.

B. **Polyarticular JRA (RF-Negative)**
   1. This form accounts for up to 30% of all JRA and

can affect any joint.
2. It has a 9:1 predilection for girls and can present at any age.
3. RF is negative and the ANA is only positive 25% of the time.
4. It is not associated with sacroiliitis or iridocyclitis.
5. Severe arthritis develops in approximately 10% of patients.

C. **Polyarticular JRA (RF-Positive)**
1. This form accounts for up to 10% of all JRA and may affect any joint.
2. It usually presents in older children.
3. There is an 8:1 female to male ratio and a prevalence of HLA-DR4.
4. RF is positive with ANA positive in 75% of patients.
5. Iridocyclitis and sacroiliitis are rare.
6. RF is positive (100%) as is ANA (75%).
7. More than 50% have severe arthritis.

D. **Pauciarticular JRA Type I**
1. This form affects up to 40% of children with JRA.
2. Up to 80% of children affected are young female children.
3. Synovitis is noted in large joints (knees, elbows, ankles).
4. Iridocyclitis may be chronic in a third of patients.
5. The RF is negative, but ANA is positive in most patients.
6. HLA-DR5, -DR6, and -DR8 are seen frequently in affected patients.

E. **Pauciarticular JRA Type II**
1. This form of JRA accounts for 10% of those affected.
2. Males predominate 9:1 over females.
3. It presents later in childhood and is associated with HLA-B27.
4. It affects joints primarily in the hip girdle, and unlike other forms of JRA, sacroiliitis is common.
5. Acute iridocyclitis does occur approximately 10% of the time.
6. Spondyloarthropathy can be debilitating.

F. **Systemic Onset JRA**
1. Systemic onset JRA is seen in up to 20% of those affected.
2. It has a 6:1 male predominance and can occur at any age.
3. ANA and RF are usually negative.
4. One quarter of patients with this form of JRA may have severe, debilitating arthritis.
5. The systemic signs and symptoms include fever, rash, hepatosplenomegaly, pleuritis and pericarditis, abdominal pain, anemia, and myalgia.

G. The differential diagnosis is extensive and includes osteomyelitis, septic joint, arthritis associated with other disease (parvovirus B19, Lyme disease, gonorrhea, rubella, malignancy, SLE), acute rheumatic fever, joint trauma, Legg-Calve-Perthes disease, slipped capital femoral epiphysis, or toxic synovitis.

H. Therapy
1. The goals of treatment are to preserve function, avoid iatrogenic illness, and treat systemic manifestations.
2. Nonsteroidal anti-inflammatory drugs are first line drug therapy.

8.2.2 Other Spondyloarthropathies

A. **Reiter's Disease**
1. This is the combination of urethritis, conjunctivitis, and arthritis.
2. The arthritis typically involves large joints.
3. There is an association with HLA-B27.
4. It primarily affects males.

B. **Juvenile Ankylosing Spondylitis**
1. This arthritis presents early with hip and leg involvement. Eventually the sacroiliac joints and back become symptomatic.
2. It affects predominantly males at any age.
3. There is an association with HLA-B27.

C. Inflammatory bowel disease can present as a pauciarticular large joint arthritis.

D. Psoriasis is associated with an arthritis that occurs primarily in females.

E. **Reactive arthritis** is a sterile joint inflammation occurring after infection with *Yersinia*, *Salmonella*, *Shigella*, and *Campylobacter*.

8.2.3 Systemic Lupus Erythematosus (SLE)

A. SLE is a condition characterized by a multisystem inflammatory process. Its etiology is unknown.
1. SLE can present in childhood (20%), usually in females over 8 years of age.
2. Symptoms may be precipitated by illness and include fever, malaise, arthritis, arthralgia, weight loss, debility, and rash.
3. Diagnosis is often delayed due to the nonspecific nature of symptoms.

B. Organ Systems Affected
1. Skin
   a. Patients may present with the typical "butterfly" malar rash. It is photosensitive and may spread to involve the rest of the face, scalp, neck, and chest.
   b. They may also have erythematous macules over the trunk and extremities.
   c. Mucosal ulcerations may occur in the mouth and the nose.
   d. Purpura may be present.
2. Central nervous system may be affected with manifestation of seizure, personality change, neuritis, en-

cephalitis, and stroke.

3. Pulmonary fibrosis may occur, resulting in restrictive lung disease.
4. Cardiovascular
   a. Myocarditis and pericarditis may be life threatening.
   b. Raynaud phenomenon (see section 8.2.8) may occur.
5. Gastrointestinal. Abdominal pain, vomiting, and hepatosplenomegaly are common.
6. Hematologic
   a. Anemia is common.
   b. idiopathic thrombocytopenic purpura may occur (thrombocytopenia).
   c. Patients may have a positive Coombs test secondary to anti-erythrocyte antibody.
   d. Thrombosis may occur due to alterations in clotting function.
7. Renal
   a. Nephritis may occur.
   b. Some patients may progress to end stage renal disease.
   c. Blood urea nitrogen and creatinine may be elevated.
8. Lymphadenopathy is present.
9. Growth retardation is common in children due to the disease or its treatment.

C. Diagnosis
   a. History and physical examination leading to clinical suspicion of SLE are the most important diagnostic tools.
   b. All patients with SLE have a positive ANA.

D. Therapy
1. Drug therapy is with nonsteroidal anti-inflammatory drugs and systemic corticosteroids.
2. Immunosuppressive drugs may be required.
3. Anticoagulation may also be necessary if lupus anticoagulant is present.
4. Individualized treatment of specific organ dysfunction is necessary.

E. **Neonatal Lupus**
1. This condition is seen in infants of mothers with SLE, Sjögren's syndrome, or other rheumatic disease. The mothers may actually be well (and undiagnosed) when the infant is born.
2. The etiology is unknown, but infants have anti-rho or anti-la antibody.
3. Signs and symptoms include congenital heart block, thrombocytopenia, leukopenia, liver disease, and skin rash. Symptoms usually remit over the first year of life with the exception of the cardiac conduction disturbance.
4. Not all infants born to mothers with rheumatic disease are affected, suggesting a genetic predilection.

8.2.4 Vasculitis

A. **Henoch-Schönlein purpura** (HSP) is an immunoglobulin A mediated, leukocytoclastic vasculitis affecting multiple organ systems including skin, kidneys, joints, and the gastrointestinal tract.
1. It can occur at any age, but is most common in 2 to 8 year olds.
2. Etiology
   a. Etiology is unknown, but the fall through spring seasonal prevalence suggests an infectious cause.
   b. Many conditions have been identified as possible triggers for HSP. These are infection (*Mycoplasma*, group A β-hemolytic streptococcus, cold exposure, insect bites, immunizations (yellow fever), allergies, and drug sensitivities to name a few.
3. Signs and Symptoms
   a. The rash (urticaria, erythematous macules, petechiae, purpura) is present in 100% of those affected. Children under 2 years old may experience painful subcutaneous edema.
   b. Other symptoms may present before the rash and result in confusion in diagnosis, and include arthritis (no permanent damage) in 85%, abdominal pain, gastrointestinal bleeding, nephritis (microscopic hematuria in 50%, end-stage renal failure <1%), nephropathy, central nervous system disease (seizure, irritability, rarely stroke), myocardial infarction (rare), testicular torsion (rare), and pulmonary hemorrhage (rare).
4. The most serious conditions included in the differential diagnosis are meningococcemia, Rocky Mountain spotted fever, and child abuse.
5. Treatment
   a. Therapy is primarily supportive with nonsteroidal anti-inflammatory drugs for arthritis and arthralgias.
   b. Steroids can be considered for renal disease or significant gastrointestinal bleeding.
   c. Affected children should undergo periodic urinalysis for hematuria throughout their lifetimes.

B. **Kawasaki disease** is discussed in section 10.6.1.

8.2.5 Dermatomyositis

A. Dermatomyositis is an inflammatory condition affecting the skin and subcutaneous tissue, gastrointestinal tract, and striated muscle.

B. Females are affected more frequently than males and are usually over 2 years old (Usually 8 to 9 years old).

C. Signs and Symptoms
1. Weakness is prominent.
   a. Proximal muscle groups are affected first.
   b. Gower's sign is present. In order to rise up from sitting on the floor, the child must "crawl" up

his own body using it for support.

2. Musculature is stiff and sore.
3. Skin involvement includes violaceous (**heliotrope**) erythema of the eyelids, potentially a butterfly malar rash as seen in SLE, nailbed telangiectasia, erythematous scaling over extensor joints, and skin atrophy. The skin may appear tight and glossy.
4. Gastrointestinal manifestations include impaired swallowing function and evidence of hepatopathy.
5. Fever, lymphadenopathy, arthritis, and joint contractures also occur.

D. Treatment is with steroids. Immunosuppressive agents are used if corticosteroid treatment fails.

8.2.6 Scleroderma

A. This is a fibrosing disease of skin that may also involve the gastrointestinal tract, heart, lungs, kidneys, and joints.

B. It is rare in children.

C. The most common childhood manifestations are morphea (focal cutaneous lesions) and linear scleroderma. Systemic scleroderma can occur.

D. Prognosis is good in the absence of systemic disease.

E. Joint contractures are a complication of disease.

F. There are no specific laboratory tests for diagnosis. Diagnosis is made by history and physical examination.

G. There is no specific treatment.

8.2.7 Erythema Nodosum

A. This condition is characterized by shiny, red, hot, ovoid 1 to 3 cm nodules over the shins.

1. The lesions occur in crops.
2. They fade in 1 to 2 weeks leaving a brown macule.

B. Associated symptoms include fever, malaise, and arthralgia.

C. Hilar adenopathy may be noted on chest x-ray.

D. The disease was previously linked to tuberculosis. Now, it is more commonly associated with group A β-hemolytic streptococcus. Other associated conditions include sarcoidosis, inflammatory bowel disease, leptospirosis, Cat-scratch disease, Ebstein-Barr virus, tularemia, psittacosis, histoplasmosis, coccidioidomycosis, yersinia, and drug use (sulfonamides, birth control pills).

8.2.8 Raynaud Phenomenon

A. This phenomenon is characterized by blanching of the fingers and toes secondary to vasospasm, followed by cyanosis, then hyperemia.

B. It is precipitated by cold exposure, pressure, or emotional stress.

C. It is rare in children.

122. Human leucocyte antigen-B27 is associated with which of the following conditions B 8.1.3

A. systemic lupus erythematosus
B. spondyloarthropathy
C. dermatomyositis
D. celiac sprue
E. insulin-dependent diabetes mellitus

123. A 6-year-old girl presents with pain and effusion of her right knee. She has a negative rheumatoid factor and a positive antinuclear antibody. She is noted to have iridocyclitis as well. What is her probable diagnosis B 8.2.1

A. polyarticular juvenile rheumatoid arthritis (rheumatoid factor-negative)
B. pauciarticular juvenile rheumatoid arthritis type I
C. pauciarticular juvenile rheumatoid arthritis type II
D. systemic onset juvenile rheumatoid arthritis

124. Which of the following findings is not associated with Reiter's disease C 8.2.2

A. conjunctivitis
B. urethritis
C. meningitis
D. arthritis

125. Which of the following organisms is not commonly associated with a reactive arthritis with sterile joint effusion C 8.2.2

A. *Campylobacter*
B. *Shigella*
C. *Staphylococcus*
D. *Yersinia*

126. Which antibody is associated with neonatal lupus E 8.2.3

A. anti-double stranded deoxyribonucleic acid
B. anti-rho
C. anti-cytoplasmic
D. anti-la
E. B and D

127. A 5-year-old presents with knee and ankle pain, lower extremity purpuric rash, and abdominal pain. A urinalysis reveals microscopic hematuria. The diagnosis is B 8.2.4

A. Rocky Mountain spotted fever
B. Henoch-Schönlein purpura
C. Kawasaki disease
D. systemic lupus erythematosus

128. Heliotrope erythema of the eyelids is seen most often with which of the following conditions C 8.2.5

A. Henoch-Schönlein purpura
B. systemic lupus erythematosus
C. dermatomyositis
D. Rocky Mountain spotted fever
E. Kawasaki disease

129. Erythema nodosum is associated with which of the following D 8.2.7

A. cat-scratch disease
B. group A β-hemolytic streptococcus
C. birth control pill use
D. all of the above
E. A and B

9 RESPIRATORY DISORDERS

9.1 GENERAL CONCEPTS

9.1.1 Respiratory Distress in Infancy

A. Infants are obligate nasal breathers.
   1. Complete occlusion of the nares can result in life-threatening apnea.
   2. Nasal obstruction can also interfere significantly with feeding in older infants since it is difficult to maintain an effective suck without patent nares.

B. In evaluating the symptoms of respiratory diseases in infants, remember to investigate the possibility of symptoms due to over-the-counter cold remedies. Sleep disturbances and irritability may be a side effect of the medication, not a manifestation of the condition.

C. Airway resistance to airflow is inversely proportional to the fourth power of the radius of the airway. Therefore, a given degree of tissue swelling causes more obstruction to air flow in the smaller child or infant.

D. The number of alveoli increases until age 10 to 12 years but the number of bronchi do not increase after birth. Therefore, diseases which affect lung development can cause permanent ventilation perfusion mismatches if alveolar growth does not match that of the pulmonary vasculature development.

E. Males have smaller peripheral airways than females before school age, thus, pulmonary disease in male infants and children may be more severe than in females of the same age.

F. As soon as they can pick up objects, infants and toddlers are at risk for aspiration because they tend to put all small objects in their mouths.

G. Cardiac failure in infancy often presents as respiratory distress.
   1. Hepatomegaly in the infant with respiratory distress is the clue to congestive heart failure.
   2. Cardiac failure can be confirmed by cardiomegaly on chest x-ray.
   3. Cyanosis due to congenital right-to-left shunts does not improve with 100% oxygen inhalation while that of respiratory disorders generally will.

9.1.2 Structural and Functional Derangement

A. **Airway obstruction**
   1. Upper airway obstruction is usually manifest by inspiratory stridor and increased inspiratory effort (retractions).
   2. Obstruction below the glottis is usually manifest by expiratory stridor and may be accompanied by prolonged expiratory phase and wheezing.
   3. If the child is not hoarse, the obstruction is likely subglottic or tracheal.

B. **Gas exchange**
   1. Oxygen diffuses 20-times less readily across the capillary/alveolar surface than does carbon dioxide. Therefore, hypoxemia occurs relatively early in disorders of gas exchange.
   2. Hypercapnia is a manifestation of a much more severe derangement of gas exchange.

9.1.3 Diagnostic Modalities

A. **Arterial Blood Gas Analysis**
   1. **PaO_2** values below 85 mm Hg while breathing room air are abnormal except in the very young infant. Respiratory failure is generally present when the value decreases below 50 mm Hg.
   2. **$PaCO_2$** values above 45 mm Hg indicate hypoventilation, severe ventilation/perfusion mismatch, or compensation for chronic metabolic acidosis.
   3. **O_2 saturation**. Because of the nature of the oxyhemoglobin dissociation curve, oxygen saturation does not decrease appreciably until arterial PO_2 decreases to about 60 torr (mm Hg).
   4. **The PAO_2-PaO_2 (alveolar-arterial) difference** is a measurement of gas exchange in the alveolus.
      a. It is not influenced by minute volume. Increases in the difference are indicative of shunts between the pulmonary and systemic circulations.
      b. Alveolar PO_2 (PAO_2) can be estimated by the formula: $PAO_2 = FiO_2(P_B - 47) - PaO_2/R$. [$FiO_2$ = inspired percent of oxygen, P_B = barometric pressure, R = carbon dioxide production/oxygen consumption ratio usually 0.8]
   5. **Pulse oximetry** is a noninvasive method of monitoring O_2 saturation. Values are lowered by local vasoconstriction.
   6. **Radiography**
      a. Chest x-ray is a method for evaluation of structural aspects of the heart and lungs. It also can demonstrate radiopaque esophageal and airway foreign bodies.
      b. Lateral neck soft tissue x-ray is useful for evaluating causes of upper airway obstruction through demonstration of the tracheal air column and soft tissue structures.
      c. Contrast Studies. Pulmonary arteriogram, bronchograms, thoracic aortograms, and barium swallows are sometimes useful in differentiating gastrointestinal problems from pulmonary problems.
      d. Radionuclide lung scans facilitate evaluation of pulmonary ventilation and perfusion.
   7. **Pulmonary Function Tests** (PFT)
      a. School age children are usually able to cooperate sufficiently to perform these tests.
      b. PFTs are useful in identifying obstructive, restrictive, or diffusion abnormalities. Serial PFTs can be used to quantify response to therapy.
      c. The more commonly used PFTs are peak expi-

ratory flow rate (PEFR), forced vital capacity (FEV), forced expiratory volume in one second (FEV_1), and FEV_1/FEV ratio.

8. Flexible **bronchoscopy** and rigid bronchoscopy can be utilized for direct visualization of the airways.
   a. Flexible bronchoscopy can be performed in the ambulatory setting with mild sedation.
   b. Rigid bronchoscopy requires general anesthesia. This is the method used for removal of airway foreign bodies.
9. **Lung biopsy** may be required for histologic or culture diagnosis. The procedure can be accomplished by needle aspiration or by open tissue resection.
10. **Sweat chloride** is elevated in cystic fibrosis. False positive results are caused by adrenal insufficiency, malnutrition, ectodermal dysplasia, hypothyroidism, nephrogenic diabetes insipidus, mucopolysaccharidosis, type I glycogen storage disease, intravenous fluid use, oral steroids, and fucosidosis.

9.1.4 Pathophysiologic Manifestations

A. Symptoms
   1. **Cough**. A persistent cough is never normal in the neonate. A sudden onset of a paroxysmal cough should suggest foreign body aspiration.
   2. Sputum Production. As a rule children swallow the mucus they produce and hence "do not produce" sputum.
   3. **Chest pain** may be a clue to the location of pathology, but be aware of referred pain in evaluating the patient.
   4. **Pleurisy**. Pain associated with and exacerbated by inspiration. It may be difficult to differentiate from chest wall pain in children and can be a cause of splinting with respiration.

B. Physical Findings
   1. Respiratory Features
      a. **Tachypnea** is a respiratory rate exceeding 60 in the newborn, 40 from 1 to 6 months, 30 from 1 to 3 years, 25 from 4 to 8 years, 22 from 9 to 14 years, and 20 for children >14 years.
      b. **Grunting**. An expiratory grunt is a compensatory mechanism for loss of lung volume. It is never a normal finding. It may indicate pleural involvement and is seen sometimes with intraabdominal problems such as peritonitis.
      c. **Flaring** of the nasal alae is a sign of increased airway resistance.
      d. Subcostal **retractions** and intercostal retractions occur during inspiration and are a sign of significant respiratory distress.
      e. Stridor is indicative of upper airway obstruction.
      f. **Breath Sounds**. Normally the inspiration-to-expiration ratio is 2:1. This ratio is reversed in conditions resulting in bronchiolar obstruction.
      g. **Crackles (Rales)**. The term crackles is now preferred to rales. They are produced on inspiration by opening of small airways or alveoli.
      h. **Rhonchi and wheezes** are expiratory noises which are prolonged rather than discrete sounds. Wheezes are higher pitched and may be musical in quality.
      i. **Thoracic Configuration**. Chronic air trapping can produce a barrel-shaped chest.
      j. **Apnea** is cessation of spontaneous respiratory activity for at least 20 seconds.
   2. **Tracheal deviation** may reflect a pneumothorax or atelectasis. It can also be a clue to foreign body aspiration.
   3. **Cervical venous distention** (CVD) is seen in conditions causing persistent increased intrathoracic pressure and in cardiac tamponade.
   4. **Clubbing** of the nails is widening of the tissue of the distal digits. It can be recognized in its mild form by comparing the depth of the finger at the distal interphalangeal joint to the depth at the base of the nail. If the distance is equal, clubbing is present. It is usually seen in children with bronchiectasis or cystic fibrosis.
   5. **Cyanosis** is bluish discoloration of the skin evident when oxygen saturation is less than 85%.
      a. Central cyanosis is reflective of decreased oxygenation of the blood.
      b. Peripheral cyanosis is due to an increased arterial-venous oxygen difference and reflects local vascular stasis. The oxygen saturation is normal in peripheral cyanosis.
      c. Methemoglobin will produce cyanosis when it exceeds more than 15% of the total hemoglobin.

9.1.5 Differential Diagnosis of Respiratory Symptoms

A. The differential diagnosis for respiratory symptoms is vast. A fairly complete list of diagnoses is presented here to demonstrate the magnitude of diagnostic possibilities.

B. **Respiratory Distress – Upper Airway Disease**
   1. Congenital causes include vascular ring, laryngeal web, vocal cord paralysis, laryngomalacia, tracheomalacia, micrognathia, and glossoptosis.
   2. Infectious causes include croup, epiglottitis, bacterial tracheitis, peritonsillar abscess, retropharyngeal abscess, and diphtheria.
   3. Trauma such as foreign body ingestion or aspiration, inhalation injury, aspiration injury, and subglottic stenosis can cause distress.
   4. Allergic causes are angioneurotic edema and spasmodic croup.

C. **Respiratory Distress – Lower Airway Disease**
   1. Congenital causes include cystic fibrosis, emphysema, diaphragmatic hernia, and cystic adenomatoid

malformation.

2. Infectious causes are pneumonia, bronchiolitis, pleural effusions, and empyema.
3. Allergic disease such as asthma and anaphylaxis can cause distress.
4. Circulatory causes include congestive heart failure, pulmonary edema, pulmonary embolism, polycythemia, and severe anemia.
5. Traumatic etiologies include bronchopulmonary dysplasia, foreign body, pneumothorax, pulmonary contusion, diaphragmatic rupture, near drowning, and spinal cord injury.
6. Neoplasms (lung tumors, mediastinal masses) cause respiratory distress.
   - **a.** Anterior mediastinal masses: thymoma, thymic hyperplasia, thymic cyst, teratoma, lymphoma, vascular tumor, intrathoracic thyroid, pleuropericardial cyst, and lymphadenopathy.
   - **b.** Superior mediastinal masses: cystic hygroma, vascular tumor, neurogenic tumor, thymic tumor, teratoma, hemangioma, mediastinal abscess, aortic aneurysm, intrathoracic thyroid, and esophageal lesions.
   - **c.** Posterior mediastinal masses: neurogenic tumors, enterogenous cysts, thoracic meningocele, and aortic aneurysm.
   - **d.** Middle mediastinal masses: lymphoma, hypertrophic lymph nodes, granuloma, bronchogenic cyst, enterogenic cyst, metastasis, pericardial cyst, aortic aneurysm, and anomalies of the great vessels.
7. Miscellaneous causes include sarcoidosis, musculoskeletal anomalies, scoliosis, and pulmonary hemosiderosis.

D. Respiratory Distress – Central Nervous System Disease

1. Infectious causes are meningitis and encephalitis.
2. Neuropathic and myopathic causes include Guillain-Barré syndrome, Werdnig-Hoffman syndrome, muscular dystrophy, myasthenia gravis, and infantile botulism.
3. Miscellaneous causes are seizures and poisoning.

E. Respiratory Distress – Metabolic Disease

1. Metabolic acidosis from inborn errors of metabolism, diabetes mellitus, sepsis, dehydration, salicylism, and toxin exposure can lead to distress.
2. Increased oxygen demand from fever or hyperthyroidism can present as distress.

F. Cough

1. Recurrent cough is commonly seen in asthma, drainage from upper airways, aspiration, and frequent upper respiratory tract infections.
2. Persistent cough is associated with postinfectious pneumonitis, asthma, chronic sinusitis, bronchiectasis, foreign body aspiration, gastroesophageal reflux, pertussis, tracheoesophageal fistula, extrinsic compression of the tracheobronchial tract, tracheomalacia, tuberculosis, and habit cough.

G. Wheezing

1. Intrinsic pulmonary causes include asthma, aspiration (foreign body, food, saliva, gastric contents), hypersensitivity syndromes (visceral larval migrans, aspergillosis, eosinophilia, smoke exposure), bronchiolitis obliterans, and cystic fibrosis.
2. congestive heart failure is the cardiovascular process most often responsible for wheezing.
3. Developmental or acquired structural abnormalities (tracheomalacia, vascular ring, lung cyst, mediastinal tumor) can cause wheezing.

H. Stridor

1. Recurrent stridor should prompt a search for spasmodic croup, respiratory infection, and laryngomalacia.
2. Persistent stridor is most often due to structural lesions of the larynx or trachea that have been mentioned previously. It may also occur with gastroesophageal reflux, cri du chat syndrome, and in vocal cord dysfunction (hysterical stridor).

9.1.6 Indicators of Serious Chronic Respiratory Disease

A. History: persistent fever and symptoms limiting activity.

B. Examination: growth failure, inadequate weight gain, clubbing, purulent sputum, and sustained hypoxemia.

C. Diagnostic Tests: persistent abnormality on chest x-ray or on PFTs.

9.2 DISEASE PROFILES

9.2.1 Laryngomalacia

A. This is the most common congenital anomaly. Affected infants have an abnormally small and/or soft larynx.

B. Stridor is the prominent symptom. It worsens with concurrent upper respiratory tract infections.

C. Laryngomalacia is diagnosed by direct laryngoscopy revealing inward folding of the supraglottic structures during inspiration.

D. Complications include difficulty feeding and severe respiratory distress rarely requiring tracheostomy.

E. Differential diagnosis includes malformations of laryngeal cartilages, intraluminal webs, neck and chest neoplasms, vascular rings, and cysts.

F. Treatment is primarily reassurance of parents.

G. Prognosis is very good. Stridor usually resolves by 18 months of age.

9.2.2 Bronchopulmonary Dysplasia (BPD)

A. BPD is seen primarily in infants who have required ventilatory support. It is suspected to result from barotrauma and oxygen toxicity (requiring FiO_2 >0.8).

It occurs more frequently in infants with hyaline membrane disease, lower gestational age, male sex, patent ductus arteriosus, pulmonary infection (*Ureaplasma urealyticum*), and pulmonary edema.

B. The pathophysiologic abnormality is airway smooth muscle hypertrophy and interstitial edema from endothelial injury.

C. Physical findings include tachypnea, wheezing, crackles, retractions, and cyanosis.

D. Diagnostic Testing
1. Chest x-ray shows characteristic fibrotic and cystic interstitial changes in the chronic stage.
2. Arterial blood gas demonstrates hypoxemia on room air.

E. Potential complications are cor pulmonale, pulmonary hypertension, and growth retardation.

F. Therapeutic Plan
1. Supplemental oxygen is provided to maintain PaO_2 in 60 to 80 mm Hg range.
2. Diuretics, bronchodilators, and corticosteroids can be used to reduce pulmonary edema, hypertension, and inflammation.
3. Calorie supplementation is necessary to support growth.
4. Influenza and pneumococcal vaccines are given at the appropriate age.

G. Prognosis is dependent upon the severity of the disease.
1. Children may require oxygen supplementation for a year after hospital discharge.
2. Some children acquire normal pulmonary function by school age.
3. Affected infants are prone to asthma.
4. In severe BPD, death may result from acute exacerbation, pulmonary hypertension, or cor pulmonale.

9.2.3 Foreign Body Aspiration

A. Foreign bodies in the larynx, trachea, or bronchus are common causes of acute or chronic respiratory symptoms in children.

B. Epidemiology
1. Approximately 90% of deaths from foreign body aspiration occur in children <5 years.
2. One half of reported incidents occur in children <2 years.
3. The male:female ratio is 2:1.
4. Commonly aspirated items include nuts, hot dogs, rattles, pacifiers, balloons, balls, and toy parts.

C. Pathophysiology
1. Obstruction of a bronchus will result in atelectasis. If it becomes chronic, bronchiectasis may occur.
2. Partial obstruction may cause emphysema, pneumothorax or pneumomediastinum through a "ball valve effect."

D. Symptoms depend upon the site of entrapment.
1. A large percentage of patients have no acute symptoms.
2. Upper airway involvement may lead to complete obstruction or loss or abnormality of the voice.
3. Acutely the child may experience sudden onset of cough, dysphagia, stridor, dyspnea, cyanosis, and choking.
4. The classic triad (wheezing, cough, decreased breath sounds) is absent in 50% of documented cases.

E. Physical findings include tracheal deviation, unilateral wheezing, localized decreased breath sounds, crackles, and tachypnea.

F. Diagnostic Findings
1. Chest X-Ray
   a. One third will have a normal x-ray.
   b. Mediastinal shift is toward the lesion if atelectasis is present and away if a ball valve obstruction occurs. Inspiratory and expiratory films may help identify a ball valve effect.
   c. Subcutaneous air or pneumomediastinum may be present.
2. Pulse oximetry may reveal hypoxia.
3. Arterial blood gas, if obtained, may have an increased pCO_2 or decreased pO_2 depending on the level of obstruction.

G. Differential diagnosis includes any condition that may cause upper or lower airway obstruction.

H. Therapeutic Plan
1. Total obstruction (aphonic and not breathing). Use four back blows followed by four chest compressions. Remember abdominal thrusts and blind finger sweeps of the mouth are not used on infants.
2. Symptoms dictate timing and nature of medical response. Rigid bronchoscopy is the procedure of choice for removal.

9.2.4 Apnea of Infancy

A. Apnea is a pause in respiration for >20 seconds or a shorter interruption of breathing associated with pallor, cyanosis, alteration in mental status, or bradycardia.

B. Prematurity is the single largest risk factor for apnea. The incidence of apnea increases the earlier in gestation an infant delivers.

C. Differential diagnosis is extensive and includes the following:
1. Infants may have normal, periodic pauses in respiration normally (periodic breathing).
2. Central nervous system disorders associated with apneic events include seizures, meningitis, encephalitis, intracranial hemorrhage, increased intracranial pressure, encephalopathy, Guillain-Barré syndrome,

and central hypoventilation.

3. Pulmonary disorders include pneumonia (especially respiratory syncytial virus), pulmonary hemorrhage, and pulmonary edema.
4. Cardiovascular disease such as dysrhythmia or shock.
5. Gastrointestinal disorders such as gastroesophageal reflux, tracheoesophageal fistula, or swallowing disorders may predispose to apnea.
6. Metabolic disease includes hypoglycemia, hypocalcemia, hyponatremia, and inborn errors of metabolism.
7. Musculoskeletal disorders such as infant botulism and congenital myopathy.
8. Miscellaneous causes include severe anemia, poisoning, and hypothermia.

D. Diagnostic evaluation is tailored to the likely etiology in a given infant.

E. Treatment

1. Treat the underlying illness when possible.
2. Monitor infant with apnea and bradycardia monitors.
3. Apnea of prematurity responds to caffeine and theophylline.
4. Obstructive sleep apnea improves with nasal continuous positive airway pressure (CPAP).

9.2.5 **Cystic Fibrosis** (CF)

A. CF is an autosomal recessive disease with abnormal control of chloride channels in epithelial cells of the pancreas, sweat and salivary glands, intestine, and reproductive and respiratory tracts.

B. Pathophysiology. It is hypothesized that the function of the chloride channel determines the hydration of the mucous gel. Inadequate hydration of the cell surface is believed to result in inspissated secretions and organ damage in the pancreas, biliary tree, and lungs.

C. Epidemiology

1. Abnormalities of CF gene occur in 1 of 25 people of Northern European extraction. The frequency is less in other populations, and rare in African and Asian populations.
2. Heterozygous carriers are asymptomatic.
3. Approximately 70% of mutations in North Americans are a three base pair deletion resulting in the absence of phenylalanine at codon 508 (ΔF 508).
4. CF occurs in 1 in 2500 live births.

D. Presenting symptoms include failure to thrive (malabsorption), recurrent respiratory disease, cough, clubbing, meconium ileus (5 to 10%), obstructive jaundice, hyponatremic dehydration, rectal prolapse (20%), family history of CF, and nasal polyps (10%).

E. Laboratory Findings

1. Sweat chloride test results show a chloride >60 mEq/L.
2. Genetic testing using polymerase chain reaction (PCR) can detect 90% of abnormal genotypes reliably.

F. Potential Complications

1. Gastrointestinal: meconium ileus, failure to thrive, intestinal obstruction, malnutrition, pancreatitis, and hepatic cirrhosis.
2. Endocrine: hyperglycemia or overt diabetes mellitus and delayed puberty.
3. Pulmonary: Recurrent respiratory tract infections, development of respiratory tract pseudomonas colonization and infection, hemoptysis, pneumothorax, allergic bronchopulmonary aspergillosis, chronic hypoxemia, and respiratory failure.
4. Cardiovascular: cor pulmonale.
5. Genitourinary: cervicitis, infertility, inguinal hernia, hydrocele, and undescended testicle.
6. Miscellaneous: vitamin deficiency associated with fat malabsorption and hyponatremia.

G. Therapeutic Plan

1. Nutritional support with pancreatic enzyme replacement, fat soluble vitamin (A,D,E,K) replacement, increased caloric intake, and careful monitoring of growth curves.
2. Prevention and treatment of pulmonary disease by postural drainage and chest percussion, deoxyribonuclease to liquify sticky deoxyribonucleic acid-mucus complexes, influenza and pneumococcal vaccines, intermittent antibiotic therapy for 2 to 4 weeks with orally, intravenously, or inhaled drugs depending on severity of exacerbation, oxygen, bronchodilators, and lung transplant.
3. Anticipate and treat complications.

H. Prognosis. Life expectancy has improved with advances in care. Median survival is 28 to 30 years.

9.2.6 **Asthma**

A. Asthma is regarded as a diffuse, obstructive lung disease with hyperreactivity of the airways to various stimuli and a high degree of reversibility of the obstructive process with or without treatment.

B. Epidemiology

1. Asthma affects 10 to 15% of male and 7 to 10% of female children.
2. About 80 to 90% of those with asthma will present before the age 5 years.
3. Asthma is the most frequent admitting diagnosis in hospitals for children.
4. Asthma demonstrates multifactorial inheritance: a child who has one parent with the disease has a risk of 25%. The risk increases to 50 to 65% if both parents are affected.

C. Pathophysiology

1. Asthma results from hypersensitivity of the large and small airways to allergic and nonspecific stimuli

resulting in release of chemical mediators from mast cells, resultant airway obstruction from bronchospasm, mucosal edema, and mucus production. Triggers vary from person to person.
2. Airway obstruction leads to nonuniform ventilation, hyperinflation, ventilation-perfusion mismatch, hypoxia, hypercarbia, acidosis, and respiratory failure.
3. Inadequate long-term treatment of the underlying lung inflammatory process can lead to permanent airway remodeling.

D. Predisposing Conditions
1. Any condition causing mucosal injury (bronchopulmonary dysplasia, respiratory syncytial virus) increases the risk of asthma.
2. Presence of atopy in the child or a family member is associated with an increased incidence of asthma.
3. Passive smoke exposure results in an increase in asthma symptoms as well as more frequent upper and lower respiratory tract infections, and otitis media.

E. Symptoms include cough (nighttime cough, exercise-induced cough), wheezing, and dyspnea.

F. Physical findings may be minimal between exacerbations but can include cough, diffuse wheezing, prolonged expiration, use of accessory muscles of respiration, and retractions.

G. Diagnostic Testing
1. Chest x-ray reveals hyperinflation, atelectasis, and possibly pneumomediastinum or pneumothorax.
2. Arterial blood gases vary with severity of disease symptoms. A normal $PaCO_2$ is not necessarily a sign of normal lung function. As children begin to tire from increased work of breathing, their $PaCO_2$ rises back to normal. This is indicative of impending respiratory failure.
3. PFTs. An increase of at least 10% in peak flow rate or FEV_1 during bronchial provocation testing or pre- and post-bronchodilator therapy is suggestive of asthma.

H. Potential Complications
1. Psychological. The patient may experience vulnerable child syndrome, limitation of physical activity, school absenteeism, or social isolation.
2. Status asthmaticus, respiratory failure, pneumothorax, and sudden death are potential physical complications.

I. Differential diagnosis includes bronchiolitis, CF, tracheomalacia, pertussis, foreign body aspiration, congestive heart failure, intrathoracic tumor, and gastroesophageal reflux.

J. Asthma Classification. In 1997 The National Heart Lung and Blood Institute of the National Institute of Health published *Guidelines for the Diagnosis and Management of Asthma* in an effort to standardize asthma management. It is necessary to understand asthma severity classifications in order to apply stepwise treatment guidelines (Table 9.2.6).
1. Mild intermittent asthma describes the patient who has symptoms <3-times per week. Exacerbations are brief with variable intensity, are asymptomatic with normal PEFR between exacerbations, have nocturnal symptoms <3-times per month, and have a PEFR ≥80% of predicted with a variability of <20%.
2. Mild persistent asthma is characterized by symptoms ≥2-times per week but <1-time per day, nocturnal symptoms >2-times per month, and a negative effect of exacerbations on activity level. PEFR is ≥80% predicted with a variability of 20 to 30%.
3. Moderate persistent asthma patients have exacerbations > 2-times per week, nocturnal symptoms >2-times per week, use short acting inhaled ß-agonists daily, decreased tolerance for physical activity, and PEFR 60 to 80% of predicted with variability >30%.
4. Severe persistent asthma describes the patient who has frequent exacerbations or continuous symptoms, frequent nocturnal symptoms, limitation of physical activities, and a PEFR <60% of predicted with a variability >30%.

Table 9.2.6 Progression of pH and blood gas changes in asthma

Severity	pH	PaO_2	$PaCO_2$
Normal	7.40	98%	40 mm Hg
Mild	mildly elevated	normal	mildly decreased
Moderate	elevated	decreased	decreased
Severe	normal	markedly decreased	normal
Respiratory Failure	<7.25	<60 mm Hg	>60 mm Hg

K. Therapeutic Plan
1. Environmental control to avoid triggers.
2. Monitoring of pulmonary function with peak flow meters and PFTs in older children.
3. Use of spacers to aid in delivery of inhaled medication.
4. Pharmacologic Treatment
   a. Bronchodilators should be considered "rescue" drugs. They include β-adrenergic drugs (albuterol, terbutaline, metaproterenol) and anticholinergic medications such as ipratropium bromide preferably delivered by aerosolization.

b. Salmeterol is a long acting bronchodilator used for maintenance therapy of asthma. Tolerance does not develop to its effects. It is NOT a rescue medication due to its long onset of action (approximately 2 hours).

c. Maintenance (daily) medications include anti-inflammatory agents such as cromolyn sodium (prevents degranulation of the mast cells and prevents exercise-induced bronchospasm in some patients), inhaled steroids (first line therapy that acts by decreasing airway inflammation), and leukotriene inhibitors (prevents inflammation by interrupting the leukotriene cascade). Theophylline preparations still play a role in asthma maintenance, but are used much less frequently by primary care providers than in the past.

d. Oral corticosteroids are used for acute flare-ups (1 to 2 mg/kg/24-hours for 5 to 7 days). Use should be minimized when possible to avoid long-term complications of growth failure, cataracts, and aseptic hip necrosis. Short term side effects include vomiting, aggressiveness, increased appetite, hyperglycemia, and psychosis.

5. Treatment for mild intermittent asthma is episodic use of short acting bronchodilators alone.

6. Children with mild persistent asthma should receive a daily anti-inflammatory medication in addition to episodic use of short acting bronchodilators.

7. Moderate persistent asthma management includes either a medium potency inhaled steroid or a low potency inhaled steroid with salmeterol plus short acting bronchodilators for acute exacerbations. Some children may require a medium to high dose steroid for adequate control with salmeterol for relief of nocturnal symptoms.

8. Severe persistent symptoms should be managed with daily high potency inhaled steroids, long acting bronchodilators, short acting bronchodilators, and possibly, oral corticosteroids. These children benefit from follow up with a pulmonologist.

9. Education regarding medication classifications and use, home monitoring of asthma, basic asthma facts, and avoidance of triggers are key to successful long-term treatment.

10. Preventive care should include pneumococcal and influenza vaccination.

11. Frequency of follow up is dependent upon severity of symptoms and ranges from 1 to 6 months.

L. Treatment goals are for patients to experience minimal, if any, daily asthma symptoms, avoidance of emergency room visits and hospitalizations, attainment of near normal PEFRs, and the least possible limitations on activities, all while avoiding adverse medication effects.

130. Inspiratory stridor and retractions are indicative of obstruction at which of the following levels — D 9.1.2

A. bronchus
B. trachea
C. bronchioles
D. glottis
E. nose

131. Which of the following arterial blood gas' is indicative of respiratory failure — A 9.1.3

A. pH 7.24, pCO_2 55, pO_2 45
B. pH 7.44, pCO_2 22, pO_2 60
C. pH 7.50, pCO_2 20, pO_2 90
D. pH 7.40, pCO_2 40, pO_2 90

132. Pulmonary function tests are useful for — D 9.1.3

A. quantitating response to therapy
B. identifying obstructive airway disease
C. identifying restrictive airway disease
D. all of the above
E. B and C

133. Which of the following are causes of false positive sweat chloride test results — D 9.1.3

A. prednisone use
B. intravenous fluid therapy
C. adrenal insufficiency
D. all of the above
E. A and C

134. Which of the following states is considered tachypnea — B 9.1.4

A. respiratory rate of 58 in a neonate
B. respiratory rate of 52 in a 2-month-old
C. respiratory rate of 38 in a 4-month-old
D. respiratory rate of 22 in a 6-year-old
E. respiratory rate of 16 in a 12-year-old

135. How long of a respiratory pause, in the absence of other symptoms, is apnea — A 9.1.4

A. 20 seconds
B. 15 seconds
C. 10 seconds
D. 5 seconds
E. It is not apnea unless other symptoms are present

136. What percent is the minimum amount of methemoglobin (in % hemoglobin) required to produce clinical cyanosis — C 9.1.4

A. >5%
B. >10%
C. >15%
D. >20%
E. >25%

137. A child's risk of asthma when both parents are affected is closest to — C 9.2.6

A. 10 to 25%
B. 25 to 40%
C. 50 to 65%
D. 70 to 90%

138. A 6-month-old presents with acute onset of coughing, associated with tachypnea and mild retractions. On exam, you note a heart murmur and expiratory wheezing. Per his mother's report, he was playing happily on the floor just before his symptoms started. What study would you do next — D 9.1.3

A. echocardiogram
B. electrocardiogram
C. cardiac catheterization
D. chest x-ray
E. bronchoscopy

139. An infant presents with noisy inspiration without evidence of cyanosis or distress. The noise gets louder when the child cries. What would be the expected finding on laryngoscopy — B 9.2.1

A. a red epiglottis
B. infolding of floppy supraglottic tissues on inspiration
C. inability to visualize the vocal cords
D. all of the above
E. none of the above

140. All of the following are risk factors for bronchopulmonary dysplasia except — C 9.2.2

A. prematurity
B. patent ductus arteriosus
C. female sex
D. *Ureaplasma urealyticum* infection
E. mechanical ventilation

141. Treatment for bronchopulmonary dysplasia includes all of the following except — A 9.2.2

A. calorie restriction
B. bronchodilators
C. diuretics
D. oxygen
E. pneumococcal vaccine

142. What is the largest single risk factor for apnea — B 9.2.4

A. meningitis
B. prematurity
C. gastroesophageal reflux
D. hyponatremia
E. respiratory syncytial virus infection

143. An infant born to two healthy individuals is found to have cystic fibrosis. What is their risk of recurrence in future children — A 9.2.5

A. 25%
B. 50%
C. 75%
D. 100%

144. A child with asthma presents in respiratory distress with tachypnea and poor air movement. He is sleepy. His arterial blood gas shows a pH 7.4, pO_2 70, and pCO_2 40. His asthma exacerbation is classified as — B 9.2.6

A. respiratory failure
B. severe
C. moderate
D. mild
E. effectively treated

145. Which of the following endocrine findings may be seen in children with cystic fibrosis

E
9.2.5

A. hyperglycemia
B. delayed puberty
C. tall stature
D. all of the above
E. A and B

146. All of the following vitamins are likely to be deficient in a child with cystic fibrosis except

D
9.2.5

A. D
B. K
C. E
D. C
E. A

147. Which of the following are potential complications of asthma or asthma therapy

D
9.2.6

A. pneumomediastinum
B. cataracts
C. school absenteeism
D. all of the above
E. A and C

148. The most common genetic defect in cystic fibrosis is

C
9.2.5

A. ΔF509
B. ΔV508
C. ΔF508
D. ΔV509

149. What chloride level on a sweat chloride test is considered indicative of cystic fibrosis

D
9.2.5

A. >10 mEq/L
B. >20 mEq/L
C. >40 mEq/L
D. >60 mEq/L

150. All of the following are true for a child with mild intermittent asthma except

C
9.2.6

A. brief exacerbations occur < 3 times per week
B. peak flows are normal between exacerbations
C. nocturnal symptoms occur once a week
D. the exacerbations are variable in intensity

151. All of the following are maintenance medications for asthma except

B
9.2.6

A. cromolyn sodium
B. albuterol
C. salmeterol
D. inhaled steroids
E. leukotriene inhibitors

152. Side effects of oral steroid use include all of the following except

A
9.2.6

A. acromegaly
B. aseptic hip necrosis
C. hyperglycemia
D. short stature
E. cataracts

153. You perform a chest x-ray on an afebrile 6-month-old with acute onset of cough, wheezing, and tachypnea, after playing on the floor in his 7-year-old brother's room. The study reveals hyperinflation of the right lower lobe that persists on expiration. There is also mediastinal shift to the left. The next diagnostic or therapeutic intervention is B 9.2.3

- **A.** flexible bronchoscopy
- **B.** rigid bronchoscopy
- **C.** back blows
- **D.** chest tube placement
- **E.** admit for observation

10 CARDIOVASCULAR DISORDERS

10.1 CIRCULATORY EMBRYOLOGY

10.1.1 Heart Embryology

A. By the time an embryo has an ovulation age of 21 days, the vascular system has begun to appear as "blood islands."
   1. "Blood islands" are scattered masses of angiogenic cell clusters which increase in number and size, acquire a lumen, and eventually form a vascular plexus.
   2. Part of the plexus differentiates into main channels.
   3. At the cephalad end of the embryo, these channels further specialize, producing a pair of heart tubes which come to lie parallel to each other and eventually fuse to form a single tube.

B. By 23 days of ovulation, age differentiation continues into formation of the bulboventricular tube, with an extra pericardial portion called the aortic sac. The cardiac loop forms and the caudal half of the bulboventricular tube begins to represent the early embryonic ventricle.

C. By an ovulation age of 25 days, the heart completely occupies the pericardial cavity.
   1. Internally, it is still a single tube, but with primitive development of the left ventricle on the left side and the bulbus cordis on the right.
   2. A portion of the bulbus cordis eventually becomes the right ventricle.

D. Further development of the primitive atria and the truncus arteriosus occurs, and by an ovulation age of about 27 days, the external shape of the heart already suggests its future four chambered condition.

E. As the heart continues to develop, cardiac septation takes place, the ventricles enlarge in size, and the medial walls of the ventricles appose and fuse, forming the major portion of the muscular ventricular septum.

F. The atrioventricular (AV) canal divides into a right and left AV orifice.

G. Vascular structures change in their alignment and blood can begin to flow from one chamber to the other.

H. Pulmonary veins soon develop along with the AV valves. Septum formation continues, the chordae tendineae are formed, arterial valves develop, and the cardiovascular system increases in size and complexity.

I. Early in embryonic development aortic arches form (1st through 4th and 6th aortic arch [the 5th aortic arch is generally not present in humans or is very rudimentary]).
   1. Aortic arches progress through a complex series of transformations.
   2. The ductus arteriosus in the prenatal child is the distal portion of the left 6th aortic arch. This obliterates after birth and is converted to the ligamentum arteriosum.

J. Because the cardiovascular system in the fetus is required during fetal life for the supply of oxygenated blood to all tissues of the fetus, the cardiovascular system develops quite precociously. The cardiovascular system is completely organized by an ovulation age of 8 weeks.

10.1.2 Fetal Circulation

A. The fetal circulation has some marked differences from circulation in the postnatal infant.
   1. Oxygenated blood is supplied to the fetal heart for distribution to the fetus from the placenta through the umbilical vein and has a PaO_2 of about 35 mm Hg.
   2. Approximately 50% of this blood flows through the liver and the other 50% bypasses the liver through the ductus venosus into the inferior vena cava and to the right atrium.
   3. Blood then flows across the foramen ovale to the left atrium, into the left ventricle, and is ejected into the ascending aorta, before supplying the upper portion of the body.
   4. Blood returning through the superior vena cava flows through the right atrium and into the right ventricle, where it is ejected into the pulmonary arterial trunk. Most of this blood flows through the ductus arteriosus into the descending aorta and supplies the lower portion of the body. A small portion of this blood will flow through the pulmonary arteries to the lungs.

B. Pulmonary resistance is much higher in the fetus than in the newborn and accounts for blood preferentially crossing the ductus arteriosus and bypassing the lungs.

C. At birth, fetal circulation stops and neonatal circulation begins.
   1. Changes that result in this include an initial fall in systemic blood pressure followed by a progressive rise, a decrease in pulmonary vascular resistance with an increase in pulmonary blood flow, increased pulmonary venus return and left ventricular outflow, closure of the ductus arteriosus and the ductus venosus, and the formation of the ligamentum venosus and the ligamentum arteriosus.
   2. The foramen ovale begins its apposition to the atrial wall and is functionally closed by 3 months of age.
   3. Until the pulmonary vascular pressures decrease after birth to a level sufficiently below that of the systemic pressures, left-to-right flow will not occur through septal defects and the murmurs generated by such flow will not be heard. This means many infants with some heart defects will be undiagnosed during their newborn nursery stay and will present later. A thorough cardiovascular exam is imperative when evaluating young infants in the of-

fice practice.

10.2 DIAGNOSTIC MODALITIES

10.2.1 The History and Physical Exam

A. The medical history and exam in infants with a cardiovascular disorder is geared toward the identification of the disorder, if unknown at the time of the interview, as well as how an individual infant is compensating for the condition.

1. Perform a general history being sure to address these important points: presence or absence of cyanosis (at rest or while active), fatigue, nocturnal dyspnea, orthopnea, failure to thrive or poor growth, volume per feed in infants, dyspnea while suckling, profuse perspiring, exhaustion after activities including feeds, and requirement for frequent feeds.
2. In addition to general information, the physical examination should document growth and development, growth percentiles and trends, respiratory symptoms (tachypnea, crackles, retractions), presence of hepatosplenomegaly, peripheral edema, cyanosis, clubbing, heart rate, character of pulses, and a detailed heart exam.
   a. Blood pressure varies by age, height, and weight (also varies by exam; repeated measurements essential for reliability). Normal (after 1 year of age) can be approximated by: systolic blood pressure = 70 + (age in years X 2) diastolic blood pressure = 2/3 of systolic pressure.

B. The Cardiac Examination

1. Visually observe for a hyperdynamic or silent precordium, precordial bulge, apical heave, or substernal thrust.
2. Palpate for thrills or bruits.
3. Auscultate heart sounds for character, splitting, intensity, murmurs, clicks, or rubs.
4. Findings Suggestive of Heart Disease
   a. Hepatomegaly. The neonate and infant rarely get pedal edema from congestive heart failure, but hepatomegaly is almost always present.
   b. Cyanosis. Three to 5 g/dl of unsaturated hemoglobin is required to see cyanosis. Thus, severe hypoxemia can be missed in patients who have severe anemia.
   c. Precordial prominence is reflective of longstanding cardiomegaly during development of the chest wall.
   d. A hyperdynamic precordium is suggestive of extra volume (as in left-to-right shunts) if the child is not febrile.
   e. Diastolic murmurs should not be heard in normal healthy children.

10.2.2 Diagnostic Testing

A. **Chest X-Ray** (CXR). Note the heart size and amount of pulmonary blood flow (heart size normally occupies 50% or less of the chest and pulmonary vessels are seen from the hilar area throughout 2/3 of the chest).

B. **Electrocardiogram** (EKG). Shows myocardial mass as it is reflected by electrical activity seen at the surface and shows cardiac rhythm.

1. As a result of fetal circulation, the newborn heart has a relative right ventricular hypertrophy. The muscle mass of the right ventricle is roughly equal to the mass of the left ventricle. Postnatally, the left ventricular muscle mass begins to increase and gradually the relative right ventricular hypertrophy resolves.
2. Most children's heart disease is structural rather than the functional heart disease seen in adults. Children's hearts are generally malformed rather than malfunctioning. These diseases are reflected in different ways in the EKG (see specific disease profiles).

C. **Echocardiography** (ECHO)

1. Forms available now include M-mode and two-dimensional ECHO, as well as pulsed continuous wave and color-flow Doppler.
2. These forms now give precise information about cardiac structure and blood flow and are an essential adjunct in evaluation of the patient when done by an experienced echocardiographer with interpretation by a pediatric cardiologist.
3. Another method of using ECHO is esophageal ECHO. In special circumstances, such as anomalous return, this can be a valuable tool.
4. ECHO is an incredibly versatile tool for prenatal diagnosis of both structural and functional congenital heart disease. It should be routinely included as a part of the prenatal ultrasound.

D. **Exercise testing** is used most commonly in patients with known heart disease to assess effective exercise on cardiac function as a guide to prescribing activity for the child. It is most helpful in children with arrhythmias, chronic volume overload of the ventricles, left ventricular outflow obstruction, and hypertension.

E. **Radionuclide studies** are a relatively noninvasive procedure that can be used to assess blood flow and is also available on a portable basis. It does not provide the information about anatomic details provided by ECHO and catheterization, but may be useful in some patients.

F. **Cardiac catheterization** is always a good tool for delineation of anatomy and understanding of directional flow in an individual's heart, and an essential tool for the measurement of PaO_2, etc. in the various chambers of the heart. This information may be necessary for planning corrective surgery for a child. It is used less frequently since the advent of ECHO.

G. **Laboratory data** (arterial blood gas, chemistries, complete blood count, fibrinogen, prothrombin time, partial thromboplastin time) may be appropriate depending on the patient's particular situation. Remember, patients who are polycythemic as a result of their heart disease frequently have other hematologic abnormalities.

10.3 HEART MURMURS

10.3.1 Grades of Murmurs

A. Grade I – Soft, heard only with difficulty.

B. Grade II – Easily heard.

C. Grade III – Loud but without a palpable thrill on the chest wall.

D. Grade IV – Loud with a palpable thrill.

E. Grade V – Heard with only one edge of the stethoscope on the chest.

F. Grade VI – Heard without the stethoscope touching the chest.

10.3.2 Cardiac Cycle Location of Murmurs

A. **Systolic murmurs** are heard between the first heart sound (S_1) and the second heart sound (S_2).

1. Systolic Ejection Murmur (SEM). There is a silent interval between S_1 and the onset of the murmur. It then crescendos to a maximum intensity and decrescendos to end before the S_2 heart sound. These murmurs arise in stenotic aortic or pulmonary valve areas and must overcome the pressure in such vessels before the flow rate is great enough to produce a murmur.
2. Holosystolic Murmur. Also called pansystolic murmurs, these are the result of immediate flow from a high pressure area to a low flow area and are heard throughout systole. Areas of such pressure differentials are from a ventricle to an atrium or from the left ventricle to the right ventricle.
3. End Systolic Murmur. Also called late systolic murmurs, these murmurs are caused by prolapse of the mitral valve toward the end of systole, allowing regurgitation of blood into the left atrium.

B. **Diastolic murmurs** are heard between the second heart sound (S_2) and the first heart sound (S_1).

1. Early Diastolic Murmur. Murmurs beginning with S_2 are due to backflow through incompetent outflow tract valves and are generated by pressure in the aorta or pulmonary vessels. They rarely can be heard beyond mid-diastole. Characteristically, they are high-pitched blowing murmurs.
2. Mid-Diastolic Murmur. These murmurs are the result of turbulent flow over the mitral or tricuspid valves during the atrial filling phase of diastole. These are usually very low-pitched rumbling murmurs.
3. Late Diastolic Murmur. These are the result of end diastolic filling into a ventricle with decreased compliance as occurs in ventricular hypertrophy. These may sound more like a click than a distinct murmur.

C. Continuous murmurs continue through S_2. They begin in late systole and continue in early diastole. A typical continuous murmur is that of a patent ductus arteriosus. The systolic component is due to increased flow across a relatively stenotic pulmonary valve and the diastolic component is generated by the flow through the ductus from the aorta to the pulmonary vessel at the beginning of diastole.

Table 10.3.5 Characteristics of murmurs in selected heart lesions

Lesion	Loudest	Quality	Radiation
Aortic stenosis	Right 3rd ICS	Harsh, SEM	Cartoids
Aortic regurgitation	MLSB	Blowing, early diastolic	Apex
Pulmonary stenosis	Left 2nd ICS	Harsh, SEM	Lung fields
Pulmonary regurgitation	Left 2nd ICS	Low pitched, early mid-diastolic	Little to none
Mitral stenosis	Apex	Low pitched, mid-diastolic rumble	None
Mitral regurgitation	Apex	Blowing, holosystolic	Left axilla
ASD	Left 2nd ICS	Harsh, SEM	Lung fields
VSD	LLSB	Harsh, holosystolic	None
PDA	Left 2nd-3rd ICS	Continuous	Lung fields
ASD = atrial septal defect; ICS = intercostal space; LUSB = left upper sternal border; MLSB = middle left sternal border; PDA = patent ducts arteriosus; SEM = systolic ejection murmur; VSD = ventricular septal defect			

10.3.3. Typical Point of Maximal Intensity of Murmurs

A. Aortic area: 2nd right intercostal space (ICS).

B. Pulmonary area: 2nd left ICS.

C. Mitral area: the cardiac apex.

D. Tricuspid area: left lower sternal border (LLSB).

10.3.4 Pitch Qualities of Murmurs

A. Blowing, high-pitched murmur sound can be simulated by holding the stethoscope in the palm and stroking then back of the hand with the pad of a finger.
B. Harsh, medium-pitched murmur can be simulated by holding the stethoscope in the palm and scratching the back of the hand with a fingernail.
C. Rumbling, low-pitched murmur resembles the sound of a bowling ball rumbling down a gutter.

10.3.5 Characteristic Heart Murmurs

A. Murmurs associated with heart lesions (Table 10.3.5).

B. Functional Murmurs
1. A **Still's murmur** is a nonradiating systolic ejection murmur of grade III or less with a vibratory quality. It is heard best at the LLSB. It increases in intensity with supine positioning.
2. A **venous hum** is a loud rumbling murmur arising from blood return to the heart through the superior vena cava. It disappears when the patient is supine.
3. **Peripheral pulmonic stenosis (pulmonary bifurcation turbulence murmur)** is a systolic flow murmur heard in the left third ICS with radiation to both

Table 10.4.2 Congenital syndromes associated with congenital heart disease

SYNDROME	HEART LESIONS
Trisomy 13 (Patau's syndrome)	VSD, ASD, PDA
Trisomy 18 (Edwards' syndrome)	VSD, ASD, PDA
Trisomy 21 (Down's syndrome)	Endocardial cushion defect
Turner's syndrome	Coarctation of the aorta, aortic stenosis
Williams' syndrome	Supravalvular aortic stenosis
Noonan's syndrome	Pulmonary valve stenosis, aortic valve stenosis
Holt-Oram syndrome	ASD, VSD
Marfan's syndrome	Mitral valve prolapse, aortic valve regurgitation, dilated and dissecting aorta
Asplenia syndrome	Complex cyanotic heart lesions, anomalous pulmonary venous return, dextrocardia, single ventricle, single atrioventricular valve
Polysplenia syndrome	Pulmonary atresia, dextrocardia, single ventricle, azygos continuation of inferior vena cava
Congenital rubella	PDA, peripheral pulmonic stenosis
Glycogen storage disease	Hypertrophic cardiomyopathyP
DiGeorge's syndrome	Aortic arch anomalies, Tetralogy of Fallot, pulmonary atresia, transposition of great vessels, truncus arteriosus
Ellis-van Creveld syndrome	Single atrium
Duchenne muscular dystrophy	Cardiomyopathy
ASSOCIATION	**HEART LESION**
CHARGE association (**C**oloboma, **H**eart lesion, **A**tresia of choanae, **R**etardation, **G**enital anomalies, **E**ar anomalies)	Tetralogy of Fallot, endocardial cushion defects
VATER association (**V**ertebral anomalies, **A**nal atresia, **T**racheoesophageal fistula, **E**sophageal atresia, **R**adial and **R**enal anomalies)	VSD
ASD = atrial septal defect; PDA = patent ductus arteriosus; VSD = ventricular septal defect	

axilla. It occurs in infants due to the relatively small caliber of the branch pulmonary artery vessels and the acute angle at the site of bifurcation.

4. Remember, innocent murmurs are uncommon in the newborn, except for physiologic peripheral pulmonic stenosis.

10.4 CONGENITAL HEART DISEASE

10.4.1 General Considerations

A. Only 40 to 50% of congenital heart disease (CHD) is diagnosed by one week of age. Only 50 to 60% of CHD is diagnosed by one month of age.

B. Incidence of CHD is 10-times higher in stillborn than in liveborn infants.

C. Incidence in the liveborn child of CHD is approximately 1% (varies from .4 to 1.0% depending on the study).

D. Most estimates probably underrepresent CHD because, the majority of the studies upon which estimates are based were done when ECHO was not available, and some entities like bicuspid aortic valve (occurs in approximately 2% of the population) are best diagnosed with ECHO.

E. Risk for recurrence is impossible to predict in the overall sense because it is different for specific lesions.
1. In general, the recurrence risk is higher if the proband has a more serious lesion, if the affected parent is the mother, or if more than one first degree relative is affected.
2. Recurrence risk for individual lesions in siblings is approximately 2 to 3%.
3. Transmission risk to the next generation is approximately 5 to 10%.

F. Some CHDs are more common in one sex than the other.
1. Aortic stenosis (AS) is more common in males.
2. Coarctation is more common in males.
3. Atrial septal defect (ASD) is more common in females.
4. Patent ductus arteriosus (PDA) is more common in females.
5. Ventricular septal defect (VSD) is equal in both sexes.

G. The most common form of CHD is VSD (30 to 40% of all CHD).

10.4.2 Genetic Abnormalities and CHD

A. Chromosomal defects account for 5 to 8% of CHD and single gene defects account for 3% of CHD.

Table 10.4.5a Palliative prcoedures for selected congenital heart disease lesions

Procedure	Anatomy Involved	Result	Indication
Blalock-Taussig shunt	subclavian artery to pulmonary artery	increased pulmonary blood flow	tetralogy of Fallot, pulmonary valve atresia
Modified Blalock-Taussig shunt	tube graft from subclavian artery to ipsilateral pulmonary artery	increased pulmonary blood flow	tetralogy of Fallot, pulmonary valve atresia
Waterston shunt	aorta to right pulmonary arter\ry	increased pulmonary blood flow	tetralogy of Fallot, pulmonary valve atresia, tricuspid atresia
Rashkind procedure	balloon atrial septostomy	increased atrial mixing, decompression of right or left atria	transposition of great arteries, tricuspid atresia
Blalock-Hanlon procedure	operative arterial septostomy	increased atrial mixing, decompression of right or left atria	transposition of great arteries, tricuspid atresia
Balloon angioplasty	valves and vessels	dilation of valves/vessels	pulmonary valve stenosis, aortic valve stenosis, coarctation of the aorta
Pulmonary artery banding	pulmonary artery	decreased pulmonary blood flow and pressure	ventricular septal defect, endocardial cushion defect, single ventricle
Glenn shunt	superior vena cava to right pulmonary artery	increased pulmonary blood flow	used as a staging procedure prior to the Fontan procedure

B. Polygenic inheritance is well described for PDA with a recurrence risk of 2.5% in siblings (recurrence risk increases to 10% if greater than one family member is affected).

C. Congenital syndromes associated with CHD (Table 10.4.2).

10.4.3 Acyanotic Congenital Heart Lesions

A. With Increased Pulmonary Blood Flow (Vascularity)

1. These are lesions associated with left-to-right shunts.
2. Examples include ASD, PDA, VSD, endocardial cushion defect, AV malformation.

B. With Normal Pulmonary Blood Flow

1. These lesions have no left-to-right shunt.
2. Examples include coarctation of the aorta, AS, pulmonic stenosis without right-to-left shunt, mitral stenosis, mitral regurgitation, and endocardial fibroelastosis.

10.4.4 Cyanotic Congenital Heart Lesions

A. With Decreased Pulmonary Flow

1. These lesions have pulmonary outflow obstruction.
2. Examples include pulmonic stenosis, pulmonary atresia, Tetralogy of Fallot, tricuspid atresia, pulmonary atresia and hypoplastic right ventricle, Ebstein's anomaly.

B. Cyanotic lesions with increased pulmonary blood flow include hypoplastic left heart syndrome, total anomalous pulmonary venous return, transposition of great vessels, single ventricle complexes, and truncus arteriosus.

10.4.5 Therapeutic Considerations

A. Certain congenital heart lesions are amenable to **prostaglandin E_1 (PGE_1)**.

1. PGE_1 acts on the ductus arteriosus to keep it patent, allowing shunting of blood flow, such that either pulmonary or systemic blood flow may be maintained.
2. Examples of ductal dependent lesions include hypoplastic left heart syndrome, complex coarctation syndromes, critical AS, hypoplastic right heart syndrome, pulmonary atresia with intact ventricular septum, tricuspid atresia, and pulmonary atresia with VSD.

B. Surgical Procedures for Selected CHD Lesions

1. **Palliative Procedures** (Table 10.4.5a)
2. **Corrective Procedures** (Table 10.4.5b)

10.4.6 Heart Failure

A. Common Causes of Heart Failure By Age

1. The fetus develops heart failure with severe anemia, supraventricular tachycardia (SVT), ventricular tachycardia, and complete heart block.
2. The premature infant may develop congestive hart failure from cardiomyopathy (asphyxia, sepsis, hypoglycemia, hypocalcemia), fluid overload, PDA, VSD, and cor pulmonale from bronchopulmonary dysplasia.
3. The full-term infant may have heart failure in association with cardiomyopathy (asphyxia, sepsis, hypoglycemia, hypocalcemia), arteriovenous malformation (vein of Galen, hepatic), left-sided obstructive lesions (hypoplastic left heart, coarctation of aorta), large mixing cardiac defects (single ventricle, truncus arteriosus), and viral myocarditis.
4. Infant-toddler heart failure may be due to left-to-right cardiac shunts (VSD), hemangioma (arteriovenous malformation), anomalous left coronary artery, metabolic cardiomyopathy, acute hyperten-

Table 10.4.5b Corrective procedures for selected congenital heart disease lesions

Procedure	Anatomy Involved	Result	Indication
Fontan procedure	right atrium or vena cava to pulmonary artery anastamosis	diverts systemic venous return directly to pulmonary circulation	tricuspid atresia, single ventricle pulmonary atresia
Mustard procedure	intra-atrial baffle	right ventricle remains systemic ventricle	transposition of the great arteries (procedure rarely used)
Norwood procedure	pulmonary artery becomes ascending aorta	use right ventricle to pump to aorta	hypoplastic left heart
Heart transplant			hypoplastic left heart, cardiomyopathy
Jatene procedure (arterial switch)	switch great arteries above the valve	anatomic correction	transposition of great arteries (replacing the Mustard procedure)

sion (hemolytic-uremic syndrome), SVT, and coronary artery aneurysms (Kawasaki disease).

5. Child-adolescent congestive heart failure is found in rheumatic fever, acute hypertension, viral myocarditis, thyrotoxicosis, hemochromatosis, hemosiderosis, cancer therapy (radiation, adriamycin), sickle cell anemia, endocarditis, cor pulmonale (cystic fibrosis), and status asthmaticus.

B. Treatment (Table 10.4.6)

Table 10.4.6 Mnemonic for treating congestive heart failure with subsequent pulmonary edema

	Mnemonic	Mechanism of Action
U	Upright position	Improve ventilation-perfusion
N	Nifedipine, nitroglycerine, nitroprusside	Afterload reduction
L	Lasix® (furosemide)	Diuresis, fluid shift
O	Oxygen	Improved O_2 saturation
A	Albuterol inhalation	Bronchodilation
D	Dopamine, dobutamine, digitalis	Inotropic agents
e'		
M	Morphine	Anxiolytic, venous pooling

10.5 DISEASE PROFILES

(Only diseases that are common, specifically unique or important, or particularly interesting are included. A textbook has more comprehensive information.)

10.5.1 Persistent Fetal Circulation (PFC)

A. This is not necessarily classified as a CHD, but presents much like cyanotic CHD. PFC typically occurs in the neonatal full term infant.

B. The etiology is uncertain in some cases, but is most commonly related to perinatal hypoxemia.

C. Persistent pulmonary hypertension results in left-to-right shunting through the foramen ovale and/or the PDA.

D. Tachypnea develops in the first few hours of life with varying degrees of respiratory distress.

E. On exam, infants appear ill and may have a systolic murmur, a loud second heart sound, and a parasternal heave.

F. Testing reveals acidosis, CXR with decreased vascular flow, and ECHO with right-to-left flow seen at the foramen ovale.

G. Differential diagnosis includes the cyanotic CHDs, most specifically, transposition of the great arteries.

H. PFC is almost universally fatal if not treated, and even when treated, has significant mortality.

I. Diagnosis is based on physical exam plus CXR and is greatly helped by ECHO and measurements of differential PaO_2.

J. Therapeutic plan includes oxygen administration, mechanical ventilation, correction of acidosis and any electrolyte abnormalities, administration of nitrous oxide, and consideration of possible use of extracorporeal membrane oxygenation (ECMO).

10.5.2 Hypoplastic Left Heart Syndrome

A. Pathophysiologic abnormality is the underdevelopment of the aortic root, aortic valve, left ventricle, or mitral valve. Either or both valves may be atretic. Systemic flow is duct dependent.

B. Symptoms including severe congestive heart failure and cardiovascular collapse occurs as the duct closes.

C. Physical findings are signs of poor peripheral perfusion (mottling of skin, prolonged capillary refill, diminished or absent pulses) and congestive failure. A nonspecific murmur may be present.

D. Testing

1. CXR findings of cardiomegaly and pulmonary congestion.
2. EKG shows regular sinus rhythm.
3. ECHO is diagnostic of the lesion.

E. Congestive failure occurs early as the duct begins to close in the first few days or weeks of life.

F. Differential diagnosis is critical AS and severe coarctation of aorta.

G. Therapeutic plan is PGE_1, supportive care, and palliative surgery, while awaiting transplant.

10.5.3 Hypoplastic Right Heart Syndrome

A. Either of the following can cause this syndrome: pulmonary atresia with intact ventricular septum or tricuspid atresia with a patent ASD.

B. Pulmonary perfusion is dependent on a PDA in pulmonary atresia. Rapid deterioration results when the ductus closes.

C. Infants present with severe cyanosis at birth.

D. A continuous PDA murmur may be heard in the pulmonary atresia defect.

E. Testing

1. CXR reveals diminished pulmonary vascularity.
2. EKG is significant for right atrial enlargement and left axis deviation (in tricuspid atresia).

3. ECHO is diagnostic of the structural defect.

F. Differential diagnosis includes severe pulmonary stenosis and Tetralogy of Fallot.

G. Treatment is with PGE_1 for palliation, supportive care, and surgical establishment of an aortopulmonary artery shunt.

10.5.4 Atrial Septal Defect (ASD)

A. This is the most common CHD newly diagnosed in adults (discounting congenital bicuspid aortic valve).

B. Alternative terminology's for this lesion are ASD, ostium primum defect, and ostium secundum defect (defect at the fossa ovalis).

C. This condition is more common in females, with a 2 to 1 ratio. Genetics is multifactorial, but some Mendelian examples are available.

D. Children are usually asymptomatic, but may have mild fatigue. If ASD persists uncorrected into adulthood, patients may develop fatigue, dyspnea, and chest pain.

E. Growth and development are usually normal. Other exam findings may include right ventricular systolic lift, accentuated first heart sound plus fixed splitting of the second heart sound, a systolic murmur at the left upper sternal border (LUSB), and a mid-diastolic rumble.

F. Testing
1. CXR: some heart enlargement and prominence of pulmonary vasculature.
2. EKG: regular sinus rhythm pattern.
3. ECHO: left-to-right shunt with resultant right-sided volume overload. ASD can usually be visualized.
4. Catheterization: increased O_2 saturation in the right side of the heart.

G. There are few findings early in life, so many individuals are not diagnosed until adulthood. As adults, they may develop pulmonary hypertension and congestive heart failure, or atrial arrhythmias.

H. Differential diagnosis includes patent foramen ovale.

I. Complications of the untreated ASD are pulmonary hypertension, congestive heart failure, atrial fibrillation or flutter, mitral valve prolapse, and infections.

J. The diagnosis is made when a murmur is noted on routine exam leading to CXR, EKG, ECHO, and possibly catheterization.

K. Treatment
1. Watchful waiting is acceptable in children, with repair prior to school age.
2. Repair adults. Repair is usually direct or with a patch repair of the defect.

10.5.5 Ventricular Septal Defect (VSD)

A. Embryologically, VSD results from incomplete development of the ventricular septum.

B. Blood flow across the lesion depends on the size of the defect.
1. Small defects have high resistance to flow across the defect with little resultant shunting. These defects tend to have louder murmurs than larger defects.
2. Moderate defects have significant left-to-right shunting with much higher pressures in the left ventricle than the right.
3. Large defects have relatively complete mixing of the blood in the ventricles, with right ventricular pressure equal to the left.

C. Symptoms also depend on the size of the defect.
1. Small defects are asymptomatic.
2. Large defects cause congestive heart failure symptoms (sweating, tachypnea, grunting respirations, fatigue with feeds). These infants tend to fail to thrive.

D. Physical findings include a systolic murmur, with or without a LLSB thrill. Children with large defects have respiratory distress, decreased weight for height, narrowly split S_2, and hepatomegaly.

E. Testing
1. CXR is normal with a small defect. Large defects show an enlarged heart with prominent pulmonary vascular markings.
2. EKG with a large defect has the QRS axis oriented to the right, bilaterally increased ventricular voltage, and increased left atrial voltage.
3. ECHO images the defect.
4. Catheterization. Reflection of left-to-right shunt found in increased O_2 saturation of blood in the right ventricle.

F. Chronologic Sequence of Manifestations
1. Most small isolated VSDs are insignificant and close spontaneously.
2. Large VSDs progress to congestive heart failure with pulmonary damage.

G. Diagnosis is based on physical exam plus CXR and ECHO. ECHO demonstrates not only the size and location of the defect, but blood flow across the defect.

H. Treatment is surgical repair of moderate or large defects. Most small defects are followed with repeat exams and close spontaneously. subacute bacterial endocarditis prophylaxis is indicated.

10.5.6 Atrioventricular (AV) Canal Defect (Endocardial Cushion Defect)

A. AV canals are generally described in two basic types:
1. Partial is comprised of an ostium primum ASD, cleft mitral valve and deficient ventricular septum, but without significant interventricular shunting.
2. Complete is comprised of an ASD, an essentially single valve from atria to ventricles comprised of tissue of mitral and tricuspid valve origin, and defi-

cient ventricular septum with shunting.

3. The complete form is much less common and much more severe than the partial form.

B. About half of children with Down's syndrome have CHD, and a large percentage of these have the AV canal defect.

C. AV canal arises from the incomplete growth of the endocardial cushions during embryogenesis.

D. Associated Conditions. Nearly all patients with asplenia syndrome have a complete AV canal. Other associated conditions include Tetralogy of Fallot, polysplenia, disorder of right ventricle, and Down syndrome.

E. Symptoms depends on the type of defect.
   1. Patients with partial AV canals have symptoms similar to patients with simple ASD, unless their mitral valve is compromised to the point that they have significant mitral regurgitation. Then, they are likely to have fatigue, dyspnea, failure to gain weight adequately, and repeated respiratory infections.
   2. Those with complete AV canals progress rapidly to congestive heart failure and generally do very poorly without corrective surgery.

F. Physical Findings
   1. Partial AV canals may produce a systolic murmur at the LUSB and a holosystolic blowing murmur at the apex.
   2. Complete AV canals produce a systolic murmur at the LUSB, a systolic murmur at the LLSB, fixed splitting of the second heart sound, hepatomegaly, and evidence of congestive heart failure.

G. Testing
   1. CXR shows cardiac enlargement with or without pulmonary congestion.
   2. EKG demonstrates superior orientation of the mean QRS axis in the frontal plane, with or without a prolonged QT interval.
   3. ECHO allows visualization of the ASD, valvular function, VSD with evaluation of shunt, and evaluation of ventricular size and ability that may influence surgical plans.
   4. Catheterization demonstrates increased O_2 saturation in the right atrium and increased right ventricular pressure (complete type).

H. Chronologic Sequence of Manifestations
   1. Partial defects progress as ASDs with an increased risk of infection secondary to mitral valve deformity.
   2. Complete defects usually progress rapidly to congestive heart failure and die if not corrected in some fashion.

I. The differential diagnosis includes simple ASD and simple VSD.

J. Patients are at high risk for endocardial infection. Many children (especially with complete AV canal) have associated systemic abnormalities.

K. Diagnosis is suspected when associated syndromes are present (asplenia syndrome, Down's syndrome) and confirmed by EKG and ECHO.

L. Treatment
   1. Medical management is appropriate in those with few symptoms.
   2. Surgical correction is indicated for significant mitral regurgitation or complete AV canal.
   3. Small infants may require pulmonary banding (to decrease pressure to lung fields) until they reach an age where surgical correction is possible.

10.5.7 Patent Ductus Arteriosus (PDA)

A. PDA results when the ductus arteriosus fails to close after birth.

B. The direction of blood flow through the duct is dependent on the relative pressures in the systemic and pulmonary circuits. It can be either left-to-right or right-to-left.

C. Physical exam
   1. Bounding pulses characteristic of large left-to-right shunts are present.
   2. A continuous machinery like murmur is present after the pulmonary pressure decreases enough for a large shunt to occur.

D. Symptoms
   1. Large left-to-right shunts can result in failure to thrive and congestive heart failure.
   2. Right-to-left shunts cause dyspnea and cyanosis.

E. Premature infants are predisposed to PDA.

F. Testing
   1. CXR shows cardiomegaly and increased pulmonary vascularity in large left-to-right shunts.
   2. EKG reveals biventricular hypertrophy. Right ventricular hypertrophy indicates development of increased pulmonary resistance.

G. Pulmonary hypertension is a significant potential complication.

H. Therapy is with surgical ligation or coil ablation of the duct before pulmonary hypertension develops.

I. Prognosis is good if corrected. If pulmonary hypertension develops, usually after a year, it is irreversible.

10.5.8 Congenital Mitral Stenosis

A. The mitral valve is funnel-shaped with thickened leaflets and short, deformed cordae tendineae.

B. Symptoms include failure to thrive and dyspnea due to congestive heart failure, cyanosis, and pallor.

C. Mitral stenosis is commonly associated with PDA, AS, and coarctation of the aorta.

D. Exam reveals a rumbling diastolic murmur followed

by a loud heart first sound. The second heart sound is split and loud.

E. Testing
1. EKG shows right ventricular hypertrophy.
2. CXR reveals both left atrial and right ventricular enlargement, and pulmonary congestion.
3. ECHO demonstrates an enlarged left atrium with thick mitral valve leaflets.
4. Treatment is with mitral valve prosthesis. Patients require anticoagulation and may suffer complications of this therapy. Prognosis without treatment is poor.

10.5.9 Aortic Stenosis (AS)

A. AS is outflow obstruction to the left ventricle.
1. Congenital AS is usually due to a bicuspid valve and may not be diagnosed until adulthood. It is also seen in association with Williams syndrome.
2. Acquired AS can be a complication of rheumatic fever.

B. Most patients are asymptomatic until adulthood, when syncope, easy fatigability, or anginal pain may occur.

C. Exam reveals a harsh systolic ejection murmur at the right 2nd ICS, radiating to carotids, and a systolic thrill at the jugular notch.

D. Testing
1. CXR shows poststenotic dilatation of the aorta.
2. EKG demonstrates left ventricular hypertrophy.
3. ECHO identifies the lesion and location.

E. Therapy is surgical repair if severity warrants. subacute bacterial endocarditis prophylaxis is indicated.

10.5.10 Coarctation of the Aorta (COA)

A. COA is narrowing of the aorta, most commonly at level of the ductus arteriosus.

B. Symptoms. COA generally presents in one of three ways.
1. Because of the position of the ductus in relation to the usual coarctation, as long as the ductus remains open in the newborn, infants are asymptomatic. Many patients with COA of the aorta remain asymptomatic throughout childhood. Their coarctation may be found incidentally on routine examinations.
2. If the ductus closes early, an infant may be diagnosed with COA in the newborn nursery based on the finding of absent femoral pulses.
3. Many infants will leave the nursery without their diagnosis being made. A certain percent of these infants will have significant enough coarctation that they will proceed to heart failure in the first month of life.
   a. These infants usually present at about two weeks of age with the symptoms of heart failure including poor perfusion and a "shocky" appearance.
   b. They require emergent care of their disease and usually surgical correction.

C. Examination
1. Femoral pulses are diminished or absent in most children with COA.
2. About 10% of patients develop congestive heart failure in infancy.
3. Older children with undiagnosed COA may have hypertension or a diminished shoe size for age.

D. Laboratory Findings
1. CXR: rib notching (>5 years of age) and an abnormal aortic knob.
2. EKG may show left ventricular hypertrophy if COA is severe and prolonged.
3. The lesion can sometimes be visualized by ECHO.
4. Magnetic Resonance Imaging (MRI)
   a. MRI may allow very good delineation of the lesion preoperatively.
   b. It is also used for follow up visualization after repairs.
   c. Patient's who had patch corrections of COA done years ago may develop the late postoperative complication of an aneurysm (particularly females during pregnancy). MRI can be very useful for this diagnosis.

E. Risk factors include male sex and Turner's syndrome.

F. Therapeutic Plan
1. Bacterial endocarditis prophylaxis is indicated.
2. Repair should be undertaken either with balloon angioplasty, or with a graft or patch surgical repair.

10.5.11 Pulmonary Stenosis (PS)

A. Pulmonic stenosis is outflow obstruction of the right ventricle.

B. Cyanosis results from decreased pulmonary perfusion, and in severe stenosis, with increased right atrial pressure from a right-to-left shunt through the foramen ovale.

C. Most are asymptomatic.

D. Examination reveals cyanosis, if severe, and a systolic ejection murmur at the 2nd left ICS radiating into the posterior lung fields.

E. Testing
1. CXR: decreased pulmonary vascularity and cardiomegaly if the stenosis is severe.
2. EKG: a degree of right axis deviation that correlates with the severity of stenosis.

F. Therapeutic Plan
1. Bacterial endocarditis prophylaxis is indicated.
2. Surgical repair or balloon angioplasty may be needed if the stenosis is severe.

G. Pathologic peripheral pulmonary stenosis is a different lesion associated with congenital rubella syndrome.

10.5.12 Tetralogy of Fallot (TOF)

A. TOF is the most common cyanotic congenital heart lesion.

B. Anatomy
1. Right ventricular outflow obstruction (pulmonary stenosis). The degree of right ventricular outflow obstruction governs the degree of hypoxemia and right-to-left shunting.
2. Dextroposition of the aorta (overrides the ventricular septum).
3. VSD.
4. Right ventricular hypertrophy.

C. Examination reveals cyanosis, harsh holosystolic murmur at the LLSB, squatting posture, and exertional dyspnea.

D. Testing
1. CXR: a boot-shaped normal size heart, decreased pulmonary vascularity, and possibly a right-sided aortic arch.
2. EKG: right axis deviation and right ventricular hypertrophy.
3 ECHO: diagnostic of the structural lesions.

E. Complications include hypercyanotic spells (tet spells).

F. Therapeutic Plan
1. Bacterial endocarditis prophylaxis is needed.
2. Surgical palliation is with a Blalock-Taussig procedure or modified Blalock-Taussig procedure.
3. Definitive surgical repair is ultimately required.

10.5.13 Persistent Truncus Arteriosus

A. Single vessel trunk arising from the heart with pulmonary arteries arising from the trunk. There is an associated large VSD present.

B. Findings relate to size of the pulmonary artery and may resemble either a PDA or TOF.

C. ECHO is diagnostic.

D. Surgical repair may be done.

10.5.14 D-Transposition of the Great Arteries

A. The pulmonary artery and aorta are "switched."
1. Pulmonary and systemic blood are recirculated through their own circuits.
2. A naturally occurring or created communication between the circuits (ASD, VSD, PDA, balloon septostomy) must exist for survival.

B. D-transposition of the great arteries is more common in males.

C. Cyanosis is present at birth.

D. CXR: an egg-on-a-string appearance of the cardiac silhouette.

E. Congestive heart failure develops early if surgical communication between the two circuits is not created.

F. Balloon atrial septostomy (Rashkin's procedure) may be lifesaving with definitive surgical correction performed later.

10.5.15 L-Transposition of the Great Arteries

A. This is also known as corrected transposition of the great vessels. The great vessels are reversed but associated defects result in blood flow sequentially through the pulmonary and systemic circuits.

B. There are usually associated anomalies which determine the exact nature of this complex lesion for any individual patient.

10.5.16 Total Anomalous Pulmonary Venous Return (TAPVR)

A. The common pulmonary vein does not get incorporated into the posterior wall of the left atrium.

B. Circulatory Pattern
1. Pulmonary venous return is not to the left atrium, but instead to one or a combination of the following routes.
   - **a.** Supracardial with flow into the innominate vein.
   - **b.** Cardiac with flow into the coronary sinus or back to the right atrium.
   - **c.** Infracardiac (infradiaphragmatic) with flow into the inferior vena cava.
2. Each of these lesions must have a right-to-left shunt, usually via the foramen ovale.
3. Pulmonary venous obstruction is often present and its severity determines the degree of cyanosis present.

C. CXR shows the typical "snowman" or "figure 8" heart shape.

D. Treatment is surgical reimplantation of the veins into the left atrium.

10.5.17 Partial Anomalous Pulmonary Venous Return (PAPVR)

A. One or more of the pulmonary veins returns to the right atrium instead of to the left atrium, sometimes associated with an ASD.

B. Symptoms depend on the number of veins with anomalous connections.
1. Single vein malformations are usually asymptomatic.
2. Multiple veins cause symptoms of fatigue and dyspnea.
3. Increased return the right side of the heart leads to congestive heart failure.

C. Findings on exam include right ventricular systolic lift and widely split (but not fixed splitting) of the second heart sound.

D. Testing
1. CXR: some enlargement of right side of the heart and increased pulmonary vasculature.
2. EKG may demonstrate evidence of right volume overload.
3. ECHO: increased right-sided flow is seen. Visual-

ization of anomalous vein(s) is possible.

4. Catheterization may be able to directly enter the anomalous veins and visualize return

E. Treatment in patients with large right-sided return, large right-to-left shunts through associated ASDs, or pulmonary hypertension with congestive heart failure require surgical correction.

10.6 ACQUIRED CARDIAC DISEASE

10.6.1 Kawasaki Disease (Mucocutaneous Lymph Node Syndrome)

A. This is not truly a "heart" disease, but rather, a rheumatic disease with "heart" sequelae.

B. The etiology is unknown, but a viral etiology is strongly suspected based on cyclic occurrence and seasonal occurrence (winter and spring).

C. Pathophysiology is inflammation (increased lymphocytes, cytokines, complement components) with endothelial damage.

D. Japanese ancestry and young age (85% of cases are in children <5 years of age) are identified risk factors.

E. Kawasaki disease occurs in three phases and has specific criteria for diagnosis (five of six criteria needed for diagnosis).

1. The acute phase (~10 days) includes conjunctivitis, fever, rash, changes in oral mucous membranes, distal edema and erythema, and lymphadenopathy.
2. The subacute phases (~ days 11 to 21) usually has decrease in fever, arthritis, and skin desquamation.
3. The convalescent phase may have thrombocytosis and arthritis, and is generally the phase when the development of coronary artery aneurysms is seen.

F. Criteria for diagnosis includes fever >5 days and at least 4 of the following 5 signs.

1. Mucosal changes (strawberry tongue, erythematous lips, general oral mucosal injection).
2. Cervical lymphadenopathy.
3. Rash.

10.6.2 Rheumatic Fever (RF)

A. RF is a systemic illness related to an immune reaction precipitated by group A β-hemolytic streptococcus infection.

B. RF is more common in children 5 to 15 years of age, but can occur at all ages, though rarely in infancy (group A streptococcus infections are rare in infants).

C. Diagnosis is based on clinical presentation. Diagnosis requires the finding of two major or one major and two minor **Jones criteria** and documentation of a recent streptococcal infection.

1. Major criteria include polyarthritis, carditis, chorea, and subcutaneous nodules.
2. Minor criteria include fever, arthralgias, elevated erythrocyte sedimentation rate or C-reactive protein, and prolonged PR interval.

D. Patients who develop chronic rheumatic heart disease may develop mitral regurgitation, mitral stenosis, a combination of mitral stenosis and mitral regurgitation or aortic regurgitation with or without AS.

E. Therapeutic Plan

1. Give aspirin in anti-inflammatory doses.
2. Provide prophylactic penicillin therapy (oral or parenteral).
3. Provide symptomatic care.

10.6.3 Arteriosclerosis

A. Arteriosclerosis and coronary artery disease are rare in infants and children, but as our nation becomes more obese and less active, these diseases are being seen in a steadily younger population.

B. Predisposing Conditions

1. Positive family history of heart attacks or strokes in family members less than 60 years of age.
2. Family members who have hypertension.
3. Obesity
4. Family history of hyperlipidemia.

C. Prevention

1. It is quite rare that arteriosclerosis or coronary artery disease requires treatment in someone who is still a child, but the prevention of these diseases should certainly start in the pediatric age group.
2. Medical attention should be directed at identifying children who are high risk for the development of arteriosclerotic disease and encouraging the practice of good dietary and exercise habits in the entire population.
3. Known familial hypercholesterolemia requires treatment with diet and/or drugs.
4. Any child who is high risk for the development of coronary artery disease or arteriosclerosis should certainly avoid obesity, cigarette smoking, be monitored for the development of hypertension and have a diet with reduced saturated fats and cholesterol.

10.6.4 Hypertension (HTN)

A. Secondary HTN is much more common than essential HTN in infants and children.

1. The vast majority of children who have secondary HTN have it as a result of a renal abnormality.
2. The term essential HTN implies that no known underlying disease is present, and certainly essential HTN is not a single entity.
3. Blood pressure is persistently above the 95th percentile for age on repeated measurements with an appropriately sized cuff.

B. Risk factors for HTN include family history, salt intake (in some individuals), stress, and obesity.

C. Children with HTN are usually not symptomatic unless the disease is sustained, and then, they may have headaches, dizziness, changes in vision, or seizures.

D. Potential complications include myocardial infarction, stroke, and renal failure.

E. Treatment Plan
   1. Treatment begins with weight reduction, limitation of salt intake, a reasonable exercise program, and may proceed to pharmacologic therapy.
   2. The most important management of HTN for the pediatric population is prevention. These methods are essentially the same as the prevention of other cardiovascular disease and include a diet low in saturated fats, appropriate body weight for age and size, limited salt intake, and a healthy exercise regimen.
   3. Treat the underlying disease if one is identified.

10.6.5 Cardiomyopathies

A. Most primary cardiomyopathies in children are of the dilated type and are usually related to myocarditis, a primary cardiomyopathy, or the use of drugs, particularly adriamycin.

B. Predisposing Conditions
   1. Family history of primary cardiomyopathies.
   2. Use of drugs associated with the development of cardiomyopathy.
   3. Viral infection (coxsackie B virus).

C. Most patients with cardiomyopathies present in congestive heart failure.

D. Complications are the development chronic cardiomyopathy or death.

E. Management is supportive care initially, with consideration of heart transplant for those patients who develop chronic cardiomyopathies.

10.7 ARRHYTHMIAS

10.7.1 Atrioventricular (AV) Block

A. AV block is uncommon in children.
   1. First degree block has prolongation of the PR interval, but there is AV conduction.
   2. Second degree block is where some atrial impulses are not conducted to the ventricles.
   3. Third degree block (complete heart block) occurs when no atrial impulses are conducted to the ventricles. The atria and ventricles function independently.

B. Congenital Complete AV Block
   1. Complete heart block can occur in the pediatric population. It arises most common as a congenital disease.
   2. Etiology
      a. The majority of congenital complete heart block and the vast majority of pediatric complete heart block is secondary to autoimmune disease. In these autoimmune diseases, the conduction system is damaged by immunoglobulin G antibodies.
      b. Other causes include complex CHD, abnormal embryonic development of the conduction system, myocarditis, long QT syndrome and prior history of surgical repair of a congenital heart lesion.
   3. Congenital AV block is most commonly seen in infants of mothers with systemic lupus erythematosus, and it may also be seen in mothers with rheumatoid arthritis, dermatomyositis or Sjögren's syndrome.
   4. Symptoms
      a. Patients with congenital complete heart block may have ventricular rates lower than 50 beats per minute, may develop evidence of fetal hydrops or may develop heart failure. Some infants with congenital complete heart block do not present at birth, but develop heart block within the first 3 to 6 months of life.
      b. Older children who have complete heart block are frequently asymptomatic, but may have attacks of syncope. Their systolic blood pressure is usually elevated.
   5. Diagnosis is suspected clinically and confirmed by EKG. On EKG, the P waves and the QRS complexes have no constant relation.
   6. Complications include development of congestive heart failure, death, chronic HTN, and syncope.
   7. Management depends on the severity of the disease. Newborns or older children with complete heart block may require cardiac pacing.

10.7.2 Supraventricular Tachycardia (SVT)

A. SVT of Infancy
   1. SVT of infancy is a specific condition in which SVT develops in utero or early in life. It requires emergent management and care. The infant is usually severely ill and in heart failure.
   2. Treatment
      a. Acute treatment with adenosine or cardioversion may be necessary. Other interventions with proven effectiveness include vagal stimulation (gagging, deep abdominal exam) and induction of the diving reflex (smother the face with a bag of ice and water).
      b. Chronic management with digitalis or beta blockers is usually essential.
      c. In infants, verapamil is a contraindicated drug because its use may result in profound hypotension and myocardial depression.
   3. SVT in the neonate and infant is often initially mistakenly diagnosed as sepsis.
   4. Children are at increased risk of SVT of infancy if they are males or if they have Wolf-Parkinson-White (WPW) syndrome.
   5. Most SVT of infancy resolves by one year of age and digitalis is usually discontinued at about that

time.

B. SVT After Infancy

1. Children or adults may have or develop SVT after infancy if they have an abnormal point of origin of electrical impulses in their atria. Many of these individuals have WPW syndrome.
2. Pharmacologic management is usually attempted in these individuals but episodes of breakthrough SVT with eventual development of congestive heart failure may occur.
3. Electrical cardiac mapping with catheter ablation of abnormal foci of electrical activity is now frequently done and has been very successful for the correction of this problem.

154. When in gestation does the cardiovascular system begin to develop — C 10.1.1

A. day 6
B. day 11
C. day 21
D. day 31

155. At what gestational age is organization of the cardiovascular system complete — B 10.1.1

A. 7 weeks
B. 8 weeks
C. 9 weeks
D. 10 weeks

156. Why are murmurs of left to right flow not heard immediately after birth in newborns with congenital septal defects — D 10.1.2

A. they are present, just not audible with the stethoscope
B. left to right flow cannot occur until left ventricular filling is adequate to dilate the ventricular defect
C. murmurs are not heard until flow reverses across the defect
D. left to right flow cannot occur until the pulmonary vascular pressure is less than the systemic vascular pressure
E. murmurs are not audible until the ductus closes

157. What would be the estimated systolic blood pressure in a normal 10-year-old — A 10.2.1

A. 90
B. 100
C. 110
D. 60

158. What is the most common sign of congestive heart failure in infants — D 10.2.1

A. cyanosis
B. palpable cardiac thrills
C. pedal edema
D. hepatomegaly

159. What is the minimum amount of unsaturated hemoglobin (g/dl) required to see clinical evidence of cyanosis — A 10.2.1

A. 3
B. 5
C. 7
D. 9
E. 11

160. Which of the following should not be seen in normal children (without congenital heart disease) — C 10.2.1

A. systolic murmur
B. venous hum
C. diastolic murmur
D. hyperactive precordium

161. Cardiomyopathy may develop in children in association with which of the following — E 10.6.5

A. folate deficiency
B. adriamycin administration
C. coxsackie B virus
D. all of the above
E. B and C

162. A child presents to your office for an examination. You note a systolic heart murmur that you can hear with only the edge of your stethoscope resting on the child's chest. What grade of murmur is present — E 10.3.1

A. I
B. II
C. III
D. IV
E. V

163. A 5-year-old child presents with exercise intolerance and has a grade IV/VI systolic ejection murmur at the right upper sternal border that radiates to the carotids. What is the defect — C 10.5.9

A. atrial septal defect
B. ventricular septal defect
C. aortic stenosis
D. pulmonary stenosis
E. venous hum

164. A 7-year-old presents for a preparticipation sports physical exam. You note a loud systolic murmur in the second intercostal space that disappears when he turns his head or lies down. What is your diagnosis — E 10.3.5

A. atrial septal defect
B. ventricular septal defect
C. aortic stenosis
D. pulmonic stenosis
E. venous hum

164. If a child has congenital heart disease, what is the average recurrence risk of a similar heart defect for future siblings of the affected child — B 10.4.1

A. impossible to predict
B. 3%
C. 10%
D. 15%
E. 30%

166. Which of the following is the most common congenital heart disease lesion — B 10.4.1

A. aortic stenosis
B. ventricular septal defect
C. pulmonic stenosis
D. patent ductus arteriosis
E. hypoplastic left heart

167. Which heart lesion is associated with VATER syndrome — E 10.4.2

A. atrial septal defect
B. endocardial cushion defect
C. pulmonic stenosis
D. patent ductus arteriosis
E. ventricular septal defect

168. What is the most common heart defect in patients with trisomy 21 — C 10.4.2

A. patent ductus arteriosis
B. ventricular septal defect
C. endocardial cushion defect
D. pulmonic stenosis
E. atrial septal defect

169. All of the following are forms of cyanotic congenital heart disease except — D 10.4.4

- **A.** tetralogy of Fallot
- **B.** truncus arteriosus
- **C.** transposition of the great arteries
- **D.** ventricular septal defect
- **E.** tricuspid atresia

170. A child develops a heart murmur, cyanosis, and respiratory distress on day of life #2. Emergent treatment should include which of the following agents or procedures, while awaiting cardiology consultation for definitive diagnosis — A 10.4.5

- **A.** prostaglandin E_1
- **B.** prostaglandin F_2
- **C.** atrial septostomy
- **D.** echocardiography
- **E.** epinephrine

171. What is the palliative surgical intervention for transposition of the great vessels — A 10.4.5

- **A.** Rashkind's procedure
- **B.** Blalock-Taussig shunt
- **C.** pulmonary artery banding
- **D.** Glenn shunt
- **E.** Waterston shunt

172. What is the definitive surgical procedure for treatment of transposition of the great vessels — C 10.4.6

- **A.** Fontan procedure
- **B.** Norwood procedure
- **C.** Jatene procedure
- **D.** heart transplant
- **E.** Blalock-Taussig shunt

173. Current treatment of congestive heart failure includes all of the following except — D 10.4.5

- **A.** diuretics
- **B.** albuterol
- **C.** nitroglycerine
- **D.** extremity tourniquets
- **E.** dopamine

174. An infant, delivered through thick meconium, develops tachypnea, retractions, and metabolic acidosis 12 hours after birth. Chest x-ray shows decreased pulmonary vascularity. His room air oxygen saturation is 72%. Appropriate therapy includes all of the following except — C 10.5.1

- **A.** oxygen
- **B.** mechanical ventilation
- **C.** prostaglandin E_1
- **D.** nitrous oxide
- **E.** extracorporeal membrane oxygenation

175. Which of the following conditions is the most common congenital heart disease diagnosed in adulthood — B 10.5.4

- **A.** pulmonic stenosis
- **B.** atrial septal defect
- **C.** patent ductus arteriosus
- **D.** ventricular septal defect
- **E.** subacute bacterial endocarditis

176. The Jones criteria for diagnosis of acute rheumatic fever include all of the following except — D 10.6.2

- **A.** polyarthritis
- **B.** prolonged PR interval
- **C.** chorea
- **D.** a positive throat culture
- **E.** subcutaneous nodules

177. Findings consistent with untreated coarctation of the aorta include — D 10.5.10

- **A.** small shoe size for age
- **B.** hypertension
- **C.** rib notching on chest x-ray
- **D.** all of the above
- **E.** B and C

178. Which of the following is the most common cyanotic congenital heart disease — B 10.5.12

- **A.** truncus arteriosus
- **B.** tetralogy of Fallot
- **C.** total anomalous pulmonary venous return
- **D.** tricuspid atresia
- **E.** pulmonary atresia

179. Which congenital heart disease has a characteristic "snowman" cardiac silhouette on chest x-ray — A 10.5.16

- **A.** total anomalous pulmonary venous return
- **B.** tetralogy of Fallot
- **C.** truncus arteriosus
- **D.** transposition of the great vessels

180. Which congenital heart disease has a boot shaped cardiac silhouette on chest x-ray — B 10.5.12

- **A.** total anomalous pulmonary venous return
- **B.** tetralogy of Fallot
- **C.** truncus arteriosus
- **D.** transposition of the great vessels

181. Which congenital heart disease has an "egg on a string" cardiac silhouette on chest x-ray — D 10.5.14

- **A.** total anomalous pulmonary venous return
- **B.** tetralogy of Fallot
- **C.** truncus arteriosus
- **D.** transposition of the great vessels

182. All of the following are criteria for the diagnosis of Kawasaki disease except — C 10.6.1

- **A.** palmar erythema
- **B.** rash
- **C.** fever <5 days
- **D.** cervical adenopathy
- **E.** strawberry tongue

183. Which of the following medications is contraindicated in the child with supraventricular tachycardia — C 10.7.2

- **A.** erythromycin
- **B.** adenosine
- **C.** verapamil
- **D.** digoxin
- **E.** propranolol

184. The cardiac complication associated with Kawasaki disease is E 10.6.1

- **A.** myocarditis
- **B.** coronary artery aneurysms
- **C.** acquired aortic outflow obstruction
- **D.** mitral insufficiency
- **E.** both A and B

185. Recommended therapy for Kawasaki disease is B 10.6.1

- **A.** steroids
- **B.** intravenous immunoglobulin
- **C.** observation
- **D.** antibiotics
- **E.** acetaminophen

186. A 6-month-old presents with failure to thrive, tachypnea, diaphoresis with feeds, a left lower sternal border systolic heart murmur, and hepatomegaly. Chest x-ray shows cardiomegaly. Which of the following conditions is the most likely diagnosis A 10.5.5

- **A.** ventricular septal defect
- **B.** atrial septal defect
- **C.** patent ductus arteriosis
- **D.** pulmonic stenosis
- **E.** aortic stenosis

187. What is the most common etiology for hypertension in children B 10.6.4

- **A.** congenital heart disease
- **B.** renal disease
- **C.** congenital adrenal hypoplasia
- **D.** increased salt intake
- **E.** obesity

188. Which type of heart block results in the atria and ventricles functioning independently E 10.7.1

- **A.** first degree heart block
- **B.** second degree heart block
- **C.** third degree heart block
- **D.** congenital atrioventricular block
- **E.** C and D

11 HEMATOLOGY

11.1 GENERAL CONCEPTS

11.1.1 Embryology

A. Prenatal Hematopoiesis
   1. **Hematopoiesis** is the body's system of producing blood cells. The system arises from the mesodermal layer of the embryo and is active at three weeks postconception.
   2. By two months of fetal life active hematopoiesis is present primarily in the liver. The liver continues hematopoietic activity until about two weeks after birth.
   3. By six months gestation, primary production shifts to the bone marrow.
   4. The fetal spleen, thymus, and lymph nodes also participate in hematopoiesis.

B. Postnatal Hematopoiesis
   1. In infants, the medullary spaces of most bones contain hematopoietic tissue.
   2. As childhood progresses, the marrow in long bones is replaced by fatty tissues. This "yellow" marrow can be recruited to produce blood cells if needed, but primary blood cell production in older children and adults occurs in the ribs, sternum, vertebrae, pelvis, skull, clavicles, and scapula.

11.1.2 Pathophysiology

A. Red Blood Cells (RBCs)
   1. RBC production requires pluripotential stem cells, erythropoietin stimulation, and multiple nutrients, such as iron, folate, vitamin B_{12}. An abnormality in these areas can cause an increase, or more commonly, a decrease in RBC production.
   2. Hemoglobin (Hgb) is the most important component of RBCs.
      a. This oxygen-carrying protein is crucial to tissue metabolism.
      b. Hgb is composed of four polypeptide chains bound to two heme groups which reversibly bind O_2.
      c. During fetal life, Hgb F, $\alpha_2\gamma_2$, predominates (70% at birth) and is gradually replaced by Hgb A, $\alpha_2\beta_2$, (90% by 6 to 12 months of age).
   3. RBCs extrude their nucleus during maturation, but remain metabolically active, fueled largely by glycolysis.
   4. Fetal RBCs typically survive 90 days while mature RBCs survive approximately 120 days.

B. Platelets
   1. Platelets are produced from bone marrow megakaryocytes and have a lifespan of 7 to 10 days.
   2. They work in concert with numerous serum proteins in the delicate balance of hemostasis. Any abnormalities in this balance manifest as a coagulation disorder.

11.2 DIAGNOSTIC MODALITIES

11.2.1 History

A. As with all aspects of medicine, this component is most important.

B. It should include questions about fatigue, pallor, bleeding, bruising, diet, infections, development, illnesses, and family history, particularly of bleeding disorders or gallbladder disease.

11.2.2 Physical Exam

A. Multiple physical findings may be present with abnormalities of the hematopoietic system.

B. Findings are not exclusive to hematologic abnormalities, but may give important clues for diagnosis.
   1. Anemia may be suggested by tachycardia, skin pallor with pale palmar creases and conjunctiva, and heart murmur.
      a. If tachypnea is present, the child may have congestive heart failure secondary to severe anemia.
      b. Koilonychia (spooning of the fingernails) occurs with iron deficiency.
      c. Glossitis suggests vitamin B_{12} deficiency as a cause of anemia.
   2. RBC hemolysis can present with jaundice, scleral icterus, malaise, or lethargy.
   3. Petechiae, bruising, and purpura are seen in thrombocytopenia as well as in coagulopathy.
      Another important clue is mucosal bleeding (nose and mouth).
   4. Plethora is present in patients with polycythemia.
   5. Hemoglobinopathy may have associated maxillary hyperplasia.
   6. Splenomegaly may occur in sequestration of abnormal cells in the spleen as in sickle cell disease or with extramedullary hematopoiesis as in thalassemia. It may also be present with malignancy.

11.2.3 Laboratory

A. Complete Blood Count (CBC). The CBC provides invaluable information to the examiner.
   1. Hemoglobin Concentration (Hgb) and Amount of RBCs Packed in a Given Volume of Blood (Hct). The value indicate polycythemia (higher) or anemia (lower) when compared to age appropriate norms.
   2. RBC Indexes
      a. Mean Corpuscular Volume (MCV). The average volume of RBCs.
      b. Mean Corpuscular Hgb (MCH). The weight of Hgb in average RBCs.
      c. Mean Corpuscular Hgb Concentration (MCHC). The average concentration of Hgb in a given volume of packed RBCs.
      d. Red cell Distribution Width (RDW). A measure of heterogeneity of RBC sizes.

3. Platelet count.

B. Reticulocyte Count. This is a measure of newly produced (nucleated) RBCs. The normal level is 1 to 2%. It may be elevated in hemorrhage or hemolysis.

C. Peripheral Smear. Manual observation gives invaluable information regarding morphology and color of cells.
   1. Anisocytosis means size is variable.
   2. Poikilocytosis means varied cell shapes.
   3. Acanthocytes are spiculated cells.
   4. Hypochromia is a pale appearance of cells.

D. Iron studies are useful in identifying iron deficient or overload states and include serum iron, serum ferritin (reflection of iron storage in tissues), total iron binding capacity (TIBC), and percent saturation of TIBC.

E. Free erythrocyte porphyrins (FEP) measure heme precursor.

F. Erythrocyte osmotic fragility test identifies increased fragility of incubated RBCs.

G. Hgb electrophoresis allows quantitative determination of Hgb variants.

H. Bone marrow aspirate and biopsy permits assessment of cellularity, distribution, and maturation of cells, including abnormal cells.

I. Tests for coagulopathy
   1. Prothrombin time (PT) reflects the function of factors II, V, VII, and X.
   2. Partial thromboplastin time (PTT) reflects the function of factors VIII, IX, XI, and XII.
   3. Mixing Study. Normal plasma is added to patients plasma. If repeat PTT normalizes, a deficiency state is present.
   4. Bleeding time allows assessment of vascular and platelet function. Normal is 4 to 8 minutes.
   5. Levels of individual coagulation factors can be assayed.

11.2.4 Interpretation of Laboratory Studies in Anemia

A. RBC Morphology and Indexes
   1. Microcytic, Hypochromic Anemia
      a. Low FEP is seen in thalassemia.
      b. High FEP with high or normal ferritin can be seen in lead poisoning, chronic disease, pyridoxine deficiency, and sideroblastic anemia. If ferritin is low consider iron deficiency.
   2. Macrocytic, normochromic anemia is seen with Megaloblastic anemia (folate, vitamin B_{12} deficiency), aplastic or hypoplastic anemia, Fanconi's anemia, hypothyroidism, congenital dyserythropoietic anemia, and hepatic disease.
   3. Normocytic, Normochromic Anemia (Low Reticulocyte Count)
      a. If the platelet count is low consider leukemia, metastatic tumor to the bone marrow, aplastic anemia, and lipid storage disease.
      b. If the platelet count is high or normal, consider renal disease, infection, inflammation, chronic disease, hypothyroidism, Diamond-Blackfan anemia, transient erythroblastopenia, congenital dyserythropoietic anemia, and protein malnutrition.
   4. Normocytic, Normochromic Anemia (High Reticulocyte Count)
      a. If the indirect bilirubin is normal, blood loss is the most likely cause.
      b. If the indirect bilirubin is high and the Coombs' testing is positive, autoimmune hemolytic anemia, isoimmune hemolytic anemia (Rh or ABO incompatibility), and incompatible transfusion are possible etiologies.
      c. If Coombs' testing is negative and fragmented cells are present on the peripheral blood smear, consider hemolytic-uremic syndrome or disseminated intravascular coagulation.
      d. If fragmented cells are absent, perform osmotic fragility testing. If abnormal, spherocytosis, stomatocytosis, elliptocytosis, and vitamin E deficiency are diagnostic possibilities.
      e. If fragility testing is normal perform Hgb electrophoresis. Abnormal electrophoresis will reveal sickle cell disease, Hgb SC disease, or Hgb S-β-thalassemia.
      f. Normal electrophoresis with normal fragility and a negative Coombs' test suggests glucose-6-phosphate dehydrogenase deficiency, pyruvate kinase deficiency, elliptocytosis, or stomatocytosis.

11.3 Disease Profiles

11.3.1 Pancytopenias

A. Aplasia of the bone marrow or acquired damage to its hematopoietic elements results in profound depression of all the formed elements of blood. Clinically the consequences of thrombocytopenia and neutropenia are most striking, but anemia occurs as well.

B. Constitutional Aplastic Pancytopenia (Fanconi's Syndrome)
   1. Fanconi's syndrome is an autosomal recessive disorder with variable penetrance associated with chromosomal fragility in all cells of the body including the hematopoietic system.
   2. Two thirds of affected patients have associated anomalies such as absence of radii and thumbs, short stature, hyperpigmentation of the skin, or cardiac and renal abnormalities.
   3. Onset of pancytopenia occurs on average at 6 to 8 years of age.
   4. Laboratory testing reveals severe pancytopenia, macrocytic RBCs, bone marrow hypocellularity, an increase of Hgb F, to 5 to 15%, and 10 to 70% ab-

normal chromosome configurations (normally, changes seen are <10%).

5. Bone marrow transplantation is definitive therapy, however, many patients exhibit improvement with androgenic steroids. Supportive care with platelet and RBC transfusions and antibiotics is critical.

C. Acquired Pancytopenia
   1. Multiple etiologies have been documented for acquired pancytopenia including:
      a. Replacement of normal marrow by other tissue (neuroblastoma, acute lymphoblastic leukemia).
      b. Infectious agents (parvovirus, hepatitis).
      c. Antibiotic exposure (chloramphenicol, sulfonamides).
      d. Chemical exposure (benzene).
      e. Malignancy therapy (methotrexate, 6-mercaptopurine, ionizing radiation).
      f. In about 50% of cases, no etiologic agent is identified and the pancytopenia is termed idiopathic.
   2. Children typically present with hemorrhage secondary to thrombocytopenia. They may have features of an underlying malignancy. Anemia and infection become apparent later.
   3. Laboratory testing shows severe pancytopenia and a normal chromosome configuration.
   4. Treatment
      a. Bone marrow transplantation is the treatment of choice.
      b. Some success with immunotherapy (antithymocyte globulin, dexamethasone, cyclosporin) has been reported.
      c. Supportive care with platelet and RBC transfusions, and antibiotics is usually necessary.
   5. The prognosis is poor. Unfortunately about two thirds of patients die within six months of diagnosis.

11.3.2 Anemia

A. Anemia is defined as the reduction of the Hgb or hematocrit (Hct) below two standard deviations of the mean. Anemia is not a disease itself, but a symptom of an underlying problem.
   1. It is important to recognize that normal values vary with age.
   2. As a general rule, physiologic disturbances are minor until Hgb falls below 7 to 8 g/dL. Physiologic adjustments to anemia include tachycardia, increased cardiac output, and a shift of the oxygen-dissociation curve to the right, providing more efficient transfer of oxygen to the tissues.
   3. Manifestations such as pallor and fatigue may be subtle if the onset of anemia is gradual. Symptoms may progress to cardiac dilatation and congestive heart failure if not treated appropriately.
   4. Clinically anemias are classified according to morphologic appearance of the RBC and MCV (hypochromic microcytic, macrocytic, normochromic normocytic) as discussed in section 11.2.4.
   5. Anemia arises from decreased production of RBCs or increased destruction of RBCs.

B. **Congenital Pure RBC Anemia (Diamond-Blackfan syndrome)**
   1. This is an isolated deficiency of RBC precursors in bone marrow with a presumed genetic basis suggested by familial occurrences.
   2. About half of affected infants appear pale in the first week of life and profound anemia is evident by 2 to 6 months of age. Occasionally it is associated with phenotypic abnormalities such as triphalangeal thumbs and Turner's syndrome.
   3. Laboratory testing reveals macrocytic, normochromic anemia, low reticulocyte count, increased serum erythropoietin, increased Hgb F, increased serum iron, decreased TIBC, and markedly reduced RBC precursors on bone marrow examination.
   4. Over half of patients respond to corticosteroid therapy. Those who do not respond may require blood transfusions at 4 to 8 week intervals.
   5. Long-term complications from corticosteroid therapy and hemosiderosis secondary to multiple RBC transfusions are quite problematic. These complications include growth retardation, delayed puberty, diabetes mellitus, hepatosplenomegaly, secondary thrombocytopenia, congestive heart failure, and often death.
   6. Aggressive iron chelation therapy and attempts at corticosteroid weaning optimize care.
   7. Spontaneous remission may occur.

C. **Transient Erythroblastopenia of Childhood** (TEC)
   1. This severe reversible anemia is of unknown etiology, but likely has an autoimmune basis with serum inhibitors directed at erythroid stem cells.
   2. TEC presents as a slow, insidious development of anemia in previously normal child between 6 months and 5 years of age.
   3. Laboratory findings include normochromic normocytic anemia, decreased reticulocytes, increased serum iron and iron saturation, and normal Hgb F.
   4. Transfusions may be necessary to prevent severe anemia from causing cardiac decompensation. Typically, no treatment is required and spontaneous recovery occurs in 2 to 4 weeks.

D. **Acquired Pure RBC Anemias**
   1. Multiple etiologies can create isolated reduced RBC precursors, including erythropoietin inhibiting antibodies, erythroblast antibodies, inhibitors of heme synthesis, viral infections, and an ill-defined association with thymomas.
   2. Clinical features are dependent on etiology, but typically have slow onset of anemia. If the child also has an underlying hemolytic anemia causing de-

creased mature RBC survival time, they may experience a dramatic aplastic crisis.

3. Laboratory testing demonstrates a normochromic, normocytic anemia, decreased reticulocytes, increased serum iron, and reduction in RBC precursors on bone marrow exam.
4. Treatment depends on the etiology and may require supportive RBC transfusions, thymoma resection, or immunosuppressive medications.
5. Prognosis is also dependent on etiology, with spontaneous recovery in two weeks if the anemia is secondary to viral infections.

E. Anemia of Chronic Disease

1. This condition occurs as a complication of chronic systemic diseases associated with infection, inflammation, or tissue breakdown.
   a. RBC life span is moderately decreased secondary to increased RBC destruction by the reticuloendothelial system.
   b. There is relative failure of the bone marrow response reflecting both hypoactive marrow and inadequate erythropoietin production.
   c. Abnormalities of iron metabolism may worsen the anemia.
2. Few symptoms of mild to moderate anemia occur with the important features attributable to the underlying disease (systemic lupus erythematosus, juvenile rheumatoid arthritis, renal diseases, osteomyelitis, ulcerative colitis).
3. Laboratory findings include normochromic, normocytic anemia (Hgb 6 to 9 g/dL), occasionally hypochromic, microcytic anemia secondary to abnormal iron metabolism, decreased or normal reticulocyte count, increased FEP, decreased serum iron, increased ferritin (acute phase reactant), and normal TIBC.
4. Treatment is by management of the underlying disease.

F. Physiologic Anemia of Infancy

1. "Anemia" is a misnomer as events leading to low Hgb are normal physiologic adaptations to extrauterine life. Full-term infants experience a drop in Hgb to about 9 g/dL at 6 to 8 weeks of age.
2. Multiple adaptations create this effect.
   a. Newborns are relatively polycythemic secondary to erythropoietin stimulation from low intrauterine oxygen levels.
   b. At birth, the partial alveolar pressure of oxygen (P_aO_2) dramatically increases and erythropoietin production ceases. Decreased hematopoiesis therefore contributes to "anemia."
   c. Erythropoietin production is restimulated as Hgb falls.
   d. Other contributing factors are the relatively short life span of fetal RBCs and the dramatic increase in blood volume during the first 2 months of life.
3. Infants are asymptomatic unless other processes aggravating anemia are present, such as blood loss, hemolysis, or nutritional deficits.
4. No treatment is required.

G. Folic Acid Deficiency (Megaloblastic Bone Marrow)

1. Folic acid deficiency impairs deoxyribonucleic acid synthesis. Ribonucleic acid synthesis is less affected allowing cytoplasmic maturation to progress which accounts for the macrocytic appearance of RBCs.
2. Folic acid deficiency can arise for multiple reasons including inadequate intake (infants fed goat's milk), increased demand (pregnancy, malignancies, chronic hemolysis), impaired absorption (Crohn's disease, celiac disease), and abnormal metabolism due to drug use (sulfamethoxazole and trimethoprim, pyrimethamine, phenytoin, methotrexate, oral contraceptives).
3. Anemia appears 3 to 6 months after the onset of deficiency. It may manifest with failure to thrive, irritability, or chronic diarrhea.
4. Laboratory findings show macrocytic anemia, hypersegmented neutrophil nuclei, serum folic acid level of 3 ng/ml (normal 5 to 20 ng/ml), RBC folate level <150 ng/ml (normal 150 to 600 ng/ml), and an increased lactate dehydrogenase level.
5. Treat the underlying condition. Folic acid supplementation produces a hematologic response within 72 hours. Transfusions are rarely required.

H. Vitamin B_{12} Deficiency (Megaloblastic Bone Marrow)

1. Vitamin B_{12} deficiency impairs deoxyribonucleic acid synthesis leading to a macrocytic anemia.
2. Deficiency occurs with inadequate intake or abnormal absorption. Dietary deficiency is rare, but can occur in the breast-fed infant of a strict vegetarian. Absorption problems are much more common given the complex nature of vitamin B_{12} metabolism.
3. Vitamin B_{12} Function
   a. Vitamin B_{12} must bind with intrinsic factor produced by gastric parietal cells. This complex then must reach the terminal ileum where calcium is required for its site-specific absorption. Transcobalamin is then necessary to transport vitamin B_{12} in the plasma.
   b. Abnormalities in this sequence can create a deficiency. Examples include absence of intrinsic factor (juvenile pernicious anemia), gastric mucosal atrophy or achlorhydria, abnormal terminal ileum (regional enteritis, tuberculosis), absent terminal ileum (surgical resection), competition for vitamin absorption (bacterial overgrowth, tapeworm *Diphyllobothrium latum* infestation), and intestinal absorption defect (Imerslund syndrome).

4. Onset of anemia occurs at 9 months to 10 years of age as body stores are depleted. It may present with diarrhea, irritability, anorexia, listlessness, or neurologic manifestations such as ataxia, paresthesias, hyperreflexia, clonus, and Babinski's sign. The classic finding of a smooth, red, painful tongue is noted on exam.
5. Laboratory examination demonstrates macrocytic anemia, hypersegmented neutrophil nuclei, serum vitamin B_{12} level <100 pg/ml, elevated lactate dehydrogenase level, increased urinary excretion of methylmalonic acid, and an abnormal Schilling's test (evaluates intestinal vitamin B_{12} absorption).
6. Vitamin B_{12} supplementation is definitive therapy with a monthly maintenance dose of 1 mg given intramuscularly. If neurologic involvement is present, 1 mg intramuscularly, given daily for two weeks is necessary. If transcobalamin deficiency is present, massive parenteral doses of vitamin B_{12} are required.

I. Orotic Aciduria (Megaloblastic Bone Marrow)

1. Orotic aciduria is an autosomal recessive deficiency of orotate phosphoribosyl transferase or orotidine-5-phosphate decarboxylase. These enzymes are essential in the production of pyrimidines without which deoxyribonucleic acid and ribonucleic acid synthesis is impaired. Abnormality is present in all cells, but most dramatic in the hematopoietic system.
2. Failure to thrive and developmental delay are frequently noted, along with symptoms of anemia.
3. Laboratory findings are macrocytic anemia, neutropenia, and orotic acid crystals in urine.
4. Administration of pyrimidine precursors, found beyond the metabolic pathway block, normalizes RBC production.

J. Iron Deficiency

1. Iron is necessary for Hgb synthesis, and in its absence, a dramatic anemia can ensue.
2. Deficiency can occur with blood loss or insufficient dietary intake.
   a. Blood loss can occur at any age and for any reason, but commonly occurs during infancy from the gastrointestinal tract secondary to cow's milk protein intolerance.
   b. Dietary insufficiency often occurs in infancy if milk or cereals without iron fortification are ingested.
   c. The propensity for infants to develop a deficiency is related to the precarious balance of iron metabolism in the first months of life.
3. In the normal newborn, iron stores are sufficient for blood formation for the first 6 to 9 months. Thereafter, a diet of 8 to 15 mg/day of iron is required because only 10% of ingested iron is absorbed. If an infant's body store of iron is low (secondary to prematurity or hemorrhage) or if iron-fortified foods are not offered, a child is at risk for anemia.
4. Iron deficiency anemia often has an insidious presentation, pallor being the most important clue. Irritability and anorexia are present in severe cases.
5. Laboratory findings demonstrate hypochromic, microcytic anemia, decreased serum ferritin (<10 ng/ml), decreased serum iron (<30 mcg/dL), increased TIBC (>350 mcg/dL), decreased % saturation TIBC (<15%), increased FEP (>50 mcg/dL), normal or slightly increased reticulocyte count, and guaiac positive stool (1/3 of cases).
6. Oral administration of elemental iron, 6 mg/kg/day in three divided doses, produces a responsive reticulocytosis within 72 hours. Iron replacement should be continued at least 6 weeks after the RBC count has normalized in order to replace body stores. Equally important is attention to the underlying etiology.

K. Sideroblastic Anemia

1. Ill-defined abnormalities in iron or heme metabolism inhibit Hgb synthesis, creating anemia. Iron accumulates in mitochondria of erythroid precursors creating the typical appearance of RBCs with a perinuclear collar of hemosiderin granules, termed a ringed sideroblast. Sideroblastic anemia an be X-linked recessive or acquired.
2. The inherited trait is symptomatic by late childhood and splenomegaly is a common finding. The acquired disorder presents in alcoholics or adults with inflammatory or malignant processes.
3. Laboratory findings include hypochromic, microcytic anemia, increased serum iron, normal or increased FEP, RBC stippling, and ringed sideroblasts on bone marrow exam.
4. Some cases are responsive to pyridoxine (vitamin B_6) therapy in doses of 200 to 500 mg/day. No other findings of pyridoxine deficiency are observed in these patients.

L. Lead Poisoning

1. Environmental exposure to lead can be toxic to the central nervous system, renal and hematopoietic systems. Severity of toxicity is directly related to the level of lead absorption.
2. The hematopoietic system is affected by lead's inhibition of two enzymes (ferrochelatase and porphobilinogen) necessary in the pathway of heme synthesis. This inhibition creates elevations of aminolevulinic acid and FEP along the metabolic pathway which are utilized in diagnosis.
3. The most significant source of environmental lead is household dust and dirt, because substantial reductions of lead in food, air, and drinking water have

been mandated.

4. Symptoms are generally nonspecific, but occur most frequently in toddlers. Neurologic manifestations such as seizures, behavior problems, mental retardation, irritability, and acute encephalopathy are possible. In addition, recurrent episodes of vomiting, abdominal pain, and constipation herald gastrointestinal involvement.
5. Laboratory findings include hypochromic, microcytic anemia, venous lead level >10 mcg/dL, increased FEP, increased plasma and urine aminolevulinic acid, increased reticulocytes, and basophilic stippling on the peripheral smear. Cerebrospinal fluid studies show pleocytosis, increased protein, and increased opening pressure in cases of toxic encephalopathy.
6. Treatment
   a. Chelation therapy is indicated for children with significantly elevated lead levels. The exact level warranting medical intervention is controversial, but generally is considered to be >25 mcg/dL. Agents such as ethylenediaminetetraacetic acid (EDTA), 2,3-dimercaptosuccinic acid (DMSA), and dimercaprol (BAL) can be utilized.
   b. Close follow-up is mandatory because serum lead levels can rebound into the toxic range as chronic lead deposited in the bones is leached into the soft tissues after treatment.
   c. A complete evaluation of the child's environment is required in order to eliminate additional exposure.

M. Hereditary Spherocytosis

1. Spherocytosis is an autosomal dominant condition with 25% of cases caused by sporadic new mutations.
2. Pathophysiology
   a. Spectrin, a structural protein, is defective. Without this protein support structure, the cell loses its biconcave disc shape and becomes spherical.
   b. The spherical shape makes the RBC less deformable when passing through small vasculature and consequently is often trapped in the splenic sinusoids where hemolysis occurs.
   c. The RBC membrane is excessively permeable to sodium. This creates a metabolic crisis because more adenosine triphosphate is needed to drive the cation pump and maintain the normal electrical gradient. The spleen is a metabolic trap for the RBC. The necessary oxygen and glucose for adenosine triphosphate production are low, leading to hemolysis of defective cells.
3. Clinical Features (Varies with Age)
   a. Newborns often have severe anemia and jaundice.
   b. Older children present with pallor and splenomegaly.
   c. Adolescents often present with pigmented gallstone cholecystitis secondary to chronic hemolysis.
   d. Occasionally in the face of a superseding viral infection (parvovirus), patients may present with aplastic crisis as the bone marrow is unable to maintain its accelerated replenishment of destroyed RBCs.
4. Laboratory findings include normochromic, normocytic anemia, spherocytes, elevated MCHC, reticulocytosis (5 to 20%), unconjugated hyperbilirubinemia, and osmotic fragility.
5. Treatment
   a. Supportive care with transfusions as needed and careful attention to increased bone marrow nutrient needs such as folate and iron.
   b. Splenectomy is the definitive treatment but usually is deferred until 6 years of age. Splenectomy reduces RBC destruction and the associated complications, but RBC spherocytes remain.
   c. Pneumococcal vaccination to allow development of immunity prior to splenectomy is the standard of care.

N. Hereditary Elliptocytosis

1. This is an autosomal dominant condition with abnormal spectrin dimer interactions creating elliptical-shaped RBCs. It is generally benign except when spherocytes are also present, creating a moderate chronic hemolysis. The elliptocytosis gene is linked with the Rh locus.
2. Clinical features are variable with only about 10% of patients experiencing ongoing hemolysis. Features such as neonatal jaundice, splenomegaly, cholelithiasis, and medullary expansion of bones may be present.
3. Laboratory findings include normochromic, normocytic anemia, elliptocytes and poikilocytes on the peripheral smear, increased reticulocyte count, and unconjugated hyperbilirubinemia.
4. Asymptomatic patients require no intervention, however those with ongoing hemolysis benefit from pneumococcal immunization followed by splenectomy at 6 years of age.

O. Paroxysmal Nocturnal Hemoglobinuria

1. Ill defined inciting etiology, but mechanism is related to an acquired deficiency of decay accelerating factor. This factor normally is present in the RBC membrane. In its absence, the alternative complement pathway is triggered by C3b causing intravascular hemolysis.
   a. Episodes of hemolysis often occur at night, pre-

sumably when the serum partial pressure of CO_2 rises and the pH falls.

b. Chronic leukopenia, thrombocytopenia, and aplastic pancytopenia may be present.

2. Clinical Features
   a. Nocturnal and morning hemoglobinuria is the classic feature often accompanied by abdominal, back, and head pain.
   b. Serious complications such as thrombosis, thromboembolic phenomenon, or pyogenic infections may also be initial manifestations.
3. Laboratory findings include nocturnal hemoglobinuria, positive Ham test (increased lysis in acidified serum), positive sucrose lysis test (increased lysis in isotonic low ionic strength solutions), decreased decay accelerating factor, and decreased RBC acetylcholinesterase activity.
4. Treatment
   a. Supportive care with transfusions as needed.
   b. Iron supplementation is often needed due to its excessive loss in the urine.
   c. Patients with thromboses may benefit from anticoagulation therapy.
   d. Splenectomy is not useful because the hemolysis is intravascular. Bone marrow transplantation has been utilized with some success.

P. Stomatocytosis

1. This is a rare hereditary condition with extreme RBC membrane permeability to cations (sodium) and resulting hemolytic anemia. A similar abnormality may be acquired with other conditions such as liver disease.
2. Clinical features are generally mild, but occasionally patients can have severe hemolysis and subsequent anemia and jaundice.
3. Laboratory studies reveal swollen cup-shaped RBCs with central slit or stoma on the peripheral smear.
4. Splenectomy may be palliative but not curative in the patient with severe hemolysis.

Q. Pyruvate Kinase Deficiency

1. This is an autosomal recessive decrease in RBC pyruvate kinase content or activity.
2. Pathophysiology
   a. Pyruvate kinase catalyzes the final step in the glycolytic pathway leading to eventual adenosine triphosphate production.
   b. Adenosine triphosphate production is inadequate to operate the cation pump essential to maintain normal cellular Na^+ and K^+ balance. Intracellular K^+ is lost and Na^+ accumulates. As a result the RBC lifespan is markedly reduced.
3. Clinical Features
   a. Variable presentations exist ranging from severe neonatal hemolysis with anemia, jaundice, and possibly kernicterus, to a mild well-compensated hemolysis noted first in adulthood.
   b. Pallor and splenomegaly are usually present.
   c. The midwestern Amish have a high incidence of severe hemolytic disease.
4. Laboratory findings include decreased RBC pyruvate kinase activity, reticulocytosis, and unconjugated hyperbilirubinemia.
5. Treatment
   a. Supportive care with RBC transfusions as needed.
   b. Recurrent hemolytic episodes may require splenectomy after 6 years of age. The reticulocyte count often paradoxically increases further after splenectomy due to their prolonged survival in the circulation.

R. Glucose-6-Phosphate Dehydrogenase (G6PD) Deficiency

1. This is an X-linked recessive disease with over 100 variants identified. The normal enzyme is designated G6PD B^+ with two primary variants identified as G6PD A^- found in African Americans and G6PD B^- found in Mediterranean and Oriental ethnic groups.
2. Pathophysiology
   a. G6PD is an enzyme of the pentose phosphate pathway. This pathway functions to produce the reduced form of nicotinamide-adenine dinucleotide phosphate (NADPH) which is necessary in the conversion of glutathione from the oxidized to reduced state.
   b. Reduced glutathione is essential for the inactivation of any oxidant compound in the RBC. Oxidant compounds cause heme and globin chains to dissociate by oxidation of sulfhydryl groups. The denatured globin then precipitates as a Heinz body which in turn damages the RBC membrane.
   c. A deficiency of G6PD thus leads to accelerated splenic removal and intravascular lysis of RBCs.
3. Clinical Features
   a. Patients typically present with a drug-induced episodic hemolytic anemia. Common inciting drugs are sulfonamides, antipyretics, napthaquinolones, and antimalarials such as primaquine.
   b. Other oxidative agents may also trigger the hemolysis such as infection or ingestion of fava beans, a Mediterranean dietary staple.
   c. The degree of hemolysis varies with the inciting agent, the amount ingested, and the severity of the enzyme deficiency. Most will present 48 to 72 hours after exposure but the B^- variant will experience a more severe course while the A^- variant will commonly have self-limited hemolysis.

   d. Presentation can also occur with neonatal hyperbilirubinemia in the absence of known exposures.
4. Laboratory findings include normochromic, normocytic anemia, hemoglobinuria, and unconjugated hyperbilirubinemia, G6PD activity <10% of normal, and Heinz bodies on the peripheral smear.
5. Spontaneous recovery occurs but supportive transfusions are sometimes needed. Identification of patients with this common deficiency and prevention of oxidant exposures is optimal management.

S. **Hemolytic Disease of the Newborn**
1. Pathophysiology
   a. Hemolysis occurs with transplacental passage of maternal antibody active against RBC antigens of the infant. The D antigen of the Rh group and ABO blood type antigens are most frequently involved.
   b. Rh incompatibility arises when an Rh negative mother is exposed to an Rh positive infant. A brisk maternal immunoglobulin G (IgG) response ensues after only 1 ml of Rh positive blood exposure. This IgG in turn crosses the placenta and may cause catastrophic in utero hemolysis and hydrops fetalis.
   c. ABO incompatibility typically occurs when a B positive or more commonly A positive infant is born to an O positive mother. Maternal anti-A or anti-B antibody creates mild to moderate hemolysis in the infant. These antibodies are usually immunoglobulin M (IgM) and cannot cross the placenta, but may be present in small IgG fractions which explains the milder clinical course.
2. Clinical Features
   a. Infants with Rh incompatibility typically have severe hemolysis and subsequent multiple organ system dysfunction including the cardiac, pulmonary, and hepatic systems. The severity of involvement is dependent on the immune response by the mother.
   b. Infants with ABO incompatibility generally develop jaundice in the first 24 hours of life, but rarely experience significant complications.
3. Laboratory findings include a Coombs' positive normochromic, normocytic anemia, maternal-infant blood antigen incompatibility (Rh or ABO), unconjugated hyperbilirubinemia, and reticulocytosis.
4. Treatment
   a. Infants with ABO incompatibility require management of hyperbilirubinemia with phototherapy, and rarely, exchange transfusions.
   b. Infants with Rh incompatibility require intensive multisystem support including management of hyperbilirubinemia.
   c. Due to its devastating effects, Rh incompatibility is best managed by prevention. Administration of anti-D globulin (RhoGAM) at 28 weeks gestation and again at birth to Rh negative mothers is very effective.

T. **Autoimmune Hemolytic Anemia**
1. This condition is due to the production of abnormal IgG or IgM antibodies directed against RBCs resulting in hemolysis.
2. Pathophysiology
   a. IgG antibodies are known as warm-reactive because they are maximally reactive at 37° C. They coat RBCs but do not activate the complement cascade. RBCs are consequently destroyed by the reticuloendothelial system.
   b. IgM antibodies are known as cold-reactive because they are maximally reactive at colder temperatures. They can activate the complement system so hemolysis occurs intravascularly.
   c. The abnormal production of these antibodies is incompletely understood, but often accompanies viral infections, drug exposure, lymphomas, or autoimmune disorders such as systemic lupus erythematosus in the case of IgG. Abnormal IgM antibodies often accompany mycoplasma and Epstein-Barr virus infections.
3. Clinical features vary according to the associated disease.
   a. Children with viral infections experience acute illness with pallor, fever, jaundice, hemoglobinuria, and splenomegaly.
   b. Patients with autoimmune disorders may experience a prolonged chronic hemolysis.
4. Laboratory findings include Coombs' positive normochromic, normocytic anemia, unconjugated hyperbilirubinemia, reticulocytosis, and positive IgM cold agglutination.
5. Treatment
   a. Supportive care and transfusions as needed.
   b. Some patients will respond to immunosuppressive doses of prednisone (2.5 to 6 mg/kg/day) which can be slowly tapered.
   c. Most cases are self-limited, but some require splenectomy and additional immunosuppressive therapies.

11.3.3 Hemoglobinopathies

A. Structural abnormalities of Hgb as a result of molecular defects in the globin gene deoxyribonucleic acid are classified as hemoglobinopathies. These defects can effect single amino acids in the polypeptide structure or delete an entire globin gene. Two distinct defects can be found in the same person.

B. **Sickle Cell Disease** (Homozygous Hgb S)
1. Sickle cell disease is the result of a homozygous defect on chromosome 11 encoding for valine in-

stead of glutamic acid at the 6th position of β chains. It is most common in African Americans.

2. Pathogenesis
   a. When this Hgb is deoxygenated, a solubility problem arises because molecular polymers form and aggregate into rigid crystal-like rods. This in turn distorts the RBC into a sickle shape.
   b. These sickled RBCs are subsequently destroyed prematurely causing anemia.
   c. Their unusual shape leads to microvasculature sludging and possible obstruction. Tissue infarction follows and can occur in any organ.
3. Clinical Features
   a. Newborns are asymptomatic because they have a preponderance of Hgb F. As Hgb F levels fall and abnormal Hgb S levels rise, symptoms occur at 4 to 6 months of age.
   b. Avascular necrosis in the small bones of the hands and feet causing painful swelling called dactylitis is often the first manifestation.
   c. Acute painful episodes termed vasoocclusive crises with head, chest, back, abdominal, and extremity pain become a chronic recurrent event. Crisis occurs when hypoxia, acidosis, or infection creates increased sickling.
   d. Complications such as cerebrovascular strokes, pulmonary infarctions, splenic sequestration, renal concentrating defects, priapism, aplastic anemia, and overwhelming sepsis with encapsulated bacteria secondary to splenic dysfunction can occur.
4. Laboratory findings include normochromic, normocytic anemia, reticulocytosis, unconjugated hyperbilirubinemia, sickle cells and poikilocytes on peripheral smear, and an abnormal Hgb electrophoresis (Hgb S 80 to 95%, Hgb F 2 to 20%).
5. Treatment. Management is directed toward prevention of the multiple complications associated with sickle cell disease.
   a. Daily antibiotic prophylaxis, complete immunizations including pneumococcal vaccination, and parental education about the potential seriousness of fever are important in minimizing morbidity and mortality.
   b. Febrile patients should be examined, blood cultures obtained, and intravenous or intramuscular antibiotics administered until sepsis is ruled out.
   c. Vasoocclusive episode prevention involves avoidance of dehydration, hypoxia, and acidosis.
6. Treatment includes hydration, analgesics, and occasionally, RBC transfusions. Bone marrow transplant is curative.

C. **Sickle Cell Trait** (Heterozygous Hgb S)

1. Sickle cell trait is due to heterozygous expression of abnormal sickle Hgb encoded on chromosome 11. Because normal Hgb A is also expressed, sickling occurs only with significant hypoxic stress. sickle cell trait confers a genetic advantage because the RBCs exhibit resistance to malarial parasite invasion. Consequently this gene is frequently found in areas endemic for *Plasmodium falciparum* malaria.
2. Clinical Features
   a. Patients are generally asymptomatic, however vasoocclusive events may occur with severe hypoxia.
   b. Adolescents often will have urinary frequency secondary to a renal concentrating defect or painless hematuria.
   c. About 10% of African Americans are affected.
3. Laboratory findings include normal hematologic valves and abnormal Hgb electrophoresis (Hgb A 52 to 65%, Hgb S 32 to 45%).
4. No intervention is required unless rare vasoocclusive events occur.

D. **Hgb C Disorders** (Hgb CC, Hgb AC, Hgb SC)

1. This condition results from an abnormal β-globin gene on chromosome 11 encoding for a lysine instead of glutamic acid at the 6th position.
2. The most common presentations are homozygous HgB CC, heterozygous HgB AC, and HgB C plus Hgb S (HgB SC) disease.
3. Manifestations are dependent on the degree of expression and presence of any other abnormal globin genes.
   a. Hgb CC disease is present in 1 in 10,000 African Americans and manifests with signs of moderate hemolytic anemia and splenomegaly.
   b. Hgb AC disease is present in 3% of African Americans and is asymptomatic.
   c. Hgb SC manifests with painful episodes and other vasoocclusive symptoms much like sickle cell disease although the clinical course is usually not as severe. Hgb C participates in the molecular polymerization of deoxygenated Hgb S creating rigid rods which effectively sickle RBCs. Bone infarctions are frequent complications.
4. Laboratory Findings
   a. Hgb CC shows normochromic, normocytic anemia, target cells, spherocytes, and reticulocytosis.
   b. Hgb AC shows normal hematologic parameters with target cells on the smear.
   c. Hgb SC has a normochromic, normocytic anemia, sickle cells, target cells, reticulocytosis, and an abnormal Hgb electrophoresis (Hgb S 45 to 50%, Hgb C 45 to 50%, Hgb F 2 to 5%).

5. Supportive care is given as needed. The management of Hgb SC disease is identical to that of sickle cell anemia.

E. β-thalassemias

1. Abnormalities in transcription of messenger ribonucleic acid from the β-globin genes on chromosome 11 are the most common causes of β-thalassemias.
   a. A β° mutation denotes complete absence of production and a β^{+} mutation denotes decreased production of β chains. These mutations can occur on both chromosomes (homozygous), on one chromosome (heterozygous), or in combination with other globin chain abnormalities.
   b. When β chains are deficient, normal Hgb A cannot be produced, leading to a compensatory increases in Hgb F and Hgb A_2. When the compensatory mechanism is overwhelmed, varying stages of anemia can result.
   c. Excess α chains precipitate in RBCs as α_4 tetramers and contribute to anemia due to hemolysis.
   d. Thalassemia is often found in African or Mediterranean descendants because the abnormality is protective against *Plasmodium falciparum* malaria.
2. Clinical features are dependent on the genetic abnormality.
   a. β^{m}/β^{m} (Cooley's anemia) is complete absence of β chain production. These children present at 6 to 12 months with severe progressive anemia and hepatosplenomegaly. Compensatory extramedullary hematopoiesis creates characteristic facies with frontal bossing, maxillary hypertrophy, and an overbite. Due to hemolytic jaundice and consequent hemosiderosis, skin is often a green-brown color.
   b. β^{+}/β^{+} (thalassemia intermedia) is a marked decrease in β chain production allowing some Hgb A to be produced. The anemia is slightly less severe than Cooley's anemia, but still significant. Physical findings are very similar.
   c. β/β^{m} (β-thalassemia minor) involves production of normal β-globin chains, but only from one chromosome. Consequently a mild anemia occurs with splenomegaly and jaundice.
   d. β/β^{+} (β-thalassemia trait) is generally asymptomatic.
3. Laboratory findings include hypochromic, microcytic anemia (variable), poikilocytosis, anisocytosis, normoblasts and intracellular inclusions on the peripheral smear, unconjugated hyperbilirubinemia, increased serum iron, saturation of TIBC, increased lactate dehydrogenase level, and abnormal Hgb electrophoresis (increased Hgb F [>90% in Cooley's anemia], increased Hgb A_2, absent or decreased Hgb A).
4. Treatment
   a. Patients with $\beta^{\circ}/\beta^{\circ}$-thalassemia require repeat transfusions every 4 to 5 weeks. This chronic iron load, in addition to hyperabsorption of dietary iron, leads to hemosiderosis. To minimize cardiac, hepatic, pancreatic, and gonad complications, chelation therapy with desferrioxamine is utilized.
   b. Splenectomy is often required.
   c. Bone marrow transplantation is the definitive treatment.
   d. Less severe forms of thalassemia are not transfusion dependent.
   e. β/β°-thalassemia must be carefully distinguished from iron deficiency anemia to avoid inappropriate iron therapy.

F. α-thalassemias

1. Deletions of α-globin genes on chromosome 16 are the most common causes of α-thalassemias.
   a. Four genes are present with four forms of thalassemia identified.
   b. α chains are required for Hgb A, Hgb A_2, and Hgb F therefore production of these normal Hgbs are affected to varying degrees.
   c. Excess β chains form tetramers known as Hgb H, which is very unstable.
   d. Excess γ chains (part of Hgb F) form tetramers known as Bart's Hgb. Bart's Hgb has an extremely high oxygen affinity, therefore tissue oxygenation is severely impaired.
   e. Genetic defects are found commonly in areas endemic for *Plasmodium falciparum* malaria (Africa and Southeast Asia).
2. Clinical features are dependent on the specific genetic abnormality.
   a. α-thalassemia major is a deletion of all 4 α genes. Bart's Hgb predominates. It is incompatible with life with most affected patients dying in utero with hydrops fetalis.
   b. a-thalassemia intermedia is a deletion of 3 a genes. Hgb H comprises 4 to 20% of childhood. Patients have lifelong moderate to severe anemia with hemolysis, splenomegaly and cholecystitis.
   c. α-thalassemia minor is a deletion of 2 α genes. It presents as a mild anemia which is commonly confused with iron deficiency anemia.
   d. α-thalassemia carrier is a deletion of 1 α gene with no abnormal clinical manifestations.
3. Laboratory findings include hypochromic, microcytic anemia (variable), unconjugated hyperbilirubinemia, intracellular inclusions (unstable Hgb), and Bart's Hgb and/or Hgb H on Hgb electrophoresis.

4. Treatment is with supportive care including transfusions, splenectomy, and infection precautions.

11.3.4 Polycythemia

A. Polycythemia refers to an absolute increase in RBC volume, RBC count, Hgb and Hct. Care must be taken to determine if elevations of Hct are from polycythemia or hemoconcentration. Expansion of plasma volume with rehydration corrects hemoconcentration.

B. Erythrocytosis
   1. Overproduction of RBCs is most commonly secondary to an increased production of erythropoietin.
      a. This occurs in any situation associated with hypoxia such as cyanotic congenital heart disease, pulmonary disease, congenital methemoglobinemia, infants of diabetic mothers, small for gestational age infants, or living at high altitudes.
      b. The resultant hyperviscosity may cause thrombosis.
   2. Clinical Features
      a. Newborns often exhibit a ruddy complexion and neurologic abnormalities.
      b. Older children exhibit clubbing, cyanosis, and hyperemia of mucous membranes.
   3. Laboratory findings are alterations in Hct. Newborns have a central Hct >65% and children have a Hct >55%.
   4. Treatment
      a. In the newborn period, a partial exchange transfusion is indicated. Whole blood is removed and replaced with saline or albumin to achieve a Hct of 50%. The following formula is used for calculations:

$$\text{Vol. of Exchange} = \text{Blood Vol.} \times \frac{(\text{Observed - Desired Hct})}{\text{Observed Hct}}$$

      b. In older children periodic phlebotomies with saline replacement are also utilized.

C. Polycythemia Rubra Vera. This is a very rare disorder of childhood. The primary defect is in bone marrow hematopoietic stem cells with marked overproduction of all cell lines. In vitro, RBC precursors are active, even without erythropoietin stimulation.

11.3.5 Coagulation Disorders

A. Blood must maintain an equilibrium between the forces that control hemorrhage and protect against thromboses. This dynamic balance consists of blood vessels, platelets, protein clotting factors, and inhibitors.
   1. Abnormalities in blood vessels and/or platelets typically results in petechiae, small ecchymoses, or mucous membrane bleeding such as epistaxis, hematuria, or menorrhagia.
   2. Abnormalities in protein factors classically result in deep hemorrhage into muscles and joints.

B. **Factor VIII Deficiency (Hemophilia A)**
   1. An X-linked deficiency of factor VIII accounts for 80% of all hemophilias.
   2. Pathogenesis
      a. A cascade of reactions involving plasma proteins assists in coagulation by forming a stable fibrin clot. If a protein is missing or defective, the cascade is ineffective and bleeding occurs with even trivial trauma.
      b. Severity of bleeding depends on the degree of factor activity. Severe bleeding occurs with <1% normal activity. Mild disease occurs with 6 to 30% of normal factor activity.
   3. Clinical Features
      a. Newborn males may present with hematomas after injections or excessive bleeding with circumcision.
      b. Most patients will present in the first year of life as ambulation begins and minor trauma occurs.
      c. The hallmark of hemophilia is hemorrhage into large joints such as knees and elbows.
      d. Repeated hemarthroses may lead to a fixed immobile joint.
      e. Intracranial hemorrhages are life-threatening emergencies.
      f. Family history is helpful.
   4. Laboratory findings include prolonged PTT, normalization of PTT in a mixing study, decreased factor VIII activity, and normal platelets, PT and bleeding time.
   5. Treatment
      a. Prevention of trauma is the cornerstone of care.
      b. Medications that affect platelet function (nonsteroidal anti-inflammatory drugs) should be avoided.
      c. Episodes of hemorrhage are managed by replacement with factor VIII concentrates.

C. **Factor IX Deficiency (Hemophilia B)**
   1. This is an X-linked recessive deficiency of factor IX, interrupting the clotting cascade. Severity determined by % activity of normal.
   2. Hemophilia B is rarely diagnosed in the newborn period because factor IX levels are low, even in normal infants at birth. Manifestations are virtually identical to factor VIII deficiency.
   3. Laboratory findings include a prolonged PTT with correction in a mixing study, decreased factor IX activity, and normal platelets, PT and bleeding time.
   4. Treatment
      a. Avoidance of trauma and antiplatelet medications are important for prevention.
      b. Episodes of hemorrhage are managed by replacement with factor IX concentrates.

D. Von Willebrand's Disease

1. This is an autosomal dominant abnormality of production and function of von Willebrand's protein.
    a. This protein contains a platelet adhesive component that carries factor VIII.
    b. Abnormalities lead to abnormal platelet adhesion function and an effective decrease in factor VIII activity.
2. Episodes of bleeding are usually related to an abnormality of platelet function manifesting as menorrhagia, epistaxis, or gingival hemorrhage.
3. Laboratory findings include prolonged PTT, prolonged bleeding time, decreased factor VIII activity, normal platelets, and normal PT.
4. Treatment is with replacement of von Willebrand's factor with cryoprecipitate for episodes of hemorrhage. Replacement with factor VIII concentrate alone does not remedy the effects of abnormal platelet adhesiveness.

E. Vitamin K Deficiency. Refer to hemorrhagic disease of the newborn in section 2.3.9.

F. Disseminated Intravascular Coagulation (DIC)

1. DIC is a result of widespread intravascular activation of the clotting cascade and fibrinolytic system.
    a. DIC is initiated by systemic insults such as septic shock, neoplasms, snake envenomation, or trauma.
    b. Coagulation factors, specifically II, V, VIII and fibrinogen, are consumed.
    c. Hemolytic anemia and thrombocytopenia are present.
2. Clinical Features
    a. Symptoms of the inciting disease are most notable, however bleeding from incisions or venipuncture sites is common.
    b. Intravascular deposition of fibrin leads to tissue infarction manifesting as purpura fulminans or multiorgan system failure.
3. Laboratory findings include prolonged PT, PTT and bleeding time, decreased fibrinogen, elevated fibrin degradation products, thrombocytopenia, normochromic, normocytic anemia, and fragmented burr cells on a peripheral smear.
4. Treatment
    a. Management of the inciting insult is imperative.
    b. Hemorrhagic abnormalities are managed by replacement therapy with cryoprecipitate, fresh frozen plasma, platelets, and RBCs as needed.

11.3.6 Abnormalities of Platelets

A. Wiskott-Aldrich Syndrome

1. X-linked recessive defect in platelet formation despite normal megakaryocytes.
2. The syndrome is associated with eczema and recurrent infections. Splenomegaly, hepatomegaly, and cervical lymphadenopathy are common.
3. Laboratory findings include thrombocytopenia, small platelets on a peripheral smear, and normal megakaryocytes on bone marrow examination.
4. Treatment
    a. Splenectomy improves thrombocytopenia, but increases the risk of infection.
    b. Bone marrow transplantation has been successful.

B. Thrombocytopenia Absent Radius (TAR) Syndrome

1. Autosomal recessive absence of bone marrow megakaryocytes.
2. There is a syndromic association with absent radii. Cardiac and renal abnormalities are often associated findings.
3. Laboratory findings include profound thrombocytopenia, normal chromosome configuration, and absent megakaryocytes on bone marrow examination.
4. Treatment is with platelet transfusions as needed.

C. Kasabach-Merritt Syndrome

1. This syndrome occurs when cavernous hemangiomas of the trunk, extremities, and viscera are sites of intravascular coagulation and subsequent thrombocytopenia.
2. The hemangiomas may or may not be visible, depending upon the location, yet recurrent symptoms of thrombocytopenia and anemia occur.
3. Laboratory findings are thrombocytopenia, RBC fragments on a peripheral smear, and normal megakaryocytes on bone marrow examination.
4. Treatment
    a. Reduction of hemangioma size can be attempted with surgical excision, radiation therapy, corticosteroids, and/or interferon.
    b. Platelet and packed RBC transfusions are given as needed for supportive care.

D. Idiopathic Thrombocytopenic Purpura (ITP)

1. ITP is thrombocytopenia often associated with a preceding viral illness, however the exact etiology is unclear. It is likely an immune mechanism that triggers platelet destruction.
2. Patients present with acute onset of petechiae, epistaxis, and gingival hemorrhage about 2 weeks after a viral illness. Patient appears clinically normal except for hemorrhage. Intracranial hemorrhages are very rare.
3. Laboratory findings are thrombocytopenia and increased megakaryocytes suggestive of increased platelet production.
4. Treatment
    a. Episodes of life-threatening hemorrhage require platelet transfusions, however transfused platelets are rapidly destroyed as well.
    b. Spontaneous recovery within 8 weeks is expected, but this can be hastened with intrave-

nous gamma globulin (IVIG) or steroid therapy.

c. Some patients experience prolonged thrombocytopenia called chronic ITP (if >1 year). These patients may benefit from splenectomy.

189. Which embryologic layer does the hematopoietic system arise — B 11.1.1

A. endoderm
B. mesoderm
C. ectoderm
D. none of the above

190. All of the following are primary spaces of hematopoiesis in older children except — D 11.1.1

A. sternum
B. ribs
C. skull
D. femur
E. pelvis

191. Which hemoglobin form predominates in fetal life — A 11.1.2

A. $\alpha_2\gamma_2$
B. $\alpha_2\beta_2$
C. β_4
D. γ_4

192. What is the lifespan of a normal adult red blood cell — C 11.1.2

A. 80 days
B. 90 days
C. 120 days
D. 150 days

193. What is the normal lifespan of a platelet — A 11.1.2

A. 9 days
B. 12 days
C. 15 days
D. 20 days

194. A 5-year-old child presents with pale skin, pale mucosa, tachycardia, heart murmur, and koilonychia. What is the likely diagnosis — D 11.2.2

A. congenital heart disease
B. cystic fibrosis
C. kwashiorkor
D. iron deficiency anemia
E. rickets

195. Which of the following is associated with a normocytic, normochromic anemia and a high reticulocyte count — B 11.2.4

A. folate deficiency
B. hemorrhage
C. Diamond-Blackfan anemia
D. leukemia
E. transient erythroblastopenia of childhood

196. All of the following are complications of chronic transfusion therapy for Diamond-Blackfan syndrome except — C 11.3.2

A. short stature
B. delayed puberty
C. congenital heart disease
D. diabetes mellitus
E. death

197. Measurement of the partial thromboplastin time reflects the function of which coagulation factors — D 11.2.3

A. II, V, VII, X
B. II, VIII, IX, X
C. VIII, IX, X, XII
D. VIII, IX, XI, XII
E. IX, X, XII

198. Which of the following conditions is associated with a macrocytic, normochromic anemia — A 11.2.4

A. folate deficiency
B. iron deficiency
C. zinc deficiency
D. aplastic anemia
E. leukemia

199. Which of the following red blood cell parameters is a measure of red blood cell size heterogeneity — D 11.2.3

A. mean corpuscular volume (MCV)
B. mean corpuscular hemoglobin (MCH)
C. mean corpuscular hemoglobin concentration (MCHC)
D. red blood cell distribution width (RDW)

200. A young child has absent radii and thumbs, chronic renal failure, severe pancytopenia, and macrocytic red blood cells. What is the diagnosis — C 11.3.1

A. leukemia
B. aplastic anemia
C. Fanconi's syndrome
D. trisomy 21
E. TAR syndrome

201. Which of the following are causes of acquired pancytopenia — E 11.3.1

A. leukemia
B. parvovirus infection
C. benzene exposure
D. sulfonamide exposure
E. all of the above

202. What is the treatment of choice for acquired, persistent pancytopenia — A 11.3.1

A. bone marrow transplant
B. immunotherapy
C. steroids
D. platelet transfusion
E. intravenous immunoglobulin

203. A 3-year-old is brought to your office by Child Protective Services because of concerns of physical abuse. On exam, you note a well nourished, active toddler with multiple ecchymosis and areas of petechiae. What is your best next step in diagnosis, treatment, and disposition — D 11.3.6

A. agree with the worker that this is definitely abuse and release him to the shelter
B. it is obvious that he has meningococcemia so you hospitalize him for intravenous antibiotics
C. you determine that he has Henoch-Schönlein purpura and prescribe no treatment
D. you perform a complete blood count which reveals a platelet count of 20,000/mm^3. You recommend that the worker return the child to his family if it is a well supervised environment
E. call the oncologist to perform a leukemia work-up

204. A 3-year-old child presents with the insidious onset of anemia over a period of 2 months. Laboratory studies reveal a normochromic, normocytic anemia, decreased reticulocyte count, increased serum iron and iron saturation, and normal hemoglobin F. What is the recommended course of therapy for this child — E 11.3.2

A. immediate transfusion is indicated regardless of symptomatology
B. transfuse if overt symptoms of cardiac decompensation occur
C. administer erythropoietin
D. observe for recovery
E. B and D

205. Which of the following is considered a normal hemoglobin in an 8-week-old — C 11.3.2

A. 5 g/dL
B. 7 g/dL
C. 9 g/dL
D. 12 g/dL

206. An 11-month-old infant is noted to be pale and listless. Laboratory evaluation reveals a hemoglobin of 8 g/dl. In your history, you discover that the child has been fed goat's milk since shortly after birth. Why is the child anemic — B 11.3.2

A. iron deficiency
B. folate deficiency
C. zinc deficiency
D. lead toxicity

207. A 1-year-old with a history of prematurity and necrotizing enterocolitis presents for a well child check. Complete blood count reveals a macrocytic anemia with hypersegmented neutrophils. What is the probable cause of her anemia — A 11.3.2

A. surgical resection of her ileum
B. surgical resection of her jejunum
C. absence of intrinsic factor
D. poor calcium intake
E. poor iron intake

208. What is the genetic defect in sickle cell disease — B 11.3.3

A. glutamine substituted for valine on chromosome 5
B. valine substituted for glutamic acid on chromosome 11
C. a deletion from the short arm of chromosome 5
D. phenylalanine substituted for glutamic acid on chromosome 11

209. Which of the following statements about thalassemias are true — A 11.3.3

A. thalassemia may be protective against *Plasmodium falciparum* malaria
B. Cooley anemia is associated with β globin chains from one chromosome only
C. the genetic defect is located on chromosome 9
D. splenectomy is not performed

210. What is the definitive treatment for hereditary spherocytosis — D 11.3.2

A. pneumococcal vaccine
B. blood transfusion
C. bone marrow transplant
D. splenectomy
E. there is no treatment available

211. A 7-year-old Asian male is treated with sulfamethoxazole and trimethoprim for a sinus infection. A few days after starting the medication, his mother notices that he is jaundiced and listless. His urine is very dark. What is the most likely diagnosis for his symptoms — C 11.3.2

A. hepatitis B infection
B. hemolytic-uremic syndrome
C. glucose-6-phosphate dehydrogenase deficiency
D. serum sickness

212. An infant born to a gravida 2 para 2, type O, Rh-positive mother, is noted to be jaundiced within 12 hours of delivery. All of the following are in the differential diagnosis except — A 11.3.2

A. physiologic jaundice
B. ABO incompatibility
C. minor blood group incompatibility
D. sepsis

213. The first manifestation of sickle cell disease in an infant is often — D 11.3.3

A. acute chest syndrome
B. abdominal pain
C. stroke
D. dactylitis
E. renal failure

214. Treatment for sickle cell disease includes all of the following except — C 11.3.3

A. pneumococcal vaccination
B. parent education
C. scheduled red blood cell transfusions
D. penicillin prophylaxis
E. intramuscular antibiotics during febrile illnesses

215. All of the following statements regarding sickle cell trait are true except — E 11.3.3

A. patients may have urinary frequency
B. painless hematuria occurs
C. affected individuals may pass the trait along to their offspring
D. about 10% of all African Americans are affected
E. vasoocclusive events may occur with mild hypoxia

216. A 2-year-old presents for routine exam. You note that the child is pale, cranky, listless, and is not gaining weight well since his last appointment. A complete blood count shows a microcytic, hypochromic anemia. When you inquire about his dietary history, what is the likely response — D 11.3.2

A. "He loves to eat his sisters baby food."
B. "He eats like most kids his age."
C. "He takes a multivitamin every day."
D. "He won't eat anything, all he wants is milk."
E. "Some days he won't eat, other days you can't fill him up."

217. A 2-year-old presents with developmental delay, irritability, abdominal pain, and constipation. Laboratory evaluation is remarkable for a hypochromic, microcytic anemia with basophilic stippling on a peripheral smear. What is your diagnosis — B 11.3.2

A. iron deficiency
B. lead poisoning
C. zinc deficiency
D. anemia of chronic disease
E. sickle cell disease

218. A 9-month-old boy of Greek ancestry presents with hepatosplenomegaly, jaundice, anemia, and frontal bossing. Definitive treatment for his condition is — A 11.3.3

A. bone marrow transplant
B. repeated blood transfusions
C. deferoxamine therapy
D. splenectomy
E. supplemental iron therapy

219. A 5-year-old presents with a history of severe eczema, recurrent infection, thrombocytopenia, and hepatomegaly. What is his diagnosis — A 11.3.6

A. Wiskott-Aldrich syndrome
B. Job's syndrome
C. TAR syndrome
D. Bruton's agammaglobulinemia
E. DiGeorge's syndrome

220. Which of the following are associated with disseminated intravascular coagulation — E 11.3.5

A. II, V, VIII, fibrinogen consumption
B. burr cells
C. prolonged prothrombin time
D. snake envenomation
E. all of the above

.221 Which of the following is the most common cause of hemophilia — E 11.3.5

A. factor IX deficiency
B. hemophilia B
C. von Willebrand's disease
D. Wiskott-Aldrich syndrome
E. factor VIII deficiency

222. Which of the following laboratory studies is abnormal in a patient with hemophilia A — B 11.3.5

A. prothrombin time
B. partial thromboplastin time
C. partial thromboplastin time mixing study
D. bleeding time
E. platelets

223. Which of the following laboratory studies is abnormal in patients with von Willebrand disease — E 11.3.5

A. prothrombin time
B. partial thromboplastin time
C. bleeding time
D. all of the above
E. B and C

224. Hemorrhage in von Willebrand disease is treated with — C 11.3.5

A. factor VIII concentrate
B. platelet transfusion
C. cryoprecipitate
D. factor IX concentrate
E. all of the above

225. All of the following are findings potentially associated with Kasabach-Merritt syndrome except — B 11.3.6

A. thrombocytopenia
B. decreased megakaryocytes
C. normal physical examination
D. red blood cell fragments on peripheral smear
E. cavernous hemangiomas on the trunk

226. What hemoglobin predominates in β-thalassemia major — B 11.3.3

A. hemoglobin F
B. Bart's hemoglobin
C. hemoglobin H
D. hemoglobin AS

227. All of the following are causes of polycythemia except — C 11.3.4

A. congenital heart disease
B. congenital methemoglobinemia
C. living at sea level
D. maternal gestational diabetes

12 NEOPLASTIC DISORDERS

12.1 GENERAL CONCEPTS

12.1.1 Epidemiology

A. One percent of new cancer cases occur in children.

B. Childhood cancers differ in nature, distribution, and prognosis.
   1. Acute lymphocytic leukemia (ALL), central nervous system (CNS) tumors, and sarcomas predominate in childhood.
   2. Although overall survival rate for childhood cancers continues to improve, treatment has adverse effects on growth and development.
   3. Site of origin is variable with patient age.
      a. In children <5 years old, ALL is most common, followed by CNS tumors, lymphoma, and renal tumors.
      b. From 5 to 9 years of age, the order of incidence is ALL, followed by CNS tumor, lymphoma, and then other tumor types.
      c. In pre-teens (10 to 14 years of age), lymphoma is the most common cancer, followed by CNS tumor, ALL, then bone tumors.
      d. Between ages 15 and 19 years, lymphoma predominates, followed by ALL, gonadal tumors, then CNS tumors.
   4. Overall survival rate for childhood cancers is > 80% (1997 survey).

12.1.2 Etiology

A. Environmental exposures to physical agents (ultraviolet irradiation, ionizing radiation), chemical agents (tobacco smoke, diethylstilbestrol, pesticides, androgens, immunosuppressive agents), and microbiologic agents (Hepatitis B and C, human immunodeficiency virus, Ebstein-Barr virus, human papillomaviruses) are tumorigenic.

B. Genetics
   1. Proto-oncogenes are progenitors of tumor retroviral oncogenes. They code for proteins that participate in signal transduction, regulating cell growth, division, and differentiation. They are abnormally activated by any process leading to deregulation or amplification of gene expression. Examples of cancers arising in this fashion include leukemia and multiple endocrine neoplasias.
   2. Fusion genes are translocations or inversions of genes that encode for transcription factors.
   3. Disruption of tumor suppressor genes (antioncogenes) allows noncontrolled cell growth. Examples include retinoblastoma and skin cancers secondary to deoxyribonucleic acid damage.
   4. Recessive oncogenes ("two hit" model of cancer development) allow tumor development when both copies are inactivated. Examples include sporadic retinoblastoma, sarcomas, leukemia, breast, bone, and CNS cancers.
   5. Inherited defects in deoxyribonucleic acid repair lead to tumor formation as seen in xeroderma pigmentosa, ataxia-telangiectasia, and Bloom's syndrome.
   6. Inherited defects in immune surveillance result in failure to recognize and destroy transformed cells. Examples are Wiskott-Aldrich syndrome, severe combined immunodeficiency, lymphoma, and leukemia.

12.1.3 Common Clinical Manifestations of Cancer

A. Hematologic manifestations include pallor, anemia, petechiae, neutropenia, and thrombocytopenia as seen in leukemia or neuroblastoma.

B. Dermatologic signs are "blueberry muffin" spots seen in neonatal neuroblastoma and leukemia.

C. Thoracic masses are discussed in section 9.1.5.

D. Ophthalmologic manifestations include leukocoria (retinoblastoma), ecchymosis, and proptosis (neuroblastoma).

E. CNS disease may present with headache (pheochromocytoma, space occupying tumor), ataxia (neuroblastoma), spinal cord compression, or alteration in mental status. Stroke may occur in cancers that result in leukocytosis with sludging (leukemia).

F. Orthopedic symptoms include bone pain, limp, and arthralgia (osteosarcoma, leukemia, neuroblastoma), or tissue mass (sarcoma).

G. Gastrointestinal findings may be abdominal mass (neuroblastoma, Wilms' tumor, hepatoblastoma), or diarrhea (neuroblastoma).

H. Hypertension is seen with neuroblastoma, pheochromocytoma, and Wilms' tumor.

I. Vaginal bleeding and chronic ear discharge are seen with rhabdomyosarcoma.

J. Lymphadenopathy may be impressive with leukemia, Hodgkin's disease, and lymphoma.

K. Nonspecific symptoms of fever, weight loss, and night sweats are seen with lymphoma and Hodgkin's disease.

L. Superior vena cava syndrome (distended neck veins, plethora, head/neck edema) is seen most commonly with superior mediastinal masses.

12.1.4 Treatment

A. Treatment requires a multidisciplinary team approach with pathologists, surgeons, radiation oncologists, nutritionists, social workers, nurses, psychologists, and oncologists.

B. **Chemotherapeutic Agents**
   1. These drugs interrupt vital functions of rapidly growing cells, resulting in cell death.
   2. Unfortunately, normal cells may be susceptible to these adverse affects as well.

3. Examples of these agents are antimetabolites (methotrexate), alkylating agents (cyclophosphamide), antibiotics (adriamycin), vinca alkaloids (vincristine), enzymes (L-asparaginase), hormones (prednisone), and miscellaneous drugs (cisplatin).

C. **Bone Marrow Transplant and Stem Cell Replacement**
1. Bone marrow is harvested directly or stem cells are collected by apheresis, filtered, and administered intravenously to the recipient.
2. Types of Transplants
   a. In autologous transplants, the source of stem cells is the patient.
   b. Syngeneic transplants are collected from an identical twin.
   c. In allogeneic transplants, the bone marrow is donated by a nonidentical individual. Siblings are the best donors because of the 25% chance that they are human leucocyte antigen (HLA) identical. Alternative sources are unrelated individuals with at least 5 of 6 HLA loci matched, or umbilical cord blood.
3. Side effects include graft-versus-host disease, sterility, mucositis, pancytopenia, opportunistic infection, and liver disease.

D. **Complications of Treatment**
1. Metabolic derangement may occur as seen with tumor lysis syndrome (hyperuricemia, hyperkalemia, hyperphosphatemia), and syndrome of inappropriate secretion of antidiuretic hormone.
2. Bone marrow suppression occurs with resultant neutropenia, thrombocytopenia, and anemia, potentially requiring transfusion (with the additive risk inherent in the use of blood products).
3. Disseminated intravascular coagulation may result from sepsis secondary to immune suppression or the release of tumor necrosis factors.
4. Graft-versus-host disease occurs when immune competent T cells of transplanted bone marrow recognize the cell markers of the recipient as foreign. This affects multiple organ systems with the most common symptoms being rash, diarrhea, and abnormalities in liver function.
5. Opportunistic infection (*Pneumocystis carinii*, mycobacterial, viral, fungal) may arise due to immune suppression, splenectomy, and central line placement.
6. Infertility (alkylating agents), second cancers (alkylating agents), hepatotoxicity, pulmonary fibrosis (bleomycin), and cardiomyopathy (doxorubicin) are well recognized side effects of chemotherapeutic agents.
7. Irradiation may result in infertility, leukoencephalopathy, impaired cognition, pituitary dysfunction, and hypothyroidism.

E. Palliative care is provided when the cancer is lethal. The goal is to relieve pain, manage side effects of medications, and provide emotional support to the child and family.

12.1.5 Emergencies in Children With Cancer

A. Fever and Neutropenia
1. The child should be considered septic until proven otherwise.
2. Draw cultures and start empiric antibiotic therapy.

B. Chickenpox
1. Varicella infection can be very severe or even fatal in the immunosuppressed child.
2. Give varicella-zoster immune globulin (VZIG) within 72 hours of exposure. Start antiviral therapy if exposed or infected.

C. Increasing intracranial pressure
1. This is seen with leukemic infiltration of the CNS or CNS tumors blocking cerebrospinal fluid flow.
2. Emergency surgery for shunt placement or ventriculostomy is lifesaving.
3. Urgent irradiation of the CNS may shrink the tumor, relieving symptoms.

D. Hyperleukocytosis
1. This is seen most commonly in acute myelogenous leukemia (AML) and T cell ALL.
2. It can lead to vascular occlusion including cerebrovascular accidents.
3. Treatment is with intravenous hydration to decrease viscosity. Consult a hematologist urgently.

12.2 DISEASE PROFILES

12.2.1 Leukemia

A. Leukemia is the most common childhood cancer.

B. **Acute Lymphocytic Leukemia** (ALL)
1. ALL causes 75% of leukemia in children.
2. Peak age at onset is 4 years.
3. ALL is the first childhood cancer that was shown to be curable.
   a. Cure rate is currently 80%.
   b. Favorable prognostic indicators are age between 2 and 7-years, Caucasian race, female sex, initial white blood cell count <10,000 cells/mm^3, and normal immunoglobulin levels.
4. Diagnosis is made by bone marrow biopsy.
   a. The majority will show replacement of normal bone marrow with immature B cells.
   b. Approximately 15% demonstrate overgrowth of immature T cells.
   c. One percent show a predominance of mature B cells.
5. Chromosomal abnormalities are present in 80% of children with ALL.
6. Most children are symptomatic for only a short period before diagnosis. The symptoms include anor-

exia, irritability, lethargy, pallor, bleeding, bruising, and fever.

7. Complete blood cell count reveals either an increase or decrease in white blood cells, blast cells in the circulation, thrombocytopenia, and anemia.
8. The differential diagnosis includes bone marrow failure, aplastic anemia, myelofibrosis, or infiltration of the marrow by other types of tumor cells.
9. Treatment is with chemotherapy.
10. Relapse after remission occurs most commonly in the bone marrow. CNS relapse occurs if the child does not receive CNS prophylaxis. Testicular recurrences are common in males.

C. **Acute Myelogenous Leukemia** (AML)

1. AML accounts for 20% of childhood leukemia.
2. The presentation is similar to ALL. AML may be associated with the occurrence of a chloroma (localized mass of tumor cells in the epidural space or orbit).
3. AML is commonly associated with abnormalities on chromosomes 7 or 11.
4. Treatment is geared to induce remission followed by bone marrow transplantation with an HLA matched, related stem cell donor. Cure rate with this regimen is approximately 70%.
5. Children with Down's syndrome (10 to 30-times the leukemia risk compared to the general population) and AML have an 80% cure rate with chemotherapy alone.

D. **Chronic Myelogenous Leukemia** (CML)

1. CML is responsible for 3% of the childhood leukemias.
2. It is characterized by a slow progression of disease toward an acute myeloid or lymphoblastic crisis.
3. CML is related to the presence of the Philadelphia chromosome (9:22 specific translocation).
4. Signs and symptoms include weight loss, anorexia, night sweats, and splenomegaly.
5. Treatment is with chemotherapy in the chronic phase of the illness. Bone marrow transplantation with an HLA identical donor offers a survival rate of 80%.

E. **Chronic lymphocytic leukemia** (CLL) is rare in childhood.

12.2.2 Lymphoma

A. **Hodgkin's Disease** (HD)

1. HD causes 5% of cancers in children <5 years of age.
2. Risk is increased by preexistent immune deficiency or possible infection with Ebstein-Barr virus.
3. HD arises in lymphoid tissue. Four histologic subtypes exist. These are lymphocytic predominance, nodular sclerosing, mixed cellularity, and lymphocyte depleted.
4. HD most commonly presents as a painless, firm, cervical or supraclavicular lymph node. It may also present as an anterior mediastinal mass with airway obstruction, pericardial or pleural effusion. Other organ systems are rarely involved as well.
5. Metastasis is via local or hematogenous spread to liver, spleen, bone, bone marrow, and brain.
6. The Reed-Sternberg cell is a multinucleated cell of uncertain origin that is considered a hallmark for HD on pathologic specimens.
7. Ann Arbor Staging System
    a. Stage I: single lymph node region or single extralymphatic organ involvement.
    b. Stage II: two or more lymphoid regions on the same side of the diaphragm, or localized involvement of an extralymphatic site and a lymph node region on the same side of the diaphragm.
    c. Stage III: lymph node regions on both sides of the diaphragm, with or without localized involvement of extralymphatic organs or sites, or spleen involvement.
    d. Stage IV: disseminated involvement of one or more extralymphatic organs or tissues, with or without associated lymph node enlargement.
    e. Stages are identified as either A or B based on the absence or presence of systemic symptoms of weight loss and fever.
8. Treatment is with radiation therapy and/or chemotherapy.
9. Survival is 90% in patients with early disease stage and >70% in those with more advanced disease.

B. **Non-Hodgkin's Lymphoma** (NHL)

1. This lymphoma results from malignant proliferation of immature B cells, T cells, and indeterminate cells predominantly outside of the bone marrow.
2. Its incidence is approximately 6% of childhood cancers.
3. Immune deficiency and Ebstein-Barr virus (Burkitt's lymphoma) predispose to the development of NHL.
4. Three subtypes exist.
    a. Lymphoblastic lymphomas are usually of T cell origin. They usually present as intrathoracic tumor, chest pain, dysphagia, pleural effusion, and superior vena cava syndrome. Most affected children have cervical or axillary lymphadenopathy.
    b. Small noncleaved cell lymphoma is predominantly of B cell origin and presents 80% of the time as an abdominal mass. Symptoms include pain, distention, obstruction, change in bowel habits, and bleeding. Other sites of involvement include CNS, bone marrow, lymph nodes, and jaw (<20% in the USA, >70% in Africa secondary to the high incidence of Burkitt's lym-

phoma).

c. Large cell lymphoma can be of any cell type and presents with symptoms referable to the site of origin in the abdomen or mediastinum. Other sites of involvement include skin, soft tissue, and bone. CNS disease is not frequent.

5. Staging System
   a. Stage I: single tumor or single nodal anatomic area excluding the mediastinum and abdomen.
   b. Stage II: single tumor with regional lymph node involvement (≥2 node regions), or ≥2 tumors, with or without lymph node involvement, on the same side of the diaphragm.
   c. Stage III: 2 extranodal tumors on opposite sides
6. Treatment is with chemotherapy, with or without CNS chemotherapy, or radiation.
7. Survival is from 70 to 90% depending upon the cell type of NHL.

12.2.3 Bone Tumors

A. **Osteosarcoma** is a tumor formed by bone mesenchymal tissue cells.
1. Incidence peaks during the adolescent growth spurt.
2. The most common location is the metaphysis of long bones.
3. Patients present with pain and swelling in the region of the tumor. Often there is a history of preceding injury.
4. The classic radiographic finding is the "Sunburst" appearance of the bony tumor.
5. The tumor commonly metastasizes to other bony sites and to lung.
6. Treatment is with surgery and chemotherapy.
7. Cure rate is 70% in the absence of metastasis, otherwise it is <20%.

B. **Ewing's sarcoma** is an undifferentiated tumor of uncertain origin.
1. Its incidence peaks in the second decade of life.
2. The most common locations for tumor are the diaphysis of long bones and flat bones.
3. Patients present as in osteosarcoma.
4. The classic finding on radiography is the laminar "onion skin" appearance of the tumor.
5. Metastasis occurs to lung and bone.
6. Treatment is with surgical resection of the primary tumor, chemotherapy, and irradiation.
7. Without metastasis, survival is 60%. With metastasis, it is 20 to 30%.

12.2.4 CNS Tumors

A. Location
1. Two thirds of childhood brain tumors occur below the tentorium.
2. One third of brain tumors begin above the tentorium.

B. **Astrocytoma**
1. These tumors arise from astrocytes.
2. Tumors are classified as high- or low-grade astrocytoma, or brainstem glioma.
   a. High-grade tumors are usually supratentorial while low-grade tumors are infratentorial.
   b. Brainstem glioma's location is self-explanatory.
3. Symptoms occur based on tumor size and location, and include focal neurologic deficits, increased intracranial pressure from mass effect and hydrocephalus, seizures, ataxia, nystagmus, and cranial nerve palsies.
4. Prognosis is very good for completely resected low grade astrocytomas and poor for brainstem gliomas.

C. **Medulloblastoma**
1. This is the most common malignant brain tumor in the pediatric population.
2. It is usually cerebellar in location.
3. Symptoms include symptoms of increased intracranial pressure and abnormalities of cerebellar function.
4. This tumor metastasizes to other sites in the CNS through cerebrospinal fluid flow.
5. Prognosis is good for completely resected small tumors. Long-term survival is poor if metastasis occurs.

D. Treatment
1. Surgery is effective for removing or debulking tumors when the lesions are accessible (not located in close proximity to areas of vital brain function). ventriculoperitoneal shunt placement may be necessary for treatment of tumor associated hydrocephalus.
2. Radiation therapy can be used to shrink tumors. This may be definitive treatment or adjunctive therapy used in combination with surgery and chemotherapy.
3. Chemotherapy may prolong survival in brain tumor patients. Remember though, an intact blood-brain barrier does limit the use of systemic chemotherapy. Therapy can be introduced via the intrathecal route as well.

12.2.5 Other Tumors

A. **Wilms' Tumor**
1. Wilms' is the most common renal tumor in childhood and accounts for 6% of childhood cancers.
2. Genetics
   a. Thirty percent of tumors are noted to have deletions of gene loci on chromosome 11.
   b. Single deletions of the p13 locus are associated with *W*ilms' tumor, *A*niridia, *G*enitourinary malformation, mental *R*etardation (WAGR) and Denys-Drash syndrome (Wilms, nephropathy, genital abnormalities). Deletions of the 11p15 locus are associated with Wilms' tumor in Beckwith-Wiedemann syndrome.

c. Wilms' tumor has an association with congenital anomalies of the genital tract, hemihypertrophy, and sporadic aniridia.
3. Wilms' tumor is usually a solitary tumor (>90%).
4. Signs and symptoms are a palpable flank mass with or without abdominal pain, vomiting, hypertension, and either microscopic or gross hematuria.
5. Staging System (National Wilms' Tumor Study Group)
   a. Stage I: tumor is limited to the kidney.
   b. Stage II: tumor extends beyond the kidney but can be completely excised.
   c. Stage III: postsurgical residual tumor is limited to the abdomen.
   d. Stage IV: hematogenous metastasis has occurred (usually to lung).
6. Treatment is with excision, chemotherapy, and radiation.
7. Survival rates range from 55 to 98% depending upon the pathology and stage of the tumor.

B. Neuroblastoma

1. Neuroblastomas are tumors derived from cells of neural crest origin.
2. They account for 8% of childhood cancers and are the most common form of solid tumor outside the cranium.
3. The median age at diagnosis is 2 years.
4. Tumors develop at sites of sympathetic nervous tissue such as the adrenal gland or retroperitoneal sympathetic ganglia. The majority are in the abdomen.
5. Cell differentiation on pathologic study reveals ganglioneuroma, ganglioneuroblastoma, and neuroblastoma.
6. Signs and symptoms include fever, irritability, diarrhea, failure to thrive, "blueberry muffin" rash, abdominal mass, periorbital ecchymosis (raccoon eyes), proptosis, hepatosplenomegaly, symptoms of spinal cord compression, hypertension, and opsoclonus-myoclonus paraneoplastic syndrome (chaotic eye movements, myoclonus, ataxia).
7. Staging System
   a. Stage 1: tumor confined to organ or structure of origin.
   b. Stage 2: tumor extends beyond structure of origin but does not cross midline with (stage 2B) or without (stage 2A) ipsilateral lymph node involvement.
   c. Stage 3: tumor extends across midline, with or without bilateral lymph node involvement.
   d. Stage 4: disseminated disease.
   e. Stage 4S: age <1 year with dissemination to the liver, skin, or bone marrow, with a primary tumor that would be classified as stage 1 or 2.
8. Treatment is with surgery, radiation, and chemotherapy, depending on the stage at diagnosis.
9. Survival is best in children <1 year of age with stage 1,2, or 4S disease (approximately 90%). Survival rates with other stages are significantly worse at 25 to 30%.

C. Rhabdomyosarcoma

1. This is the most common pediatric soft tissue sarcoma, causing 5 to 8% of childhood cancer.
2. It arises from embryonic mesenchymal tissue.
3. These tumors occur in the head and neck region, genitourinary tract, extremities, and trunk, in that order of frequency.
4. Neurofibromatosis is associated with an increase in risk for rhabdomyosarcoma.
5. Signs and symptoms are a palpable painful or painless tissue mass with symptoms attributable to displacement of normal structures.
6. Four tumor subtypes exist. These are: embryonal, botryoid (grape-like), alveolar, and pleomorphic. The remainder of tumors are undifferentiated.
7. Treatment is by tumor resection, chemotherapy, and radiation.
8. Prognosis for survival is 80% in children who have complete resection of their tumor. Survival decreases to 60% when incomplete resection is achieved.

D. Retinoblastoma

1. Retinoblastoma arises in the nucleated layers of the retina.
2. The incidence is 1;180,000 and is bilateral in 20 to 30% of patients.
3. Up to 40% are heritable and are associated with a gene on chromosome 13.
4. Children present with leukocoria (white papillary reflex) and occasionally strabismus, glaucoma, hyphema, or orbital inflammation.
5. Treatment used to be enucleation of the affected globe. Now, treatment is primarily with local tumor control and chemotherapy.
6. Cure rates exceed 90%.

E. Gonadal and Germ Cell Tumors

1. **Gonadoblastoma**
   a. Gonadoblastoma is associated with gonadal dysgenesis.
   b. It may contain malignant germ cell tumor elements.
   c. Resection is the mainstay of treatment.
   d. Undescended testes are a risk factor.
2. **Teratoma**
   a. These tumors are collections of multiple tissue types that occur outside their normal body regions.
   b. They are most common in the sacrococcygeal region.
   c. They are malignant in <10% of children younger than 2 months of age and >50% of children 2

months of age or older.

d. Treatment is with surgical resection and chemotherapy if malignant.

3. Other genitourinary tumors include germinomas (ovary, testes) and embryonal carcinoma (testes).

F. **Liver Tumor**

1. Liver tumors account for 1% of malignancies in children.
2. Hepatoblastomas present as an abdominal mass associated with weight loss, anorexia, vomiting, and abdominal pain.
3. Hepatocellular carcinoma presents with acute abdominal crisis (rupture, hemoperitoneum).
4. Treatment is surgical resection and chemotherapy, with survival rates of 60 to 90% in hepatoblastoma and 30% in hepatocellular carcinoma.

G. **Gastrointestinal Tumors**

1. This group includes salivary gland tumors, nasopharyngeal carcinoma, gastric carcinoma, pancreatic carcinoma, and colonic polyps.
2. **Polyposis** is the most common tumor in the gastrointestinal group in children.
   a. Familial adenomatous polyposis is an autosomal dominant condition with a 100% risk of colon cancer occurrence. Colectomy is recommended.
   b. Generalized juvenile polyposis is an autosomal dominant precancerous condition.
   c. Isolated polyps rarely cause cancer.

H. **Carcinomas**

1. Clear cell carcinomas of the vagina and cervix are rare except in the case of prenatal exposure to diethylstilbestrol.
2. Carcinoma of the adrenal gland has a bimodal peak with disease in children occurring in those <5 years of age. Symptoms may be that of adrenal excess.
3. Skin cancers are of most concern in children with giant hairy nevi, 10% of whom will develop a malignant melanoma.

12.2.6 Benign Tumors

A. **Hemangiomas** are the most common benign tumor of infancy.

1. They are characterized by abnormal collections of vasculature that grow rapidly over the first year of life then involute slowly to resolution by approximately 10 years of age.
2. Usually hemangiomas are asymptomatic, but complications can include obstructive amblyopia with lesions that occlude vision, airway compromise, high output heart failure, or Kasabach-Merritt syndrome (thrombocytopenia, microangiopathic anemia, coagulopathy) with large lesions.
3. Treatment is usually observation alone, or may include steroids and interferon in life or sight threatening tumors.

B. **Cystic hygromas** are painless soft tissue masses composed of malformed lymphatic tissue. Treatment is usually staged surgical resection.

C. **Histiocytosis X (Langerhans' cell histiocytosis)** is a proliferation of dendritic cells of the monocyte-macrophage line.

1. Eosinophilic granuloma is uncommon in children and is usually limited to a single painful bone lesion.
2. Hand-Schüller-Christian disease involves the bone and the skin. It may present as the classic triad of skeletal lesions, diabetes insipidus, and exophthalmos.
3. Letterer-Siwe disease involves the skin, liver, spleen, lymph nodes, bone marrow, and lungs. Patients often die of sepsis or organ dysfunction.

D. Benign bone lesions do occur. The most common are osteochondroma, multiple hereditary exostosis, and nonossifying fibroma.

228. What is the most common form of cancer in children less than 5 years of age — A 12.1.1

A. acute lymphoblastic leukemia
B. brain tumors
C. renal tumors
D. acute myeloid leukemia
E. Ewing's sarcoma

229. What is the overall survival rate for childhood cancer — C 12.1.1

A. 50%
B. 65%
C. 80%
D. 90%

230. The genetic defect that leads to cancer in xeroderma pigmentosa is — B 12.1.2

A. disruption of tumor suppressor genes
B. inherited defects in deoxyribonucleic acid repair
C. presence of proto-oncogenes
D. presence of recessive oncogenes
E. none of the above

231. Blueberry muffin spots are associated with — E 12.1.3

A. leukemia
B. Hodgkin's disease
C. neuroblastoma
D. all of the above
E. A and C

232. Leukocoria is associated with which of the following tumors — B 12.1.3

A. neuroblastoma
B. retinoblastoma
C. ganglioneuroma
D. pheochromocytoma
E. leukemia

233. Which is included in the treatment team for children with cancer — E 12.1.4

A. pediatricians
B. surgeons
C. oncology nurses
D. social workers
E. all of the above

234. Which of the following chemotherapeutic agents is an antimetabolite — E 12.1.4

A. cyclophosphamide
B. adriamycin
C. vincristine
D. prednisone
E. methotrexate

235. Which tumor is associated with prenatal exposure to diethylstilbestrol — B 12.2.5

A. rhabdomyosarcoma
B. cervical clear cell carcinoma
C. ovarian cancer
D. seminoma
E. none of the above

236. Syngeneic transplants are obtained from whom — D 12.1.4

A. nonrelated donors
B. umbilical cord blood
C. nonidentical siblings
D. identical siblings
E. organ donors

237. All of the following are seen in tumor lysis syndrome except — A 12.1.4

A. diabetes insipidus
B. hyperuricemia
C. hyperkalemia
D. hyperphosphatemia
E. syndrome of inappropriate secretion of antidiuretic hormone

238. Which of the following symptoms are seen in graft versus host syndrome — D 12.1.4

A. skin rash
B. elevated hepatic transaminases
C. diarrhea
D. all of the above
E. none of the above

239. Which chemotherapeutic agent is associated with pulmonary fibrosis — C 12.1.4

A. adriamycin
B. methotrexate
C. bleomycin
D. vincristine
E. prednisone

240. What is appropriate treatment for the chemotherapy recipient who is exposed to chicken pox — E 12.1.5

A. reassurance
B. intramuscular varicella-zoster immune globulin
C. varicella vaccine
D. antiviral therapy
E. B and D

241. All of the following are favorable prognostic indicators in acute lymphoblastic leukemia except — B 12.2.1

A. age of 5 years
B. male sex
C. female sex
D. initial white blood cell count $< 10{,}000$ cells/mm^3
E. Caucasian race

242. The mainstay of treatment for retinoblastoma is currently — B 12.2.5

A. enucleation of the affected globe
B. local tumor control and chemotherapy
C. laser therapy alone
D. observation

243. What age is a hemangioma expected to involute — C 12.2.6

A. 1 year of age
B. 4 years of age
C. 10 years of age
D. 15 years of age

244. A 13-year-old male who has survived 1 year following treatment for acute lymphoblastic leukemia, presents for a routine sports exam. You note a small testicular mass. The most likely diagnosis is A 12.2.1

A. recurrence of leukemia
B. seminoma
C. hydrocele
D. appendix testis
E. hernia

245. What is the incidence of leukemia in children with Down's syndrome compared to the general population B 12.2.1

A. 5- to 10-times
B. 10- to 30-times
C. 40- to 50-times
D. 50- to 60-times

246. Which leukemia is associated with the Philadelphia chromosome D 12.2.1

A. acute lymphoblastic leukemia
B. acute myeloid leukemia
C. chronic lymphoblastic leukemia
D. chronic myeloid leukemia

247. A 4-year-old child presents with a supraclavicular lymph node that has been present for approximately 8 weeks. Biopsy shows a predominance of abnormal looking lymphocytes with the presence of Reed-Sternberg cells. Additional evaluation should include E 12.2.2

A. complete blood count
B. liver function tests
C. bone marrow biopsy
D. computed tomography scan of the chest and abdomen
E. all of the above

248. A 5-year-old with Hodgkin's disease is noted to have disease isolated to a group of cervical lymph nodes without other nodal or organ involvement on staging exam. His chance for long term survival is A 12.2.2

A. 90%
B. 80%
C. 70%
D. 60%
E. 50%

249. Which of the following conditions predispose to the development of non-Hodgkin's lymphoma C 12.2.2

A. Epstein-Barr virus
B. immune deficiency
C. both
D. neither

250. A child with non-Hodgkin's lymphoma undergoes evaluation for staging of his disease. Testing reveals involvement of intraabdominal viscera and an intrathoracic mass. No central nervous system or bone marrow involvement is identified. What stage is this C 12.2.2

A. I
B. II
C. III
D. IV

251. Which tumor is characterized by a sunburst appearance on plain x-ray — A 12.2.3

A. osteosarcoma
B. Ewing's sarcoma
C. osteochondroma
D. rhabdosarcoma

252. An 8-year-old girl presents with a painful mass on her left chest. When an x-ray is performed, a bony lesion with an onion skin appearance is noted. She most likely has — B 12.2.3

A. osteosarcoma
B. Ewing's sarcoma
C. rhabdosarcoma
D. osteochondroma

252. Where does Ewing's sarcoma usually metastasize to — E 12.2.3

A. lung and liver
B. liver and bone
C. liver and kidney
D. kidney and bone
E. lung and bone

254. Which of the following central nervous system tumors has the best prognosis — D 12.2.4

A. medulloblastoma
B. brainstem glioma
C. high-grade astrocytoma
D. low-grade astrocytoma

255. Which of the following is not a component of WAGR syndrome — A 12.2.5

A. growth retardation
B. Wilms' tumor
C. genitourinary malformation
D. mental retardation
E. aniridia

256. What is the region of the body most likely to be affected with teratoma — A 12.2.5

A. sacrococcygeal
B. ovary
C. brain
D. testis
E. liver

257. What is the occurrence risk of cancer in individuals with familial adenomatous polyposis — A 12.2.5

A. 100%
B. 90%
C. 80%
D. 60%
E. 40%

258. What is the incidence of chromosomal abnormalities in acute lymphoblastic leukemia — D 12.2.1

A. 20%
B. 40%
C. 60%
D. 80%
E. 100%

259. A 3-year-old female is brought to the emergency room for evaluation of vaginal bleeding. On your exam you notice bleeding from the vaginal orifice and what appears to be an intravaginal tissue mass shaped like a cluster of grapes. You diagnose — C 12.2.5

- **A.** child molestation
- **B.** intravaginal foreign body
- **C.** rhabdomyosarcoma
- **D.** uterine prolapse
- **E.** ambiguous genitalia

260. A child with Beckwith-Wiedemann syndrome is brought to your office to establish care. On exam, you note a left-sided flank mass in addition to the normal anomalies seen with this syndrome. What is your suspected diagnosis — B 12.2.5

- **A.** hemihypertrophy
- **B.** Wilms' tumor
- **C.** pancreatic tumor
- **D.** hepatomegaly

261. A child with a known liver hemangioma, presents at 4 months of age with tachypnea, difficulty feeding, intercostal space retractions, diaphoresis, and a new heart murmur. His complete blood count is normal for age. What is the likely diagnosis — D 12.2.6

- **A.** airway hemangioma
- **B.** Kasabach-Merritt syndrome
- **C.** pneumonia
- **D.** heart failure
- **E.** asthma

262. A 3-year-old child presents to the clinic with fever for 2 weeks, diarrhea, weight loss, irritability, periorbital ecchymosis, hepatosplenomegaly, and jerking eye movements. What is your diagnosis — E 12.2.5

- **A.** child abuse
- **B.** dermatomyositis
- **C.** Epstein-Barr virus
- **D.** hepatitis
- **E.** neuroblastoma

13 GASTROENTEROLOGY

13.1 GENERAL CONCEPTS

13.1.1 Gastrointestinal Tract

A. The gastrointestinal tract extends from the mouth to the anus.

B. Disease may occur in any of the number of tissues present in the system.

C. Gastrointestinal disease differs in children and adults.

1. Conditions considered relatively normal phenomena in an infant (gastroesophageal reflux) are abnormal in an older child and adult.
2. Congenital disease can cause life-threatening consequences in a child, yet if not diagnosed until adulthood, are less likely to have severe manifestations.
3. Children are less likely to be cooperative for invasive testing (colonoscopy, endoscopy) than adults.
4. Disease processes may have a different presentation or natural course in children.
5. Treatments used in adults may not be safe or approved for use in children.

D. Function

1. The three major physiological functions are motility, absorption and secretion, and immunologic protection.
2. Some gut functions develop early in fetal life, but others mature postnatally and some are not fully developed until preschool age.
3. The uniqueness of the human gut is seen in its ability to adapt to a variety of nutrient sources and to utilize them for further growth and development.

13.1.2 Embryology

1. The gastrointestinal tract is formed during the fourth week of gestation. It begins as a small, 4 mm hollow tube.
2. The epithelial tissues of the gut are derived from the endodermal layer, and the muscles and connective tissues are derived from the mesodermal layer of the embryo during invagination of the embryonic disc.
3. The foregut comprises the esophagus, stomach, duodenum, liver, gallbladder, and pancreas.
4. The midgut is composed of jejunum, ileum and the ascending, and transverse colon.
5. The hindgut comprises the descending and rectosigmoid colon.

A. The third trimester is the period of maximal growth and differentiation of the gastrointestinal tract.

13.1.3 Diagnostic Modalities

A. History should include general information and specifics about pain, vomiting, weight loss, stools quantity, frequency, and quality.

B. Physical examination

1. A complete examination is indicated including the rectal exam.
2. "Red flags" on examination include documented weight loss, abdominal wall hernia, organomegaly, perianal fistula, anal fissure, perirectal ulceration, occult blood in the stool, joint swelling and tenderness, and ophthalmologic signs of systemic involvement of gastrointestinal disease.

C. Laboratory

1. Appropriate laboratory studies must be guided by history and exam results. Studies commonly include complete blood count, erythrocyte sedimentation rate, amylase, serum chemistries, stool occult blood, and stool for ova and parasites.
2. Specialized studies to be considered include sweat chloride testing, urinalysis, stool culture (bacterial, viral), hydrogen breath testing, stool pH and reducing substances, fecal fat, and esophageal pH study.

D. Radiographic and Other Studies

1. What is appropriate depends on the patient's age, history, and exam.
2. Studies include abdominal x-ray, abdominal ultrasound, endoscopy, barium enema, Meckel's scan, barium swallow, and chest x-ray.

13.2 CONGENITAL MALFORMATIONS

13.2.1 Cleft Lip and Palate

A. Cleft Lip

1. Hypoplasia of the mesenchymal layer results in failure of medial nasal and maxillary processes to join.
2. The incidence of cleft lip with or without cleft palate is about 1:1,000.
3. Genetic factors are more important in cleft lip than cleft palate.
4. The recurrence risk is 3 to 4% in siblings.

B. Cleft Palate

1. Cleft palate is due to failure of the palatal shelves to approximate or fuse.
2. The incidence of cleft palate alone is 1:2,500.

C. Treatment

1. Management requires a multidisciplinary approach.
2. Treatment is initially focused on assuring adequate nutritional intake. This may require specially designed bottle nipples that do not require the infant to compress the nipple to obtain formula.
3. Surgical repair of the cleft lip is usually performed within the first two or three months of life.
4. Palate repair is accomplished within the first year of life, several months after lip repair.
5. As the children age, they require subsequent surgeries for cosmetic improvement, palatal expansion, relief of velopharyngeal insufficiency, and bone grafting of the alveolar ridges to provide dental support.
6. Orthodontia is almost universally required to assure the best possible dental alignment.

7. Aggressive speech therapy is recommended.

D. Complications of cleft palate are recurrent ear infections requiring pressure equalization tube placement, dental decay, malocclusion, and speech deficits.

13.2.2 Pierre Robin Sequence

A. This sequence consists of micrognathia with glossoptosis and pseudomacroglossia with high-arched or cleft palate.

B. Obstruction of the air passages may occur, particularly on inspiration, and usually requires therapy to prevent suffocation.

1. Previously, treatment for airway obstruction necessitated tracheostomy.
2. Currently, airway obstruction can be treated with mandibular distraction. This surgical procedure involves fixation of external distraction devices to the mandible at the site of osteotomy. The mandible is advanced daily over approximately two weeks, bringing the hypoplastic chin forward with subsequent relief of airway obstruction.

C. Feeding problems, including aspiration and poor caloric intake, are seen, just as in nonsyndromic cleft lip and palate.

D. Complications are the same as in cleft lip and palate.

13.2.3 Esophageal Atresia

A. This abnormality generally occurs in association with tracheoesophageal fistula.

B. The most common anatomic arrangement is a blind proximal esophageal pouch that has a distal tracheoesophageal fistula (85 to 90%).

C. Incidence of this anomaly is 1 in 4,000.

D. Presentation

1. Infants present with excessive drooling, regurgitation, cough, choking, or cyanosis with feeding.
2. Abdominal distention or scaphoid abdomen may occur depending on the fistulous connection.

E. Diagnosis is by clinical exam and radiography.

F. Treatment

1. Primary repair can be done in babies as small as 1,200 g.
2. Progress is usually excellent, but complications like stricture formation at the anastomotic site can easily be managed with dilatation.
3. Infants with pure esophageal atresia or those with compromising medical conditions such as pneumonia may require staged repair.

13.2.4 Omphalocele

A. Omphalocele is herniation of abdominal contents into the base of the umbilical cord. The sac is covered by peritoneum only.

B. It is usually associated with a high incidence of other malformations such as congenital heart disease or Beckwith-Wiedemann syndrome.

C. Treatment is surgical repair.

1. If the defect is not large and repair does not create respiratory distress, primary surgical repair and closure can be performed.
2. If the defect is large or respiratory difficulty occurs when the contents are returned to the abdominal cavity, the omphalocele can be confined to a surgically created tower and slowly advanced into the abdomen.

13.2.5 Gastroschisis

A. Gastroschisis results from a defect in closure of the anterior abdominal wall. Abdominal contents extend through the defect to varying degrees.

B. The contents are not protected by the peritoneum.

C. Treatment is by surgical repair.

13.2.6 Umbilical Hernia

A. This is a defect in closure of the anterior abdominal wall musculature at the level of the umbilicus.

B. It is more common in premature and African American infants, and in infants with hypothyroidism.

C. Treatment

1. Fascial defects less than 0.5 cm usually spontaneously close by 2 years of age.
2. Defects 0.5 to 1.5 cm spontaneously close by 4 years of age.
3. Occasionally surgical repair is indicated.
4. Abdominal binders (coins taped over the defect) do not accelerate the healing rate.

13.2.7 Small Bowel Obstruction

A. Duodenal Obstruction

1. This small bowel obstruction may be complete or partial.
   a. Complete obstruction is usually due to atresia of bowel segments.
   b. Partial obstruction (stenosis) is usually due to a web, band, or annular pancreas.
2. Duodenal atresia is more common in premature infants and infants with Down's syndrome.
syndrome.
3. The classic abdominal x-ray finding is the "double bubble." Air is seen in the stomach and in the preobstructed duodenum separated by the pylorus.

B. Jejunal or Ileal Obstruction

1. The lesion may be partial or complete.
2. Polyhydramnios is present in complete atresia.
3. Bile-stained vomitus occurs within 24 to 48 hours after initiation of feedings.
4. X-ray of the abdomen shows dilated loops of small bowel with absence of air in the colon.
5. Meconium ileus with or without atresia is associated with cystic fibrosis.

C. Malrotation and Volvulus

1. Malrotation is due to a defect in development resulting in abnormal position and fixation of the bowel in the abdominal cavity. Volvulus occurs when the poorly fixed bowel twists around the superior mesenteric artery resulting in ischemia and obstruction.
2. The majority of infants with this anomaly present with symptoms within the first month of life.
3. Bilious vomiting and abdominal distention suggests obstruction. Bloody stools may also be present, but would be considered a late finding.
4. Volvulus is diagnosed by upper gastrointestinal series with small bowel follow-through.
5. It is a surgical emergency.

13.2.8 Meckel's Diverticulum

A. It is due to the presence of a vestigial remnant of the omphalomesenteric duct.

B. It is the most common anomaly of the gastrointestinal tract.

C. Gastric tissue is present in the diverticulum and leads to bleeding due to acid secretion and ulceration.

D. Presenting clinical manifestations include painless rectal bleeding, intestinal obstruction due to intussusception or volvulus, or diverticulitis (mimics appendicitis).

E. The "Rule of 2's" for Meckel's Diverticulum
1. It occurs in 2 % of the population.
2. It has a 2:1 male:female ratio.
3. It is 2 inches long.
4. It has 2 tissues, gastric and pancreatic.
5. It is 2 feet proximal to the ileocecal valve.
6. It has a bimodal presentations, < 2 years of age and at adolescence.
7. It has 2 presentations, hemorrhage and obstruction.

13.3 PATHOPHYSIOLOGIC MANIFESTATIONS OF GASTROINTESTINAL DISORDERS

Table 13.3.3B Differential diagnosis of constipation

ETIOLOGY	NEWBORN	INFANT	TODDLER AND SCHOOL-AGE CHILD
MECHANICAL OBSTRUCTION	Imperforate or stenotic anus (sometimes with VATER syndrome) Intestinal atresia Small left colon syndrome Meconium ileus Meconium plug Tumor	Anterior ectopic anus Tumors (lymphoma, rhabdomyosarcoma, neuroblastoma) Malrotation Rectal duplications Congenital or acquired strictures or adhesive peritoneal bands	Tumors (lymphoma, rhabdomyosarcoma, neuroblastoma) Malrotation Rectal duplications Congenital or acquired strictures or adhesive peritoneal bands Crohn's disease
OTHER INTESTINAL DISEASE	Hirschsprung's disease Neuronal intestinal dysplasia Primary ganglioneuromatosis Visceral myopathies and neuropathies	Hirschsprung's disease Visceral myopathies and neuropathies von Recklinghausen's disease Multiple endocrine neoplasia type IIB Myotonic dystrophy	Hirschsprung's disease Multiple endocrine neoplasia type IIB Myotonic dystrophy Dermatomyositis
ABNORMALITY OUTSIDE THE GASTROINTESTINAL TRACT	Hypothyroidism Adrenal insufficiency Hyper- or hypokalemia Hypercalcemia Hypermagnesemia	Spinal cord lesion Familial dysautonomia Hypothyroidism Hypokalemia Hypercalcemia Infant botulism Drug-induced constipation	Spinal cord lesion Autonomic neuropathy, primary or acquired Lead poisening Drug-induced constipation Hypothyroidism Hypokalemia Hypercalcemia Porphyria Pheochromocytoma Diabetes mellitus
FUNCTIONAL DISORDER	None	Dietary abnormality Slow transit	Dietary abnormality Functional fecal retention

13.3.1 Abdominal Pain

A. Warning Signs for Significant Disease
   1. The pain is localized away from the umbilicus. Apley's law states that the further the pain is from the umbilicus, the more likely that it represents identifiable disease.
   2. Changes in bowel function (constipation, diarrhea, incontinence) may signify significant bowel disease.
   3. Acute onset of constant pain that lasts minutes to days is less likely to be functional.
   4. Pain that awakens child at night or radiates to the back, shoulder, or lower extremities is pathologic unless proven otherwise.
   5. Other symptoms that imply underlying disease are vomiting (especially without diarrhea), dysuria, fever, weight loss, rectal bleeding, altered growth rate, rash, and arthralgia.
   6. Presentation at <4 years or >15 years of age is more concerning for organic pain.
   7. Family history of gastrointestinal or systemic illness (peptic ulcer disease, inflammatory bowel disease) increases the likelihood of gastrointestinal pathology.

B. Common Causes of Abdominal Pain
   1. Infants: necrotizing enterocolitis, volvulus, incarcerated hernia, Hirschsprung's disease, intussusception, infantile colic, and perforation.
   2. Child: gastroenteritis, appendicitis, Henoch-Schönlein purpura, urinary tract infection, hemolytic-uremic syndrome, constipation, ulcers, pancreatitis, and functional pain (recurrent abdominal pain).
   3. Adolescent: pelvic inflammatory disease, ectopic pregnancy, inflammatory bowel disease, testicular torsion, and biliary disease.

13.3.2 Diarrhea

A. Secretory Diarrhea
   1. This is caused by decreased absorption or increased secretion of fluid by the intestinal mucosa.
   2. The stool is watery with normal osmolality.

B. Osmotic Diarrhea
   1. This is due to malabsorption of nutrients or maldigestion of foodstuffs.
   2. Stool is watery and acidic, with increased reducing substances.
   3. Osmolality is increased.

C. Increased Peristalsis
   1. This results in decreased transit time.
   2. Stools may appear normal yet more frequent.
   3. Stooling is stimulated by the gastrocolic reflex.

D. Decreased Mucosal Area
   1. Intestinal functional capacity is decreased, limiting absorption of fluid and nutrients.
   2. Stool is watery.

E. Mucosal Damage
   1. Inflammation and infection decrease colonic reabsorption of fluid and increase intestinal motility.
   2. Stools tend to be loose and may be grossly bloody or have increased fecal leukocytes.

13.3.3 Constipation

A. Encopresis (See section 4.2.3)

B. Differential Diagnosis of Constipation (Table 13.3.3B)

C. **Table 13.3.3C** Comparison of functional fecal retention and Hirschsprung's disease

SYMPTOM	FUNCTIONAL FECAL RETENTION	HIRSHSPRUNG'S DISEASE
Delayed passage of meconium	Rare	60%
Constipation as a newborn	Rare	Almost always
Onset after age 2 years	Common	Sometimes
Fecal incontinence	Common	Almost never
Difficulty bowel training	Common	Rare
Avoidance of toilet	Common	Rare
Stool withholding behavior	Common	Rare
Stool in rectal ampulla	Common	Rare
Obstructive symptoms	Rare	Common

13.4 DISEASE PROFILES

13.4.1 Gastroesophageal Reflux (GER)

A. This is a common problem seen in the first year of life.

B. The incidence of significant reflux and complications is 1:300 to 1:10,000.

C. Pathophysiology
   1. Lower esophageal sphincter tone is persistently or intermittently diminished, allowing passage of gastric contents into the esophagus.
   2. These events are associated with and exacerbated by increased intraabdominal pressure, delayed gastric emptying, and reduced esophageal acid clearance.

D. Symptoms
1. Infants commonly present with vomiting which abates by 2 years of age in 60% of cases without treatment. Most have significant improvement by about 15 months of age.
2. Gastrointestinal bleeding and pain can occur secondary to gastric acid induced esophagitis.
3. If vomiting is severe enough to interfere with calorie intake, failure to thrive may result.
4. Apnea is a common reason for hospital visits in the infant with GER.
5. Recurrent respiratory distress, chronic respiratory disease, and aspiration pneumonia are frequent sequelae of GER.
6. **Sandifer's syndrome** is the association of pain, arching of the back, head turning, and iron deficiency anemia, associated with severe GER.

E. Diagnosis is usually by history with confirmation by upper gastrointestinal x-ray series, esophageal pH monitoring, or gastric scintigraphy.

F. Management
1. Uncomplicated GER is managed by elevating the head of the crib by 30 degrees, thickening the formula, frequent burping, and avoidance of overfeeding.
2. Complicated GER employs the methods described above in addition to antacids and H_2-blockers for esophagitis, motility agents (metoclopramide), and surgery (Nissen fundoplication) if medical treatment fails.
3. GER is a recognized contraindication to the current recommendation of supine sleep position in infants.

13.4.2 Acute Diarrhea

A. Diarrhea is an increase in the number, fluid content, or volume of stools.

B. In the United States, attack rates average 1.3 to 2.3 episodes per year between birth and 5 years of age.

C. The incidence of diarrheal illness peaks in winter.

D. There are numerous causes of acute diarrhea.
1. Local, noninvasive infectious causes include rotavirus, Norwalk virus, adenovirus, *Giardia lamblia, Cryptosporidium parvum, Escherichia coli,* and *Vibrio cholera.*
2. Systemic invasive or toxigenic causes include *Campylobacter jejuni, Salmonella, Shigella, Yersinia, Escherichia coli,* and *Clostridium difficile.*
3. Acquired causes include postinfectious diarrhea, bacterial overgrowth, immune deficiency, malabsorption, milk allergy, hepatitis, disaccharidase deficiency, drugs (laxatives, antacids, sorbitol, antibiotics), and poisoning (heavy metal, organophosphates, chemotherapy, irradiation).

E. Laboratory studies can be considered if indicated by history and examination. These are stool consistency, fecal leukocytes, stool for bacterial cultures, virology, ova and parasites, and blood chemistry if hepatitis is suspected or dehydration is evident.

F. Management
1. Treat the underlying condition if applicable.
2. Maintain hydration with either oral electrolyte containing fluids or intravenous fluid support.
3. Educate caregivers regarding home management of diarrhea including prevention.
4. Early refeeding is advisable. It will stimulate gut repair and prevent starvation diarrhea.
5. Antidiarrheal drugs are rarely indicated and not recommended.
6. Specific Treatment
   a. *Clostridium difficile* responds to oral vancomycin or metronidazole. Metronidazole is usually used because it is easier to obtain and much less expensive.
   b. First-line treatment for *Shigella* is amoxicillin or sulfamethoxazole and trimethoprim. Organism resistance has been reported to these agents necessitating treatment with third-generation cephalosporins.
   c. *Campylobacter jejuni* is treated with erythromycin.
   d. First-line therapy for *Giardia lamblia* is metronidazole.
   e. *Yersinia* is treated with sulfamethoxazole and trimethoprim, chloramphenicol, or tetracycline (>8 years of age).

13.4.3 Chronic Diarrhea

A. By definition, chronic (persistent) diarrhea lasts longer than 14 days.

B. Etiologies
1. Infectious diseases as noted in section 13.4.2.
2. Metabolic causes include endocrine tumors, neuroendocrine tumors, hyperthyroidism, diabetes mellitus, and specific disaccharide enzyme deficiencies.
3. Intestinal abnormalities include microvillus atrophy, short gut syndrome, inflammatory bowel disease, protein-losing enteropathy, and milk allergy.
4. Chronic pancreatitis, Schwachman-Diamond syndrome, and cystic fibrosis lead to diarrhea due to pancreatic enzyme insufficiency.
5. Hepatic bile acid deficiency due to cholestatic syndromes result in fat malabsorption and diarrhea.
6. The acquired causes of acute diarrhea may cause chronic diarrhea as well.
7. Nonspecific diarrhea of infancy (toddler's diarrhea) has no defined etiology. Children have no sign of illness except for diarrhea.

C. Physical exam may be normal or reveal stigmata of the underlying disease.

D. Laboratory studies are performed to confirm the suspected diagnoses.
1. Stool examination is performed for consistency, pH, reducing substances, fecal leukocytes, blood, fat globules, ova and parasites, and cultures.
2. Stool can be collected to assess for fat malabsorption (72 hour fecal fat test) or protein malabsorption (α_1-antitrypsin clearance), and electrolyte content.
3. Blood evaluation can include a complete blood count, erythrocyte sedimentation rate, C-reactive protein, a comprehensive metabolic panel, immunoglobulins, human immunodeficiency syndrome, coagulation studies, and lead levels.
4. Available urine tests are urinalysis, cultures, homovanillic acid, and vanillylmandelic acid (pheochromocytoma).
5. Specialized tests include sweat chloride (cystic fibrosis), breath hydrogen test (enzyme deficiency), and tissue biopsy.

E. Management
1. Nonspecific diarrhea of infancy (toddler's diarrhea) requires no therapy.
2. Fruit juices should be avoided.
3. In postinfectious diarrhea, although no specific therapy is indicated, adequate protein and calorie intake enhances resolution.
4. Specific therapies for other etiologies.
   - **a.** Enterokinase deficiency: protein hydrolysate formula and pancreatic enzyme replacement.
   - **b.** Short gut syndrome and microvillus atrophy: parenteral nutrition, somatostatin analogues, and prednisone (if autoimmune).
   - **c.** Protein-losing enteropathy. treat the underlying disorder.
   - **d.** Bacterial overgrowth. administer poorly absorbed antibiotics orally (metronidazole, gentamicin).
   - e. Inflammatory bowel disease: corticosteroids (most effective), sulfasalazine (except isolated small bowel Crohn's disease), calorie supplementation, and an elemental diet if the disease is resistant to treatment.
   - **f.** Exocrine pancreatic insufficiency: titrated pancreatic enzyme replacement, fat soluble vitamin (A,D,E,K) supplementation, and increase calories to between 120 and 150% of maintenance requirements.
   - **g.** Lactase deficiency: lactase replacements and avoid lactose containing products.
   - **h.** Celiac disease is treated with a gluten-free diet.

13.4.4 Inflammatory Bowel Disease

A. Chronic inflammatory bowel disease can be either **Crohn's disease (regional enteritis) or ulcerative colitis**.

B. The cause is unknown but is probably due to an immunologically-mediated chronic inflammatory process in a genetically susceptible host.

C. It begins in late childhood or adolescence with bloody diarrhea, abdominal cramps, weight loss, or growth failure.

D. Extraintestinal manifestations include arthritis, ankylosing spondylitis, skin rash, ophthalmologic inflammation, hepatitis, and fever.

E. **Table 13.4.4** Differentiating features of Crohn's disease and ulcerative colitis

FEATURES	CROHN'S DISEASE	ULCERATIVE COLITIS
Rectal bleeding	+/-	+
Rectal disease	+/-	++
Abdominal mass	+	-
Ileal disease	+	-
Perineal disease	+	-
Strictures and fistulas	+	-
Skip lesions	+	-
Transmual disease	+	-
Crypt abscesses	-	+
Granulomas	+	-
Colon cancer risk	+/-	++

F. Differential Diagnosis
1. Infections
   - **a.** Bacterial: *Yersinia, Campylobacter, Salmonella, Shigella,* and Tuberculosis.
   - **b.** Parasitic: *Entamoeba histolytica* and *Giardia lamblia.*
   - **c.** Human immunodeficiency virus related: *Cryptosporidium* and cytomegalovirus.
2. Immunologic diseases include congenital or acquired immunodeficiency, Behçet's syndrome, lymphoid nodular hyperplasia, and graft-versus-host disease.
3. Vasculitic diseases in the differential are systemic lupus erythematosus, Henoch-Schönlein purpura,

and hemolytic-uremic syndrome.

4. Malignancy such as lymphoma and adenocarcinoma can present similarly to inflammatory bowel disease.

G. Treatment.

1. Pharmacotherapy is described in section 13.4.3. Additionally, azathioprine, metronidazole, and clarithromycin are useful in the treatment of perirectal fistulas (Crohn's disease).
2. Surgical resection of affected bowel segments. Recurrence rate is high in Crohn's disease.
3. Ensure adequate protein and calorie intake.
4. Mental health intervention may be appropriate, especially for adolescents, to aid the patient and family cope with chronic disease.

13.4.5 Gastrointestinal Bleeding

A. Etiology of Upper Gastrointestinal Bleeding by Age Group (Table 13.4.5A)

B. Etiology of Lower Gastrointestinal Bleeding by Age Group (Table 13.4.5B)

C. Infectious causes of hematochezia can occur at any age and include *Salmonella, Shigella, Yersinia, Campylobacter jejuni,* enterohemorrhagic *Escherichia coli,* enteroinvasive *Escherichia coli, Clostridium difficile,* and *Entamoeba histolytica.*

D. Diagnostic Studies

1. Laboratory studies include complete blood count, erythrocyte sedimentation rate, prothrombin time, partial thromboplastin time, blood urea nitrogen, creatinine, liver transaminases, and stool studies (leukocytes, occult blood, cultures).
2. Radiological investigations include upper gastrointestinal series with or without followthrough, barium enema (single contrast for obstruction, double contrast for mucosal abnormalities), or plain abdominal x-rays to rule out obstruction.
3. Specialized tests include endoscopy, biopsy, Meckel's scan, angiography, and technetium 99 tagged red blood cell scan (bleeding scan).
4. Gastric lavage can be performed to confirm mild upper gastrointestinal bleeding.

E. Management

1. Initial stabilization with intravascular volume and blood replacement, nasogastric suction, and maintain in a nulla per os (NPO; nothing by mouth) status.
2. Gastric lavage may be both therapeutic and diagnostic.
3. Endoscopy allows direct visualization of the bleeding site for intravascular injection of vasoactive agents (vasopressin, somatostatin), sclerotherapy, and thermal or laser coagulation.
4. Balloon tamponade is used as a temporizing measure. Occasionally bleeding will not recur.

13.4.6 Malabsorptive Disorders

A. These are disorders that lead to defective assimilation of nutrients.

B. They manifest with abdominal distension, pale, foul, bulky stools, retardation of height and weight growth, and muscle weakness.

C. Causes

1. Defective digestion due to pancreatic deficiency (cystic fibrosis pancreatitis, Schwachman-Diamond syndrome) and bile salt deficiency (biliary atresia, cholestasis, hepatitis, cirrhosis, bacterial deconjugation).
2. Defective absorption due to primary absorption defects, glucose-galactose malabsorption, abetalipoproteinemia, cystinuria, and Hartnup's disease.
3. Decreased mucosal surface area as seen in Crohn's disease, malnutrition, and short bowel syndrome.
4. Small intestinal diseases leading to malabsorption include celiac disease, tropical sprue, giardiasis, lymphoma, and allergic enteritis.
5. Infestations with hookworm, tapeworm, and opportunistic infections in immunosuppressed states, such as acquired immunodeficiency syndrome, cause malabsorption.
6. Lymphatic obstruction such as lymphangiectasia, Whipple's disease, and lymphoma also lead to symptoms.

D. Diagnostic Studies

1. Laboratory evaluation includes a complete blood count, chemistries, cultures, stool for parasites, and

Table 13.4.5A Etiology of upper gastrointestinal bleeding by age group

NEONATE	INFANT	CHILD	ADOLESCENT
Swallowed maternal blood Gastritis Esophagitis Congenital blood dyscrasia Vascular malformation	Gastritis Esophagitis Stress ulcer Mallory-Weiss tear Duplication Vascular malformation	Esophageal varices Peptic ulcer disease Stress ulcer Gastritis Mallory-Weiss tear Foreign body Esophagitis	Esophageal varices Peptic ulcer disease Gastritis Mallory-Weiss tear Esophagitis Stress ulcer

measurement of serum vitamins, protein, and immunoglobulins.

2. Gut Absorptive Function
   a. Fat absorption can be quantitated by measurement of fecal fat content and fasting serum carotene.
   b. Carbohydrate absorption is evaluated by measuring stool for reducing substances and breath hydrogen testing.
   c. Protein absorption is measured by documenting enteric protein loss and fecal α_1-antitrypsin clearance.
3. Radiologic imaging includes basic x-rays, ultrasound, and barium studies as well as specialized studies such as retrograde pancreatic and biliary tree studies.
4. Endoscopy and biopsy are used for tissue diagnosis.

13.4.7 α_1-Antitrypsin Deficiency

A. Clinical illness results when patients with this illness have a low level of α_1-antitrypsin protease.

B. Affected children present with neonatal cholestasis which resolves usually without diagnosis, failure to thrive, hepatomegaly, or with cirrhosis.

C. Patients may also have chronic lung disease.

D. No specific treatment for the deficiency is available, but end-stage liver disease can be treated with transplantation.

13.4.8 Pancreatitis

A. This is inflammation of the pancreas caused by activation of pancreatic enzymes and autodigestion of the organ.

B. Numerous predisposing factors have been identified. They include trauma, surgery, infection (mumps, mycoplasma), biliary obstruction, congenital abnormalities, drugs, diabetes mellitus, hyperlipidemia, and rheumatologic disease.

C. Most patients present with abdominal pain that radiates to the back, nausea, and vomiting.

D. Physical examination may reveal a tender, distended abdomen with decreased bowel sounds. Depending on the mechanism of their disease and the severity of the pancreatitis, some patients may present in shock.

E. Laboratory findings show elevated serum amylase and lipase levels.

F. Complications of acute pancreatitis include hyperglycemia, hypocalcemia, peritonitis, abscess formation from secondary infection, hemorrhage, and pseudocyst.

G. Therapy
1. The child is made NPO.
2. Low intermittent nasogastric suction is performed.
3. Intravenous fluids to maintain hydration and hyperalimentation if the child remains NPO for more than a few days.
4. Pain control with meperidine. Morphine sulfate may be associated with spasm of the sphincter of Oddi so is not usually used in the presence of pancreatitis.
5. Surgery may be required to address disease complications.

13.5 SURGICAL GASTROINTESTINAL DISEASE

13.5.1 Pyloric Stenosis

A. Pyloric stenosis is gastric outlet obstruction secondary to hypertrophy and hyperplasia of the pyloric sphincter. The antral musculature is involved as well.

B. It usually occurs in males (1:150). Multifactorial inheritance is likely, but it sometimes occurs in mini-epidemics.

C. Symptoms include gradual onset of nonbilious vomiting progressing to projectile episodes. The baby is hungry and will feed voraciously even right after the vomiting episodes.

D. Complications
1. Prolonged vomiting gives rise to failure to thrive.
2. Gastritis with or without hemorrhage may occur.
3. The classic electrolyte disturbance associated with pyloric stenosis is hypochloremic metabolic alkalosis with or without dehydration.

Table 13.4.5B Etiology of lower gastrointestinal bleeding by age group

NEONATE	INFANT	CHILD	ADOLESCENT
Anal fissure Upper gastrointestinal bleeding Volvulus Necrotizing enterocolitis Swallowed maternal blood Infectious colitis Milk allergy Blood dyscrasia Duplication	Anal fissure Intussusception Meckel's diverticulum Infectious diarrhea Milk allergy Duplication Pseudomembranous colitis	Polyps Anal fissure Meckel's diverticulum Infectious diarrhea Henoch-Schönlein purpura Hemolytic-uremic syndrome Intussusception Pseudomembranous colitis	Polyps Hemorrhoids Inflammatory bowel disease Infectious diarrhea

4. Hyperbilirubinemia is sometimes seen as well.

E. Diagnosis
1. A careful history is suggestive of the disease.
2. Palpation of the pyloric "olive" is diagnostic. Unfortunately the olive is palpable only about half of the time. Successful palpation requires a vast amount of patience, a relaxed anterior abdominal wall, and an empty stomach.
3. Peristaltic waves may be transmitted to the anterior abdominal wall and may be visible on exam.
4. Confirmation of the diagnosis is by ultrasound examination of the pylorus or an upper gastrointestinal x-ray series demonstrating a thin line of barium traversing the pylorus (string sign).

F. Management
1. Correction of electrolyte and acid-base abnormalities followed by surgical pyloromyotomy.
2. Nonsurgical treatment with a cholinergic blocking agent has been abandoned.

13.5.2 Hirschsprung's Disease

A. This is the absence of intramural neural ganglia in the rectum leading to constipation.

B. Pathogenesis
1. Research suggests that Hirschsprung's disease results from arrest of vagal neural crest cell migration due to abnormalities of the extracellular matrix of the distal bowel.
2. Extrinsic nerve axonal processes still enter the bowel, proliferate, and stimulate unopposed contraction, resulting in functional obstruction of the aganglionic bowel segment.

C. Epidemiology
1. It is a rare condition with an incidence of 1:5,000 live births.
2. Males are predominantly affected (80%).
3. A family history can be obtained in 7% of cases.
4. Risk of disease to a sibling of an affected patient is 2.5%.

D. Associations are noted with Waardenburg's syndrome, Smith-Lemli-Opitz syndrome, trisomy 21, and 13 short arm deletion syndrome.

E. Presentation
1. Newborns demonstrate delayed passage of meconium with constipation in the first several days, ultimately with the development of symptoms of intestinal obstruction.
2. Older infants have a history of constipation and may present with toxic megacolon.

F. Diagnosis
1. Unprepped barium enema examination reveals a small distal colon with a dilated segment of bowel above the "transition zone." The dilated bowel is the normal bowel.
2. Anorectal manometry evaluates response of the anal sphincter to inflation of a balloon in the rectum (negative response in Hirschsprung's disease).
3. Suction rectal biopsy can be performed. If the specimen is insufficient for diagnosis, full thickness rectal biopsy is indicated.

G. Management
1. The only effective treatment is resection of the affected segment of bowel.
2. Infants who do not require urgent surgery can be managed for a short period of time with daily rectal saline washes.

13.5.3 Appendicitis

A. Appendicitis is the most common condition leading to abdominal surgery in childhood.

B. The classic presentation of symptoms is fever, anorexia, malaise, and periumbilical abdominal pain that ultimately localizes to the right lower quadrant.

C. Diagnosis is made based on history and physical. Adjunctive tests such as a complete blood count', urinalysis, ultrasound, abdominal c-ray, and computed tomography scanning can be used to support or confirm the diagnosis.

D. Treatment is by surgical excision of the inflamed appendix.

E. The most frequent complication is perforation. This occurs most commonly in children under 2 years of age or those with an atypical presentation leading to a delay in the diagnosis of appendicitis.

13.5.4 Intussusception

A. This is the telescoping (invagination) of one portion of the intestinal tract into a distal segment.

B. The most common location is ileocolonic. It occurs most frequently in toddlers.

C. Intussusception occurs at the location of an anatomic lead point such as a Meckel's diverticulum, polyp, tumor, or hypertrophied Peyer's patches. The lead point is drawn into the intestinal lumen and peristalsed distally, drawing bowel with it.

D. Presentation
1. Children may demonstrate severe, colicky abdominal pain and have bouts of crying with intervening calm periods.
2. Other children become lethargic and may be mistaken for having a neurologic injury or sepsis.
3. Occasionally a right lower quadrant mass can be palpated.
4. Children may have vomiting.
5. The classic finding of bloody "currant jelly" stools is a late finding and implies significant bowel wall ischemia.

E. Diagnosis

1. History and examination are often suggestive of the condition.
2. Abdominal x-ray may demonstrate obstruction, decreased air in the right lower quadrant, or may be normal.
3. The lesion can be demonstrated by ultrasound.
4. Barium or air contrast enema will demonstrate the intussusception and often is used to reduce the defect.

F. Treatment is by surgical repair if hydrostatic reduction has failed or if the child has intestinal perforation.

13.5.5 Biliary Atresia

A. Biliary atresia is a congenital disorder of bile duct paucity in the liver.

B. The condition usually presents within the first several weeks of life as persistent jaundice with elevation of direct bilirubin above the level expected with physiologic jaundice.

C. Signs and symptoms include jaundice, acholic stools, and a firm liver on palpation.

D. Diagnosis
1. The gallbladder is not filled and is difficult to identify on ultrasound.
2. Nuclear medicine studies of hepatic uptake (hepatobiliary iminodiacetic acid [HIDA] scan) show no excretion of contrast into the small bowel.
3. Biopsy, if performed, reveals bile ductule proliferation and portal fibrosis.

E. Treatment
1. Portoenterostomy (Kasai procedure) can provide successful drainage of the biliary tract if performed before the infant is 2 months of age.
2. Liver transplantation is an option for those patients who fail portoenterostomy.

F. Choledochal cyst is a malformation of the biliary tree that presents with symptoms very similar to biliary atresia. It is amenable to surgical correction if it is an isolated defect.

263. Which of the following are physiologic functions of the gastrointestinal tract — E 13.1.1

A. motility
B. immune defense
C. secretion
D. absorption
E. all of the above

264. Mesodermal tissue gives rise to which portions of the gastrointestinal tract — B 13.1.2

A. mucosa
B. muscle
C. crypts
D. secretory cells
E. all of the above

265. A child is evaluated because of abdominal pain and weight loss. Which of the following findings is most suggestive of an underlying organic disease — C 13.1.3

A. periumbilical location of the pain
B. pain only on school days
C. uveitis
D. large, formed stools
E. a scar from a repaired inguinal hernia

266. Which of the following are potential complications of cleft lip and palate — D 13.2.1

A. speech disorder
B. failure to thrive from poor caloric intake
C. dental malocclusion
D. all of the above
E. A and C

267. A 7-week-old infant presents with persistent direct hyperbilirubinemia. On exam you note acholic stool, jaundice, and firm hepatomegaly. What test would you perform next to make the diagnosis — D 13.5.5

A. hepatitis virus profile
B. hepatic transaminase levels
C. liver biopsy
D. hepatobiliary iminodiacetic acid (HIDA) scan
E. kidney, ureter, bladder (KUB) x-ray

268. A newborn infant has coughing, cyanosis, and respiratory distress that began with the first feed and now persists. He also is noted to be drooling excessively and has abdominal distention. What is his likely diagnosis — C 13.2.3

A. choanal atresia
B. respiratory distress syndrome
C. tracheoesophageal fistula
D. sepsis
E. necrotizing enterocolitis

269. A 6-year-old presents with a 1 day history of periumbilical pain that is now localized to the right lower quadrant. He also has fever, malaise, anorexia, and nausea. What is the most frequent complication of this condition — D 13.5.3

A. sepsis
B. thrombosis
C. postoperative infection
D. perforation
E. hypovolemic shock

270. Which of the following abdominal wall birth defects is covered by peritoneum alone — A 13.2.4

A. omphalocele
B. gastroschisis
C. umbilical hernia
D. ventral abdominal wall hernia

271. A child presents for a well child exam. Her mother is concerned about the "lump on her belly button." You palpate a <5 mm fascial defect at the base of the umbilicus. Your advice to the infant's mother is — B 13.2.6

A. tape a quarter over the defect
B. reassure her that the defect will close on its own
C. she must take her child to see the surgeon for repair next week
D. she will have an "outee" when she gets older

272. Which gastrointestinal disorder is associated with the "double bubble" sign on x-ray — D 13.2.7

A. pyloric stenosis
B. ileal atresia
C. jejunal atresia
D. duodenal atresia
E. tracheoesophageal fistula

273. A 3-week-old infant presents with a history of bilious emesis and abdominal distention of 1 days duration. What test will you order to make the diagnosis — D 13.2.7

A. pyloric ultrasound
B. kidney, ureter, bladder (KUB) x-ray
C. barium enema
D. upper gastrointestinal series with follow through
E. endoscopy

274. A 3-week-old infant presents with a history of vomiting that has become projectile over the past week. He appears dehydrated. What is his acid-base and electrolyte status — D 13.5.1

A. hyperchloremic, metabolic alkalosis
B. hyperchloremic, metabolic acidosis
C. hypochloremic, metabolic acidosis
D. hypochloremic, metabolic alkalosis

275. Which gastrointestinal abnormality is associated with the "string sign" on radiologic exam — B 13.5.1

A. duodenal atresia
B. pyloric stenosis
C. Hirschsprung's disease
D. intussusception
E. appendicitis

276. All of the following are included in the "rule of 2's" for Meckel's diverticulum except — C 13.2.8

A. it occurs in 2% of the population
B. it has 2 tissues, gastric and pancreatic
C. it has a 2:1 female to male predominance
D. it is located 2 feet proximal to the ileocecal valve
E. it has 2 presentations, hemorrhage and obstruction

277. What is the most common type of tracheoesophageal fistula — B 13.2.3

A. isolated fistula between the esophagus and trachea
B. proximal esophageal blind pouch with a distal tracheoesophageal fistula
C. proximal and distal fistulas between the esophagus and trachea
D. H-type tracheoesophageal fistula

278. An 18-month-old child presents with lethargy, a palpable abdominal mass, and bleeding from the rectum. He seemed to have had abdominal pain 1 day prior to presentation. What is the most likely diagnosis — A 13.5.4

A. intussusception
B. Meckel's diverticulum
C. volvulus
D. colonic polyp
E. Henoch-Schönlein purpura

279. A child presents with a 3 week history of watery diarrhea. Laboratory study reveals that the stool is acidic, with high osmolarity, and is positive for reducing substances. What type of diarrhea is this child having — C 13.3.2

A. secretory diarrhea
B. diarrhea secondary to increased peristalsis
C. osmotic diarrhea
D. diarrhea secondary to direct mucosal injury
E. diarrhea secondary to decreased mucosal area

280. A 4-month-old child presents with a few day history of lethargy and constipation. He is not breathing well and requires mechanical ventilatory support. In your history, you discover that his grandmother has been feeding him raw honey to treat a previous history of firm stools. What is his probable diagnosis — A 13.3.3

A. infantile botulism
B. hypothyroidism
C. anal stenosis
D. ileal atresia
E. intussusception

281. Which of the following is commonly associated with functional fecal retention, but not with Hirschsprung's disease — D 13.3.3

A. constipation as a newborn
B. obstructive symptoms
C. delayed passage of meconium
D. fecal incontinence
E. all of the above

282. Which syndrome is associated with gastroesophageal reflux, arching of the back during feeding, head turning, and pain — C 13.4.1

A. Hirschsprung disease's
B. Zollinger-Ellison syndrome
C. Sandifer's syndrome
D. cystic fibrosis
E. Blount's disease

283. An 8-year-old with a recent history of mumps presents with nausea, vomiting, and abdominal pain radiating to the back. What is appropriate therapy for his condition — B 13.4.8

A. give him morphine for pain control
B. make him stop oral feedings and place a nasogastric tube to low intermittent suction
C. call a urologist to evaluate him for orchitis
D. call a surgeon to take out his gallbladder
E. send him home with instructions for frequent small amounts of oral fluid to maintain hydration

284. A 6-year-old child has received multiple courses of antibiotics for "sinusitis." He now has bloody diarrhea secondary to *Clostridium difficile.* What is the treatment of choice for his condition — A 13.4.2

A. oral metronidazole
B. intravenous vancomycin
C. oral metoclopramide
D. oral erythromycin
E. antibiotic therapy is not indicated

285. A 3-year-old has a 2 month history of watery stools a few times per day. Stool studies, hepatitis profile, complete blood count, and serum chemistries are all normal. Which of the following historical or physical findings would suggest the diagnosis of toddler's diarrhea — E 13.4.3

A. nightly abdominal pain
B. intermittent bloody stools
C. decreased height velocity
D. sibling with cystic fibrosis
E. normal weight gain

286. Which of the following findings is present in ulcerative colitis but usually absent in Crohn's disease — A 13.4.4

A. crypt abscesses
B. perianal disease
C. fistulas
D. skip lesions
E. ileal disease

287. A 1-day-old vomits blood, but is otherwise normal on exam. The initial evaluation should include all of the following except — E 13.4.7

A. evaluate the mother's breasts for cracked, bleeding nipples
B. complete blood count
C. prothrombin time and partial thromboplastin time
D. saline gastric lavage
E. immediate referral for angiography

288. A 6-year-old presents with chronic jaundice and hepatic cirrhosis. Past laboratory evaluation has ruled out infectious hepatitis as the cause and he has no history of toxin exposure. His past history is remarkable for jaundice at birth that resolved after 2 weeks of age. His family history is significant for nonsmoking family members with emphysema. What is his probable diagnosis — B 13.4.9

A. Epstein-Barr virus hepatitis
B. α-1-antitrypsin deficiency
C. cystic fibrosis
D. ulcerative colitis
E. Wilson's disease

289. A 2-month-old child is admitted to the hospital for observation, following an acute life-threatening event. His weight is only a few ounces above birth weight. His history is significant for recurrent vomiting and pain with feeding. Once an obstructive lesion is ruled out, what is the next step in treatment — B 13.4.1

A. consult a surgeon to perform a fundoplication
B. start therapy with metoclopramide and ranitidine and see him in clinic in 1 week
C. institute reflux precautions alone and follow weight gain as an outpatient
D. recommend no pharmacologic therapy as the infant will eventually outgrow his reflux
E. contact Child Protective Services for placement of the child in therapeutic foster care

290. The barium enema, performed on an infant with severe constipation and symptoms of obstruction, reveals a narrow sigmoid colon with dilatation of the proximal descending colon above the transition zone. Which segment is normal bowel — A 13.5.2

A. the dilated segment
B. the narrowed segment
C. both
D. neither

291. What is the treatment of choice for intussusception — B 13.5.4

A. surgical reduction in all cases
B. hydrostatic reduction with air or barium enema
C. colonoscopic reduction
D. intravenous fluids and hospitalization

292. Mandibular distraction is treatment for which of the following conditions — A 13.2.2

A. Pierre Robin sequence
B. cleft palate
C. laryngomalacia
D. laryngeal cleft
E. macroglossia

293. All of the following are true regarding Hirschsprung's disease except — C 13.5.2

A. males are affected more often than females
B. incidence is higher in children with Down's syndrome
C. siblings of affected patients have a 7% risk of disease
D. short-term management may include rectal saline washes
E. definitive treatment is resection of the affected portion of bowel

294. The pathophysiology of diarrhea in cystic fibrosis is — C 13.4.3

A. bacterial overgrowth
B. increased peristalsis
C. pancreatic enzyme deficiency
D. bile acid deficiency
E. disaccharidase deficiency

14 RENAL DISORDERS

14.1 GENERAL CONCEPTS

14.1.1 The Newborn

A. Nephrogenesis is not complete until 36 weeks of gestation. Therefore, premature infants have compromised renal functional capacity compared to full-term infants.

B. Fetal urine is excreted into the amniotic fluid.
   1. Oligohydramnios will result from inadequate urine output from a fetus.
   2. Inadequate amniotic fluid is associated with pulmonary hypoplasia which may be incompatible with life.
   3. **Potter's syndrome**, characterized by a typical facial appearance, low set ears, and pulmonary hypoplasia, can result from severe intrauterine oliguria or anuria.

C. Intrauterine urinary tract obstruction can cause renal dysplasia with resulting renal insufficiency from which the infant may not completely recover.

D. Serum creatinine (Cr) for the first 5 days of life in the newborn reflects the mother's Cr level, not the infant's renal function.

E. **Glomerular Filtration Rate** (GFR)
   1. The GFR at birth is 20 to 30 ml/1.73 m^2/min.
   2. The GFR doubles to 40 to 60ml/1.73m^2/min by 2 weeks after birth.
   3. The GFR should reach adult levels (120 ml/1.73m^2/min) by 2 years of age.
   4. Drugs cleared by renal excretion may cause toxicity if given to infants in doses based on expected adult level GFR.

F. Urine Concentrating and Diluting Ability
   1. Newborn kidneys can only concentrate urine to 1/2 that of adults (600 to 700 mosm/kg, instead of 1,200 to 1,400 mosm/kg).
   2. Newborns can dilute urine to adult levels (50 mosm/kg), but total water load excretion is limited by decreased GFR.

G. Electrolyte Regulation. Newborns can neither conserve nor effectively excrete excess sodium. As a result, potassium and hydrogen secretion are impaired.

14.1.2 Diagnostic Modalities

A. **Specific Gravity**
   1. 1.002 (50 mosm/kg osmolality) reflects a maximally dilute urine.
   2. 1.035 (1200 mosm/kg osmolality) reflects maximally concentrated urine.
   3. 1.010 (300 mosm/kg osmolality; isosthenuria) reflects neither concentration nor dilution of filtered serum.

B. Urine Dipsticks
   1. Dipsticks are readily available and can measure albumin, glucose, ketones, bilirubin, blood, and leukocyte esterase.
   2. Positive blood in the absence of red blood cells (RBCs) in the microscopic urinalysis occurs from free hemoglobin and myoglobin in the urine.

C. **Urine Microscopy**
   1. Useful for identifying RBCs, white blood cells, casts, crystals, and bacteria.
   2. The presence of epithelial cells should also be noted since large numbers may reflect a nonclean catch specimen.
   3. The urine must be examined as soon as possible after voiding to accurately identify microscopic components because cells and casts can lyse in the urine.

D. **Urine Electrolytes**
   1. Sodium (Na^+). Maximal conservation is reflected by a value of <20 mEq/L.
   In renal failure the urine Na^+ is >50 mEq/L.
   2. Chloride (Cl^-). Maximum conservation is reflected by a value <10 mEq/L. The significance of urine Cl^- concentrations must be interpreted in light of the patient's acid-base status.
   3. Potassium (K^+). Maximal tubular conservation is reflected in a value of <20 mEq/L.
      a. Low values may reflect a total body deficit of K^+ regardless of the serum K^+ level.
      b. Urine K^+ also reflects renin activity and tubular response to that activity. Increased renin activity (whether physiologically or pathologically elevated) will increase K^+ excretion. Renin can be elevated in response to hypovolemic states even in the presence of total body or serum K^+ deficits.

E. **Glomerular Function Tests**
   1. Blood Urea Nitrogen (BUN)
      a. BUN is dependent on dietary protein intake.
      b. BUN begins to rise when the GFR is <50% the normal value.
      c. Elevation is also caused by blood in gastrointestinal tract.
      d. Upon restoration of normal renal function, an elevated BUN level should decrease by 1/2 its value every 16 hours.
   2. Serum Cr is not influenced by protein intake. The normal value can be estimated by the formula: Cr = 0.004 x height (in centimeters).
   3. BUN/Cr Ratio
      a. Normal is 15:1 (range 10:1 to 20:1).
      b. In prerenal azotemia the ratio is >40:1.
   4. GFR. The most common method used for measuring the GFR is by calculating the Creatinine Clearance (C_{Cr}).

a. $C_{Cr} = \dfrac{\text{Urine Cr x Urine Volume}}{\text{Plasma Cr}}$

b. Corrected $C_{Cr} = \dfrac{\text{Patient's } C_{Cr} \text{ x } 1.73 \text{ m}^2}{\text{Patient's surface area}}$

c. Simplified $C_{Cr} = \dfrac{\text{K x Height (in cm.)}}{\text{Plasma Cr (in mg/dl)}}$

K = 0.45 under 1 year of age
K = 0.55 over 1 year of age

F. **Renal Tubular Function Tests**

1. Tubular function tests can help differentiate between causes of oliguria due to decreased GFR in the presence of tubules with normal functional capability (prerenal azotemia) and those accompanied by more diffuse renal damage (renal failure azotemia).
2. In prerenal azotemia the Fractional excretion of Na^+ (FENa) is low (<1%), whereas, in renal failure azotemia, it is high (>7%).
3. FENa calculation:

$$\text{FENa} = \frac{\text{Urine Na}^+ \text{ x Serum Cr}}{\text{Urine Cr x Serum Na}^+} \text{ x } 100\%$$

G. **Imaging Tests**

1. Ultrasound is noninvasive. It can identify the size, shape, and density of the kidneys, but is not helpful for assessing renal function.
2. The availability of radionuclide scanning has largely replaced the need for intravenous pyelography (IVP) in children. Besides the potential of allergic reactions to the dye, IVP's tonicity can precipitate renal failure. IVP does provide better delineation of caliceal structures than radionuclide scans.
3. Voiding cystourethrography (VCUG) is useful for identifying vesicoureteral reflux. The same information can be obtained more safely with radionuclide scanning, except for visualization of the urethra.
4. Radionuclide scanning can provide as assessment of the GFR in each kidney as well as assessment of tubular activity depending on which isotope is used. When the isotope is instilled into the bladder instead of being given intravenously, radionuclide scanning can be used for cystograms (identifying vesicoureteral reflux), but not for visualization of the urethra.

H. **Serum Complement** (especially C3). Hypocomplementemia can be found in the following conditions:

1. Poststreptococcal Glomerulonephritis. Levels should return to normal within 8 weeks.
2. Systemic Lupus Erythematosus. Decreased complement reflects exacerbation of active lupus nephritis.
3. Membranoproliferative Glomerulonephritis. The complement level remains persistently low.
4. Chronic Infections. Decreased complement reflects vasculitis which can involve the glomerular artery.
5. Vasculitis. Hereditary complement deficiencies can also be associated with vasculitis.

I. Renal biopsy may be necessary if a histologic diagnosis is needed. It is generally not needed in uncomplicated cases of lipoid nephrosis of childhood nor in acute glomerulonephritis.

14.1.3 Renal Dialysis: indications for Dialysis

A. In acute renal failure, the level of BUN and/or Cr are not the determining factors in deciding when to initiate dialysis.

B. Dialysis is initiated in acute renal failure to control the following:

1. Metabolic acidosis and electrolyte abnormalities. Hyperkalemia may not be controlled by diet alone when the GFR drops below 5 ml/min/1.73m^2.
2. Fluid overload with resultant hypertension, congestive heart failure, and pulmonary edema.
3. Uremic complications such as encephalopathy, pericarditis or pericardial effusion, and coagulation disturbances.

C. In chronic renal failure, dialysis will generally be required when the GFR falls to < 0.1 to 0.15 ml/min/kg (7 to 11 ml/min/1.73m^2).

14.1.4 Pathophysiologic Manifestations

A. **Oliguria**

1. Oliguria may be a normal physiologic response to water and/or salt depletion (prerenal oliguria) or a reflection of renal failure. The concomitant presence of azotemia reflects a process beyond the kidney's ability to compensate.
2. **Table 14.1.4A** Differentiation of prerenal versus renal oliguria

TEST	PRERENAL	RENAL
FENa	<1%	>3%
BUN/Cr ratio	>20:1	<10:1
Urine Specific Gravity	>1.015	<1.010

BUN = blood urea nitrogen; Cr = creatinine; FENa = fractional excretion of sodium

B. **Edema**

1. Edema formation requires an excessive accumulation of both Na^+ and salt.
2. The kidneys may cause edema due to ineffective excretion of Na^+ and water or through their enhanced reabsorption, either to replenish a decreased intravascular volume or in response to mineralocorticoid excesses.
3. Causes of Generalized Edema
   a. Inability to excrete a Na^+ and water load as in

glomerular lesions resulting in decreased GFR or excess salt intake.

b. Loss of plasma oncotic pressure as seen with nephrotic syndrome, protein-losing enteropathy, and chronic heart failure.

c. Decreased cardiac output as seen with congestive heart failure and pericardial effusion.

d. Excessive mineralocorticoid activity as in hyperrenin states, hyperaldosteronism, and corticosteroid excess.

e. Hepatic failure.

C. Polyuria

1. Water conservation is dependent on antidiuretic hormone (ADH) and its effect at end-organ sites on the distal renal tubules.
2. Causes of Polyuria
   a. Central diabetes insipidus (ADH deficiency) may be idiopathic or acquired (central nervous system infection, pituitary trauma).
   b. Nephrogenic diabetes insipidus may be inherited or acquired (interstitial nephritis, sickle cell disease, chronic renal failure, hypokalemia, papillary necrosis).
   c. Other causes are osmotic load (diabetes mellitus, iatrogenic hyperglycemia, mannitol), psychogenic polydipsia, diuretic use, and volume expansion (intravenous fluid administration, diuretic phase of resolving acute renal failure).

D. Hypertension

1. Renal diseases are the most common organic cause of hypertension in children. The finding of hypertension demands evaluation of renal function.
2. Hypertension may be due to salt and water retention, excess rennin, or both as the result of a renal disease.
3. In general hypertension should be further evaluated if the blood pressure is greater than 120/80 in infants, 140/90 in children, or 160/100 in adolescents, or is associated with the following signs of end-organ insult:
   a. Central Nervous System. Hypertensive encephalopathy, increased intracranial pressure, headache, seizures, or altered sensorium.
   b. Cardiovascular. Congestive heart failure, pulmonary edema, or ventricular hypertrophy.
   c. Kidney. Proteinuria or decreased GFR.

E. Hematuria and Proteinuria

1. Hematuria. RBCs exceed the normal range of 0 to 5 RBC/high powered field.
2. Proteinuria
   a. Normal protein excretion is <4 mg/m^2/hour.
   b. Nephrotic syndrome is a rate of protein excretion >40 mg/m^2/hour.
3. Differentiating the cause of proteinuria and/or hematuria can be facilitated by consideration of associated findings in the patient.
   a. Proteinuria without Hematuria or Edema
      1). Transient proteinuria.
      2). Orthostatic proteinuria.
      3). "Allergic" phenomena.
      4). Prenephrotic.
      5). Focal segmental glomerulosclerosis.
   b. Proteinuria with Edema and No Hematuria
      1). Minimal-change nephrotic syndrome.
      2). Focal segmental glomerulosclerosis.
   c. Proteinuria with Edema and Hematuria
      1). Acute glomerulonephritis.
      2). Minimal-change nephrotic syndrome.
      3). Chronic and/or progressive glomerulonephritis.
         a). Lupus nephritis.
         b). Membranoproliferative glomerulonephritis.
         c). Hereditary glomerulonephritis.
   d. Proteinuria with Hematuria and No Edema
      1). Acute glomerulonephritis.
      2). Idiopathic hypercalciuria.
      3). Immunoglobulin A (IgA) nephropathy
      4). Reflux nephropathy.
      5). Acute intestinal nephritis.
      6). Urinary tract infection.
      7). Cystic kidneys.
   e. Hematuria without Proteinuria or Edema
      1). Benign transient hematuria.
      2). Trauma.
      3). Idiopathic hypercalciuria.
      4). Nephrolithiasis.
      5). Urethral foreign body.

F. Enuresis

1. Ninety percent of children stop bedwetting by 5 years of age.
2. Urinary tract infections and idiopathic hypercalcinuria need to be ruled out.
3. See sections 4.2.1 and 4.2.2 for treatment recommendations.

G. Nephrotic Syndrome

1. Nephrotic syndrome is characterized by proteinuria, hypoproteinemia, edema, and hyperlipidemia.
2. If urinary protein loss exceeds 40 mg/m^2/hour for an adequate length of time, hypoproteinemia (liver's inability to replenish the loss), edema (decreased oncotic pressure), and hyperlipidemia (a byproduct of increased protein synthesis by the liver) will ensue.
3. Causes of Nephrotic Syndrome
   a. Primary glomerular involvement without inflammatory change can be seen with minimal-change nephritic syndrome, focal segmental glomerulosclerosis, and congenital nephritic

syndrome.

b. Primary glomerular involvement with inflammatory change is seen with poststreptococcal glomerulonephritis, membranoproliferative glomerulonephritis, membranous nephropathy, and mesangial proliferative glomerulonephritis.

c. Glomerular insults secondary to systemic diseases with vasculitis include inflammatory diseases (systemic lupus erythematosus, Henoch-Schönlein purpura, systemic vasculitis, hemolytic-uremic syndrome), and infections (hepatitis, cytomegalovirus, Ebstein-Barr virus, subacute bacterial endocarditis, shunt nephritis, malaria).

d. Malignant diseases include lymphomas, leukemias, and solid tumors.

e. Metabolic diseases include diabetes mellitus and hypothyroidism.

f. Exogenous toxins and poisons include medications, heavy metals, and venoms.

g. Hyperviscosity or hypercoagulable states such as sickle cell disease and renal vein thrombosis also can cause nephrotic syndrome.

H. **Renal failure** is the inability of the kidney to maintain water, electrolyte, and acid-base homeostasis or to eliminate waste products of metabolism. It may occur with or without decreased urine output (oliguric or non-oliguric renal failure).

1. Acute tubular necrosis is a potentially transient renal insult which, if promptly reversed by judicious fluid supplementation and/or low dose dopamine (5 mcg/kg/min), may not progress to frank renal failure.
2. Acute renal failure is a compromise of renal function to the extent that complications can develop. Complications include:
   a. Water retention leads to dilutional hyponatremia causing coma, seizures, and lethargy.
   b. Na^+ retention leads to fluid overload causing edema, hypertension, and cardiac failure.
   c. Hyperkalemia causes cardiac rhythm and conduction disturbances.
   d. Metabolic acidosis results in impaired cellular metabolism.
   e. Uremic syndrome leads to accumulation of "uremic toxins" which eventually causes anorexia, encephalopathy, pericarditis, and a prolonged bleeding time.

   Dialysis may be required to support the patient until renal function has improved.
3. Chronic Renal Failure. In addition to the complications seen in acute renal failure, chronic renal failure is characterized by:
   a. Malnutrition and Growth Failure. Dialysis can permit adequate calorie and protein intake to promote growth.
   b. Renal Osteodystrophy (Renal Rickets). In addition to added dietary vitamin D and phosphate binders such as calcium carbonate, amelioration of this complication may require parathyroidectomy.
   c. Anemia. An effective synthetic erythropoietin is available which avoids the necessity of blood transfusions for this complication.
   d. Hypertension. If present, treatment will be required to prevent additional insult to the kidney as well as other organs.
   e. Hyperkalemia. Dietary K^+ restriction is generally not needed until the GFR has decreased to less than <7 to 11 ml/min/1.73m^2. Dialysis may not be necessary until the GFR has decreased to <5 ml/min/1.73m^2.
4. End-Stage Renal Disease. Treatment will require chronic dialysis (hemodialysis or peritoneal dialysis) or renal transplant.
5. Causes of Renal Failure
   a. Prerenal failure is decreased perfusion of the kidneys with resultant impaired substrate delivery to renal cells. It can be due to hypotension (septicemia, cardiac failure, hemorrhage, neurogenic shock), hypovolemia (hemorrhage, gastrointestinal fluid loss, hypoproteinemia, adrenal failure, burns), malignant hypertension, hypoxemia (cardiac failure, respiratory failure, severe anemia), hypoglycemia, and renal artery occlusion.
   b. Renal failure is due to intrinsic parenchymal injury. Some causes are glomerulonephritis (poststreptococcal glomerulonephritis, membranoproliferative glomerulonephritis, systemic lupus erythematosus, Henoch-Schönlein purpura, hereditary nephritis), nephrotoxicity (heavy metals, nephrotoxic chemicals or drugs, hemoglobin, myoglobin, shock, ischemia), intravascular coagulation (hemolytic-uremic syndrome, disseminated intravascular coagulation, renal vein thrombosis), and cystic or hypoplastic kidneys.
   c. Postrenal failure is obstruction of urine flow from the kidneys. It is most commonly seen with uric acid nephropathy, lithiases, extrinsic tumors, vesicoureteral reflux, and structural defects.

14.2 DISEASE PROFILES

14.2.1 Glomerular Disorders

A. Glomerular injury results in two distinct types of functional lesions, inflammatory and noninflammatory.

1. Noninflammatory glomerular lesions result in protein leakage through the injured filtering interface. These are referred to as nephrotic lesions.

a. In uncomplicated cases they do not compromise the GFR. Fluid retention, hypertension, and elevated BUN/Cr are not expected.
b. The prototype of such lesions is seen in the idiopathic nephrotic syndrome of childhood.

2. In inflammatory lesions (nephritic lesions), eroded areas allow loss of particles as large as RBCs, however swollen glomeruli decrease the total filtering surface available.
a. These lesions result in fluid retention, hypertension, decreased GFR, and hematuria.
b. Poststreptococcal glomerulonephritis is the prototypical inflammatory glomerular lesion.

3. Many glomerular disorders have components of both nephrotic and nephritic lesions.

B. **Idiopathic Nephrotic Syndrome of Childhood**

1. This is the most common cause of nephrotic syndrome in children.
2. Alternate terms are nil (nothing in light) disease, minimal-change disease, and lipoid nephrosis of childhood.
3. Etiology may be an abnormality of T cell lymphocytic function resulting in increased permeability of glomerular filtering surfaces.
4. Pathophysiologic abnormality is urinary protein loss >40 mg/m^2/hour.
5. Predisposing conditions include male sex, age 2 to 6-years, and preceding viral upper respiratory tract infection.
6. Symptoms include anorexia, abdominal pain, diarrhea, and lethargy.
7. The prominent physical exam finding is edema. Proteinuria leads to hypoalbuminemia which leads to edema (periorbital, then dependent, finally generalized).
8. Laboratory evaluation reveals proteinuria, hypoalbuminemia, hyperlipidemia, normal C3, BUN, Cr, and no hematuria or RBC casts.
9. Potential complications include infections (peritonitis [*Streptococcus pneumoniae* most common], pneumonia, sepsis), cellulitis, urinary tract infection, vascular thrombosis, and steroid-induced cataracts.
10. Differential diagnosis includes other forms of renal disease: focal segmental glomerulosclerosis and mesangial proliferative glomerulonephritis.
11. The mainstay of treatment is prednisone 2 mg/kg/day until proteinuria resolves or 4 to 6 weeks, then taper.
12. Prognosis. Prognosis for recovery is very good. Up to 95% of patients with minimal-change disease respond to corticosteroids. If they do not, misdiagnosis must be considered. Relapses may occur with upper respiratory tract infections and require retreatment.

C. Focal segmental glomerulosclerosis may be indistinguishable from minimal-change disease. Only 20% with this morphologic lesion respond to corticosteroids. The remainder progress to end-stage renal disease. The disease recurs in transplanted kidneys.

D. **Mesangial Proliferative Glomerulonephritis**

1. This condition is also called immunoglobulin M (IgM) nephropathy.
2. It has features of both minimal-change disease and focal segmental glomerulosclerosis.
3. About 50% respond to corticosteroids, the others progress to end-stage renal disease.

E. **Hemolytic-Uremic Syndrome** (HUS)

1. HUS is the most common cause of acute renal failure in infants and children.
2. It has been associated with bacterial (especially *Escherichia coli* O157:H7) and viral gastrointestinal infections.
3. Pathophysiologic Abnormality
a. Renal vascular endothelial injury results from platelet deposition and consumption.
b. RBCs are broken up as they pass through the fibrin strands and renal perfusion is compromised.
c. The result is the characteristic triad of azotemia, thrombocytopenia, and microangiopathic hemolytic anemia.
4. Symptoms are fever, vomiting, diarrhea (often bloody), irritability, altered sensorium, and oliguria.
5. Physical findings are edema, pallor, petechiae, and hepatosplenomegaly.
6. Laboratory findings include elevated BUN/Cr, anemia, elevated reticulocyte count, elevated bilirubin, leukocytosis, thrombocytopenia, negative Coombs' test, helmet and burr cells on the peripheral smear, and a normal C3 level.
7. Chronologic sequence of manifestations is acute gastroenteritis followed 7 to 10 days by improvement. Patients then develop acute onset of renal failure and anemia.
8. Potential complications include problems due to acute renal failure and diffuse vasculitis and/or intravascular thrombosis.
9. Differential diagnosis includes bilateral renal vein thrombosis, lupus nephritis, and acute glomerulonephritis.
10. Treatment
a. Treatment is primarily supportive.
b. Peritoneal dialysis is indicted for acute renal failure.
c. Plasmapheresis is advocated by some, but data is not available to support its use.
d. Corticosteroids, anticoagulants, and platelet inhibitors have no proven benefit in HUS therapy and are not recommended.

11. Prognosis.
    a. Recovery of renal function can occur after 2 or more weeks of anuria. With vigorous supportive care 90% of patients will survive the acute renal failure.
    b. Hypertension, chronic renal failure, and cerebrovascular accidents or other intravascular thrombotic phenomena are worrisome potential late sequelae.

F. **Poststreptococcal Glomerulonephritis** (PSGN)
1. PSGN competes with IgA nephropathy as the most common cause of gross hematuria in children.
2. It is caused by throat or skin infection with nephritogenic strains of group A β-hemolytic streptococcus.
3. Pathophysiologic Abnormality. Inflammatory glomerular lesions cause decreased GFR and fluid retention.
4. Patients present with tea-colored urine, oliguria, lethargy, malaise, abdominal pain, flank pain, and fever. They may have edema, hypertension, and fluid overload.
5. Laboratory Findings
    a. Urinalysis shows RBC casts, hematuria, proteinuria, and white blood cells.
    b. Serum studies reveal low C3 levels, a positive Streptozyme test, elevated antistreptolysin-O (ASO) titer (post pharyngitis; not impetigo), elevated BUN/Cr, and normal proteins.
6. Renal failure is the feared complication.
7. Differential diagnosis includes the other causes of hematuria (see section 14.1.4E).
8. Treatment is with Na^+ and fluid restriction, loop diuretics, antihypertensives (if the blood pressure is elevated), and therapy for renal failure if it occurs.
9. Ninety-five percent of patients recover completely. Morbidity may result from uncontrolled hypertension.

G. **Postinfectious Nonstreptococcal Glomerulonephritis**. Other causes of acute infection-mediated glomerulonephritis include bacterial (staphylococcal shunt nephritis), viral (hepatitis B, infectious mononucleosis, cytomegalovirus infections), fungal (histoplasmosis), and parasitic (toxoplasmosis, falciparum malaria).

H. **Membranoproliferative Glomerulonephritis** (MPGN)
1. MPGN is the most common cause of chronic glomerulonephritis in older children and adults.
2. It is also called mesangiocapillary glomerulonephritis.
3. MPGN presents in the 2nd decade of life with proteinuria and hematuria.
4. Renal biopsy is required for the diagnosis because hypocomplementemia does not always occur.
5. Complications
    a. Most develop nephrotic syndrome.
    b. Many patients progress to end-stage renal disease.

I. **Membranous Glomerulopathy** (MGN)
1. MGN is the most common cause of nephrotic syndrome in adults.
2. Clinical manifestations are similar to membranoproliferative glomerulonephritis except the C3 level is normal.
3. Most cases in children resolve spontaneously.

J. **Rapidly Progressive Glomerulonephritis** (RPGN)
1. RPGN is also called diffuse crescentic glomerulonephritis.
2. If the typical glomerular crescents are not due to poststreptococcal, membranoproliferative, anaphylactoid purpura, systemic lupus erythematosus, or Goodpasture's disease, progression to end-stage renal disease can be expected within months of onset.
3. Serum C3 level is normal.
4. Diagnosis is made by renal biopsy.

K. **Hereditary Glomerulonephritis**
1. The most common form of this condition is **Alport's syndrome.**
2. Patients present at school age with asymptomatic hematuria followed by the development of proteinuria. Many have hypertension, which may be severe, and 1/3 have sensorineural hearing loss. Eye problems also occur in 15% of patients.

L. **Lupus Nephritis**
1. Nephritis is a common manifestation of systemic lupus erythematosus in childhood.
2. It is a disease characterized by remissions and relapses as it progresses.
3. Adolescent females are most commonly affected.
4. Normalization of C3 levels reflects effective immunosuppressive therapy.
5. The renal injury may progress to end-stage renal disease.
6. Complications may occur both from the disease and from the therapy it requires (corticosteroids, immunosuppressive drugs).

M. **Immunoglobulin A (IgA) Nephropathy**
1. The alternate terminology is **Berger's nephropathy**.
2. Pathogenesis of the disease is IgA deposition on glomerular basement membranes.
3. Predisposing conditions are upper respiratory tract infections, male sex, or other IgA mediated conditions (Henoch-Schönlein purpura).
4. Laboratory findings include a normal C3 level, microscopic and gross hematuria, and non-nephrotic range proteinuria.

5. Potential Complications
   a. Up to 20% develop hypertension, nephrotic syndrome, and eventual renal failure.
   b. The nephropathy recurs in transplanted kidneys.

N. **Henoch-Schönlein Purpura Glomerulonephritis**
   1. The pathophysiologic abnormality is a small vessel vasculitis which can cause decreased GFR.
   2. Signs and symptoms include a rash (urticaria, macular, papular, purpura) on the buttocks and lower extremities, abdominal pain, gastrointestinal bleed, and arthralgia.
   3. Laboratory findings include hematuria, proteinuria, normal C3 level, and normal platelets.
   4. Prognosis. When severe renal involvement occurs it is unresponsive to treatment.

O. **Sickle Cell Nephropathy**. The initial defect is usually in the concentrating ability of the tubules. Renal involvement may progress to include episodic hematuria and a nephrotic syndrome.

14.2.2 Juxtaglomerular Disorders

A. Histologically demonstrable juxtaglomerular disorders are extremely rare, but such disorders should be included in the differential diagnosis. Checking urine Cl^- is a helpful marker since these disorders are associated with hypovolemia and subsequently, have low urine Cl^- level.

B. **Bartter's Syndrome**
   1. This is due to generalized hyperplasia of the juxtaglomerular apparatus.
   2. Pathophysiologic Abnormality
      a. A defect in Cl^- reabsorption in the ascending loop of Henle results in urinary K^+ wasting when excess sodium chloride presents to the distal tubule and is reabsorbed in exchange for K^+.
      b. Hypokalemia stimulates prostaglandin and renin synthesis.
      c. The elevated prostaglandin contributes to a defect in platelet aggregation and the elevated renin stimulates aldosterone production which exacerbates the hypokalemia.
   3. Signs and symptoms include muscle weakness, polyuria, constipation, carpopedal spasm, dehydration, growth failure, and normal blood pressure.
   4. Laboratory findings include severe hypokalemia, defective platelet aggregation, hypochloremic metabolic alkalosis, elevated renin, elevated aldosterone, elevated prostaglandin E_2, elevated urine K^+, and elevated urine Cl^-.
   5. Differential diagnosis is licorice abuse, pyelonephritis, diabetes insipidus, chronic vomiting, chronic diarrhea, laxative abuse, and diuretic use.

14.2.3 Interstitial Disorders

A. **Acute Interstitial Nephritis**
   1. This is a disorder of unknown etiology characterized by interstitial inflammation and edema.
   2. Acute interstitial nephritis most often due to drug therapy, and in such cases, may be a hypersensitivity reaction. It is also seen in association with infections and other disorders, including renal transplant rejection.
   3. Staining of the urinary sediment for eosinophils may be helpful in identifying this entity, but diagnosis is made by renal biopsy.
   4. Chronic interstitial nephritis occurs once the interstitial edema of acute interstitial nephritis is replaced by fibrosis. The condition is progressive and end-stage renal failure ensues.

14.2.4 Tubular Disorders

A. **Renal Tubular Acidosis** (RTA)
   1. RTA is a heterogeneous group of disorders all of which have hyperchloremic metabolic acidosis and tubular dysfunction.
   2. Renal failure is not an expected component of this group of disorders.
   3. **RTA Type I** (Distal Renal Tubular Acidosis)
      a. RTA type I may be primary or secondary due to obstructive uropathy, pyelonephritis, sickle cell nephropathy, lupus nephritis, medullary sponge kidney, renal transplant rejection, or toxins.
      b. The pathophysiologic abnormality is defective hydrogen ion secretion in the distal tubule which results in up to 15% of the filtered sodium bicarbonate ($NaHCO_3$) load being lost in the urine.
      c. Signs and symptoms include failure to thrive, anorexia, vomiting, and dehydration.
      d. Laboratory findings are hyperchloremic metabolic acidosis, mild hypokalemia, and alkaline urine.
      e. Potential complications include hypercalciuria, nephrocalcinosis, and renal stones.
      f. Treatment with 2 to 3 mEq/kg/24hr $NaHCO_3$ is therapeutic and distinguishes RTA type I from the proximal type (RTA type II), which may require >10 mEq/kg/24hr of $NaHCO_3$.
      g. Prognosis is good if renal injury can be avoided.
   4. **RTA Type II** (Proximal Renal Tubular Acidosis)
      a. RTA type II may be primary, a component of Fanconi's syndrome, or due to tubular immaturity in premature infants.
      b. The pathophysiologic abnormality is a lowered renal threshold for bicarbonate reabsorption in the proximal tubule. If serum acidosis drops below this threshold, the urine becomes acidic.
      c. Laboratory findings include hyperchloremic metabolic acidosis and hypokalemia.
      d. Rarely, nephrocalcinosis will occur in affected patients.
      e. Treatment is with high (>5 mEq/kg/24hr) doses of $NaHCO_3$.

f. Prognosis is excellent if the condition is an isolated lesion, otherwise it is dependent on the underlying disorder.

5. **RTA type III** is RTA type I with an associated bicarbonate tubular leak.
6. **RTA Type IV** (Mineralocorticoid Deficiency RTA)
    a. The serum metabolic abnormality is hyperchloremic acidosis with hyperkalemia.
    b. Nephrocalcinosis is rare.
    c. Etiologies include adrenal failure, congenital adrenal hyperplasia, primary hypoaldosteronism, pyelonephritis, interstitial nephritis, obstructive lesions, nephrosclerosis, diabetes mellitus, and pseudohypoaldosteronism.

B. Diffuse Proximal Renal Tubular Dysfunction (Fanconi's Syndrome)

1. Fanconi syndrome's is a defect in tubular function with hyperchloremic acidosis, glycosuria, aminoaciduria, and depressed tubular reabsorption of phosphate.
2. Etiologies
    a. Inherited disorders: cystinosis, Lowe's syndrome, galactosemia, tyrosinemia, hereditary fructose intolerance, glycogen storage disease type I, and Wilson's disease.
    b. Systemic disorders: rubella syndrome, amyloidosis, and Sjögren's syndrome.
    c. Toxins: heavy metals, outdated tetracycline, and lindane.
    d. Organ dysfunction: hyperparathyroidism and interstitial nephritis.
3. Prognosis is dependent on the underlying disorder.

C. Nephrogenic Diabetes Insipidus. All forms are diagnosed by lack of response to vasopressin.

14.2.5 Urologic Causes of Azotemia

A. Posterior urethral valves should be considered in any male child with azotemia.

B. Hypospadias. Avoid circumcisions since the foreskin is used in repair of the lesion.

C. Cryptorchidism. This should be surgically corrected (orchiopexy) by age 2 years of age.

D. Testicular torsion is a true surgical emergency because delayed correction can lead to loss of the testicle.

E. Other causes include hydronephrosis, urolithiasis, neurogenic bladder, and urethral stenosis.

F. Diagnosis can be made by physical examination and radiologic imaging studies.

295. At what gestational age is nephrogenesis complete — D 14.1.1

A. 24 weeks
B. 27 weeks
C. 32 weeks
D. 36 weeks
E. 40 weeks

296. A newborn is noted to have flattened facial features, low set ears, and severe respiratory distress. His prenatal history is significant for oligohydramnios. What is his probable diagnosis — B 14.1.1

A. trisomy 21
B. Potter's syndrome
C. Noonan's syndrome
D. trisomy 18
E. Eagle-Barrett syndrome (prune-belly syndrome)

297. Which of the following cause a positive result for blood on a urine test strip in the absence of blood on microscopic urinalysis — E 14.1.2

A. bilirubin
B. myoglobin
C. concentrated urine
D. hemoglobin
E. B and D

298. All of the following are causes for elevated blood urea nitrogen except — D 14.1.2

A. glomerular filtration rate < 50% of normal
B. increased dietary protein
C. blood in the gastrointestinal tract
D. intravenous fluid hydration

299. A patient's blood urea nitrogen is 40 mg/dL. Approximately how long will it take for the blood urea nitrogen to decrease to 20 mg/dL once renal perfusion is restored — B 14.1.2

A. 48 hours
B. 16 hours
C. 4 hours
D. 1 hour

300. What is the renal abnormality seen in patients with Lowe's syndrome and Wilson's disease — A 14.2.4

A. diffuse proximal renal tubular dysfunction
B. renal tubular acidosis type I
C. renal tubular acidosis type II
D. membranoproliferative glomerulonephritis
E. none of the above

301. Which of the following conditions is seen with renal transplant rejection or drug hypersensitivity — B 14.2.3

A. poststreptococcal glomerulonephritis
B. acute interstitial nephritis
C. membranoproliferative glomerulonephritis
D. Henoch-Schönlein purpura

302. What specific gravity reflects neither concentration nor dilution of the urine — C 14.1.2

A. 1.002
B. 1.030
C. 1.010
D. 1.020

303. A child presents with oliguria. He has been vomiting for approximately 2 days. Prerenal azotemia from dehydration can be distinguished from renal failure by — B 14.1.2

A. urine specific gravity <1.010
B. fractional excretion of sodium <1%
C. fractional excretion of sodium >7%
D. a low blood urea nitrogen

304. Which of the following renal imaging modalities also provides an assessment of renal function — A 14.1.2

A. nuclear renal scan
B. renal ultrasound
C. voiding cystourethrography
D. nuclear cystogram
E. intravenous pyelography

305. Which of the following renal diseases is associated with a decrease in circulating complement — D 14.1.2

A. poststreptococcal glomerulonephritis
B. membranoproliferative glomerulonephritis
C. systemic lupus erythematosus
D. all of the above
E. none of the above

306. Renal dialysis is indicated for renal disease with all of the following except — B 14.1.3

A. fluid overload with pulmonary edema
B. hyperkalemia controlled by diet
C. glomerular filtration rate <0.1 ml/min/kg
D. uremic encephalopathy

307. What is the rate of protein excretion in patients with nephrotic syndrome — A 14.1.4

A. >40 mg/m^2/hour
B. 30 mg/m^2/hour
C. <4 mg/m^2/hour
D. >50 mg/m^2/hour

308. Which of the following conditions is associated with proteinuria and edema, but no hematuria — C 14.1.4

A. glomerulonephritis
B. hypercalciuria
C. focal segmental glomerulosclerosis
D. urinary tract infection
E. nephrolithiasis

309. What is the recommended course of treatment for hemolytic-uremic syndrome — D 14.2.1

A. steroids
B. anticoagulants
C. platelet inhibitors
D. dialysis for renal failure
E. none of the above

310. Which of the following syndromes is associated with renal disease and hearing loss — C 14.2.1

A. hemolytic-uremic syndrome
B. meningitis
C. Alport's syndrome
D. Henoch-Schönlein purpura
E. membranous glomerulopathy

311. A 5-year-old male child presents with a 1 week history of abdominal pain, diarrhea, and lethargy. On exam, you note generalized edema. Laboratory testing reveals nephrotic range proteinuria, hypoalbuminemia, hyperlipidemia, normal C3, negative antistreptolysin-O (ASO) titer, and no hematuria. What is the treatment of choice for this child's condition — C 14.2.1

A. albumin infusion
B. cholesterol lowering agents
C. prednisone
D. penicillin
E. cyclophosphamide

312. Which of the following is the most common cause of acute renal failure in infants and children — A 14.2.1

A. hemolytic-uremic syndrome
B. Henoch-Schönlein purpura
C. membranoproliferative glomerulonephritis
D. poststreptococcal glomerulonephritis
E. minimal-change nephrotic syndrome

313. A 5-year-old presents to the emergency room with vomiting, bloody diarrhea, obtundation, and oliguria. He was well until 2 days ago when he attended a backyard cookout. On exam you note petechiae, edema, and pallor. What is the probable etiology of his condition — B 14.2.1

A. *Salmonella*
B. *Escherichia coli*
C. *Shigella*
D. *Campylobacter*
E. *Yersinia*

314. A 10-year-old female presents with facial swelling, malaise, abdominal pain, fever, and tea-colored urine. On exam, you note that she is hypertensive. Laboratory studies reveal a low C3, hematuria, proteinuria, and red blood cell casts. Which of the following historical points suggest the diagnosis — E 14.2.1

A. her diabetic grandfather has nephrotic syndrome
B. she had a sore throat 2 weeks ago
C. she had her tonsils out 3 years ago
D. she had a crusting skin lesion (infected "insect bite") 2 weeks ago
E. B and D

315. An adolescent, with a history of Henoch-Schönlein purpura when he was 5 years old, presents with gross hematuria and low-grade proteinuria. He has no other symptoms. What is his probable diagnosis — A 14.2.1

A. Berger's nephropathy
B. Henoch-Schönlein purpura
C. hemolytic-uremic syndrome
D. poststreptococcal glomerulonephritis
E. rapidly progressing glomerulonephritis

316. A newborn presents with vomiting, a sunken anterior fontanelle, pale extremities, weak pulses, and respiratory distress. The infant has a urine specific gravity of 1.010, so you feel reassured that the child is not dehydrated. You proceed with your next step in evaluation and treatment which is — A 14.1.1

A. realize that the infant is in fact dehydrated, place an intravenous catheter, and give a fluid bolus
B. start a dopamine drip for suspected congenital heart disease with failure
C. give intramuscular antibiotics while waiting for collected culture results
D. get an echocardiogram
E. get a cardiology consult

317. All of the following are complications of chronic renal failure except D 14.1.4

A. growth failure
B. anemia
C. hypertension
D. hypokalemia
E. rickets

318. Which form of renal tubular acidosis is associated with defective hydrogen ion secretion in the distal tubule E 14.2.4

A. type I
B. type II
C. type III
D. type IV
E. A and C

15 ELECTROLYTE AND ACID-BASE DISORDERS

15.1 GENERAL CONCEPTS

15.1.1 Fluid Spaces

A. **Total Body Water** (TBW)
  1. Water is 70 to 75% of TBW in the newborn.
  2. After the postnatal diuresis, TBW is 65% and remains constant until puberty when it decreases to 55 to 60%.

B. **Extracellular Fluid** (ECF) is 1/3 of the TBW
  1. Sodium (Na^+) is the predominant cation of the ECF. It is present in a concentration of 140 mEq/L.
  2. ECF contains only 4 mEq/L of potassium (K^+).
  3. Regulation of the ECF volume is through the interaction of antidiuretic hormone, thirst, and the renin-angiotensin-aldosterone axis.
  4. Distribution of fluid between the two compartments of the ECF (plasma fluid and interstitial fluid) is regulated primarily by the oncotic pressure of plasma proteins.
  5. The clinical signs of dehydration are a reflection of changes in the ECF volume.

C. **Intracellular Fluid** (ICF)
  1. ICF accounts for 2/3 of the TBW.
  2. K^+ is the major cation in the ICF. Its concentration there is approximately 160 mEq/L.

15.1.2 Diagnostic Modalities

A. **Osmolality** is the mechanism which governs distribution of body fluids across the compartments' semipermeable membranes. The normal osmolality is 285 mosm/L.

B. **Osmolar Gap**
  1. This is the difference between measured osmolality and calculated osmolality.
  2. The expected osmolality can be calculated by the formula:

$$\text{Plasma osmolality} = 2 \times Na^+ + \frac{\text{Glucose}}{18} + \frac{\text{BUN}}{2.8}$$

(BUN = blood urea nitrogen)

C. **Anion Gap** reflects the amount of organic acids present in the serum. It can be calculated by the formula:

$$\text{Anion gap} = (Na^+ + K^+) - (Cl^- + HCO_3^-) = 8 \text{ to } 12 \text{ mEq/L}$$

15.2 FLUID AND ELECTROLYTE DISTURBANCES

15.2.1 Abnormal Saline Concentrations

A. Na^+ imbalance may be due to an excess or deficit of either the Na^+ or the water contained within.

B. Hypernatremia, hyponatremia, or Na^+ in the normal range merely reflects the concentration of Na^+ in the ECF, not the total body Na^+.

C. Urine Na^+
  1. This measure reflects a regulatory response to excess or depletion of total body Na^+, and to TBW.
  2. If there is a total body deficit of Na^+, the urine Na^+ concentration will be low whether the child's serum Na^+ concentration reflects hypernatremia or hyponatremia.

D. **Antidiuretic Hormone** (ADH)
  1. ADH maintains vascular perfusion by promoting reabsorption of water in the distal tubules as well as increasing the mean arterial pressure (arteriolar vasoconstriction).
  2. ADH effect may perpetuate or worsen hyponatremia if the child has severe vascular volume depletion. Vascular volume will be maintained to the extent it can via the release of ADH even if doing so results in hyponatremia in the ECF.

E. It is helpful to determine whether the Na^+ imbalance is accompanied by decreased TBW (dehydration), normal TBW, or excessive TBW.
  1. The most accurate way to determine whether TBW is decreased, normal, or increased is by noting recent weight change in the child. Unfortunately, this information is often not available.
  2. The clinical assessment of dehydration is based on parameters which reflect reduction in ECF and vascular volume. Fluid shifts into or out of the ICF space will alter the amount of TBW loss required to cause the findings associated with clinical mild, moderate, or severe dehydration.
     a. Hyponatremia is associated with a shift of fluids into the cells, thus the clinical signs which denotes the degree of dehydration will occur with less fluid loss.
     b. The converse is true in hypernatremia dehydration. By the time severe dehydration is apparent in patients with hypernatremic dehydration, the child is in danger of catastrophic vascular collapse because of the amount of TBW lost.
  3. The presence of edema indicates an increase in both Na^+ and TBW.

F. Clinical Assessment of the Degree of Dehydration (Table 15.2.1)

G. Causes of Hypernatremia
  1. Hypernatremia Associated with Decreased ECF
     a. Due to extrarenal water losses (urine $Na^+ < 10$ mEq/L): skin losses, respiratory losses, gastrointestinal losses, severe burns, and thyrotoxicosis.
     b. Due to renal water losses (urine $Na^+ > 40$ mEq/L): diuretics, renal disease, relief of urinary obstruction, and osmoreceptor failure.
  2. Hypernatremia associated with normal ECF: impaired thirst, nonrenal water losses, and renal water losses.
  3. Hypernatremia associated with increased ECF: iatrogenic saline excess, mineralocorticoid excess,

hyperaldosteronism, Cushing's disease, and steroids.

H. Causes of Hyponatremia

1. Hyponatremia Associated with Decreased ECF
   - **a.** Due to extrarenal Na^+ losses (urine Na^+ <20 mEq/L): sweating, vomiting, diarrhea, burn fluid loss, peritonitis, and pancreatitis.
   - **b.** Due to renal Na^+ losses (urine Na^+ >40 mEq/L): aldosterone deficiency, congenital adrenal hyperplasia, salt losing nephropathy, renal tubular diuretics, and osmotic diuretics.
2. Hyponatremia Associated with Normal ECF
   - **a.** Increased ADH secretion: syndrome of inappropriate secretion of ADH (SIADH), pain, physical or emotional stress, and myxedema.
   - **b.** Normal ADH secretion: water intoxication, iatrogenic water overload, psychogenic polydipsia, and sick cell disease (reset osmostat).
3. Hyponatremia Associated with Increased ECF
   - **a.** Decreased glomerular filtration rate and abnormal tubules (oliguria, urine Na^+ >40 mEq/L): renal failure.
   - **b.** Decreased glomerular filtration rate with normal tubules (oliguria, urine Na^+<20 mEq/L): decreased vascular volume, decreased cardiac output, cardiac failure, hepatic failure, and nephrotic syndrome.
4. Factitious hyponatremia: hyperglycemia, hyperlipidemia, and hyperproteinemia.
   - **a.** Since glucose remains extracellular in hyperglycemia, it draws intracellular water into the extracellular space and factitiously dilutes the measured Na^+.
   - **b.** The true serum Na^+ concentration in hyperglycemia can be calculated by assuming that Na^+ is diluted 1.6 to 1.8 mEq/L for each 100 mg/dl the glucose is above its normal 150 mg/dl.

15.2.2 Maintenance Fluid and Electrolyte Guidelines

A. Table 15.2.2A Daily fluid requirements

BODY WEIGHT	MAINTENANCE WATER REQUIRED
Up to 10 kg	100 cc/kg
11 to 20 kg	1000 cc + 50 cc/kg for each kg over 10 kg
Above 20 kg	1500 cc/kg + 20 cc/kg for each kg over 20 kg

B. Table 15.2.2B Daily electrolyte requirements

CATION	MAINTENANCE REQUIRED
Sodium	3 mEq/kg/24 hours
Potassium	2 mEq/kg/24 hours

C. Maintenance Fluids

1. Fluids can be provided by using D_5W 1/4 normal

Table 15.2.1 Clinical assessment of the degree of dehydration

PARAMETER	MILD (<5%)	MODERATE (10%)	SEVERE (15%)
Skin color	Pink	Acrocyanosis	Mottled
Tears	Present	Reduced	Absent
Mucous membrane	Normal	Dry	Parched
Eyeball	Normal	Depressed	Sunken
Fontanelle	normal	Depressed	Sunken
Level of consciousness	Alert	Lethargic	Obtunded
Pulse rate	Upper normal	Increased	Markedly increased
Capillary refill	Upper normal	Definitely prolonged	Markedly prolonged
Blood pressure	Normal	Orthostatic hypotension	Recumbent hypotension
Blood urea nitrogen	Normal	Elevated	Very high
Arterial pH	7.40 to 7.30	7.30 to 7.00	<7.10
Urine volume	Small	Oliguria	Oliguria or anuria
Urine specific gravity	<1.020	>1.030	>1.035

saline plus 20 to 30 mEq/L potassium chloride. The infusion rate can be calculated using the expected 24 hour fluid volume requirement guidelines given in Table 15.2.2A or can be directly calculated as an hourly rate by Table 15.2.2C.

Table 15.2.2C Hourly maintenance fluid rate

WEIGHT	RATE
0 to 10 kg	4 cc/kg/hr
11 to 20 kg	40 cc/kg/hr + 2 cc/kg/hr for each kg >10
>20 kg	60 cc/kg/hr + 1 cc/kg/hr for each kg >20

15.2.3 Treatment of Fluid and Electrolyte Imbalances

A. Hypernatremia

1. Hypernatremia with edema and a normal blood urea nitrogen (unless in shock) is due to salt poisoning and requires urgent dialysis.
2. The serum Na^+ in hypernatremic dehydration must be replaced slowly, over 48 hours, to avoid too rapid osmolar shifts of water into brain cells with resulting cerebral edema. For the same reason, the replacement fluid should be at least 1/4 normal saline, not dextrose, in water alone.
   a. The degree of dehydration estimated from clinical signs of dehydration relies on findings reflecting the ECF volume.
   b. In hypernatremic dehydration, the amount of fluid loss is often underestimated because the fluid shift from the intracellular space in hypertonic dehydration delays clinical manifestations of the amount of TBW lost.
   c. The actual water deficit in hypernatremic dehydration can be estimated by:

$$\text{TBW} = 0.6 \times \text{Normal wt (kg)}$$

$$\frac{\text{Normal Na}^+}{\text{Measured Na}^+} \times \text{TBW} = \text{Current TBW}$$

$$\text{Fluid deficit} = \text{Normal TBW} - \text{Current TBW}$$

B. Hyponatremia

1. Symptomatic hyponatremia rarely occurs unless the serum Na^+ is less than 120 mEq/L. Symptoms such as seizures are more the result of the rapidity of fall in Na^+ concentration than the level reached.
2. A key to assessing the approach to treatment of hyponatremia is the blood urea nitrogen.
   Hyponatremia with a normal blood urea nitrogen is

Table 15.2.3 Guidlines for Treatment of Dehydration

DEHYDRATION TYPE	WEIGHT LOSS PER SEVERITY LEVEL			REPLACEMENT FLUID	HOURS OF DEFICIT REPLACEMENT	
	Mild	Moderate	Severe		1st 1/2	2nd 1/2
Hypotonic dehydration	2%	5%	10%	D_5W 3/4 normal saline	4 hrs.	20 hrs.
Isotonic dehydration	5%	10%	15%	D_5W 1/2 normal saline	8 hrs.	16 hrs.
Hypertonic dehydration	10%	15%	20%	D_5W 1/4 normal saline	24 hrs.	24 hrs.

1. Correct shock with boluses of 20 cc/kg of normal saline or lactated Ringer's solution. If additional volume is needed, use plasminate or albumin (if hemorrhage is suspected, consider blood replacement).
2. Obtain results for blood urea nitrogen, serum creatinine, serum eletrolytes (sodium, potassium, chloride), serum bicarbonate, and serum glucose.
3. Estimate severity of dehydration.
4. Based on the severity and type of dehydration identified by electrolyte results, multiply the percent deficit (note Weight Loss Per Seveity Level above) by the patient's body weight and replace the calculated deficit in two equal parts over the appropriate time frame (note Hours of Deficit Replacement above).
5. Add potassium chloride in a concentration of 20 to 40 mEq/L to the replacement fuid requirements once adequate urine flow is demonstrated.

The above volumes and concentratoins should be added to the daily maintenance flud requirements (see Table 15.2.2A) to assure adequate replacement of ongoing needs.

due to either SIADH or water intoxication, and the treatment of either condition is water restriction, not fluid replacement, unless the hyponatremia is symptomatic.

3. Symptomatic hyponatremia may be treated with hypertonic saline (3%).
   a. The volume required to raise the serum Na^+ above 120 mEq/L (desired Na^+) can be calculated by the formula:

$$\left(\text{Desired Na}^+ - \text{Measured Na}^+\right) \times 0.6 \times \text{wt (kg)} = \text{Na}^+ \text{ Required}$$

   Note: 3% saline contains 0.5 mEq Na^+/cc.
   b. Symptomatic hyponatremia will usually respond to raising the serum Na^+ concentration 10 mEq/L. Correction of the remaining imbalance should be done more slowly.

C. Hyperkalemia

1. Physiologically significant hyperkalemia is reflected in the electrocardiogram. The earliest change in the electrocardiogram is a tenting or peaking of the T wave.
2. Treatment of Hyperkalemia
   a. Treatment can be initiated with calcium gluconate (calcium chloride can worsen the acidosis which is usually present in hyperkalemic conditions), sodium bicarbonate, insulin, glucose, or a cation exchange resin (sodium polystyrene sulfonate). These are listed in descending order of rapidity on onset of action and ascending order of duration of action.
   b. Dialysis may be needed for situations not adequately controlled by the preceding temporary measures.

D. Hypokalemia

1. Total body K^+ deficits are not necessarily reflected in serum K^+ values.
2. A urine K^+ of <20 mEq/L, however, reflects the normal kidney's effort to conserve the K^+ presented to its tubules. Urine K^+ should guide replacement of total body K^+ deficits.
3. Physiologically significant hypokalemia is reflected in the electrocardiogram with ST segment depression, T wave amplitude reduction, and U waves.
4. Except in unusual circumstances, K^+ concentration in IV fluids should not exceed 40 mEq/L.

E. Dehydration

1. Goals for the Treatment of Dehydration
   a. Adequate urine volume should be achieved in the first hour.
   b. Urine specific gravity ≤1.010 should be reached within the first few hours. When this is achieved infusion rate of fluids can be decreased to maintenance rates because the kidneys will just excrete any excess at that point.
   c. Normal electrolytes should occur in hours (hyponatremia) to days (hypernatremia).
   d. Blood urea nitrogen, if elevated, is decreased by half every 15 to 20 hours.
   e. Normal acid-base status is achieved in 1 to 3 days.
   f. Urine K^+ >40 meq/L is reached in 3 to 5 days.
2. Guidelines for Treatment of Dehydration (Table 15.2.3)

15.3 ACID-BASE DISTURBANCES

15.3.1 The Basics

A. A pH of 7.40 is the result of a ratio of bicarbonate to the partial alveolar pressure of carbon dioxide ($PaCO_2$) of 20 to 1. Changes in this ratio cause a corresponding change in the pH.

1. The $PaCO_2$ is dependent on the minute volume of respiration and can change in minutes.
2. The bicarbonate is regulated by the kidneys and changes take hours to days.

B. Any change in either of these determiners of pH is accompanied by a compensatory change in the other.

1. **Table 15.3.1B1** Compensatory changes in bicarbonate and partial alveolar carbon dioxide pressure

	HCO_3 <21	**HCO_3 21 to 26**	**HCO_3 >26**
$PaCO_2$ >45	Combined Metabolic Acidosis and Respiratory Acidosis	Respiratory Acidosis	Mixed Metabolic Alkalosis and Respiratory Acidosis
$PaCO_2$ 35 to 45	Metabolic Acidosis	Normal	Metabolic Alkalosis
$PaCO_2$ <35	Mixed Metabolic Acidosis and Respiratory Alkalosis	Respiratory Alkalosis	Combined Respiratory Alkalosis and Metabolic Alkalosis

$PaCO_2$ = partial alveolar pressure of carbon dioxide (mm Hg); HCO_3 = bicarbonate (mEq/L)

2. In mixed disorders, the pH reflects which mixed disorder pair is primary and which is secondary since compensation is never complete nor overcompensated.
3. The mechanisms for the compensatory changes depicted in Table 15.3.1B3.

C. General Acid-Base Rules of Thumb

a. A 1 mm Hg increase in $PaCo_2$ causes a 0.01 decrease in pH.
b. A 1 mEq/L decrease in bicarbonate causes a 0.02 decrease in pH.
c. A 0.1 increase in pH causes a 0.5 mEq/L decrease in K^+.
d. A 0.1 increase in pH shifts the oxygen dissociation curve to the left enough to decrease oxygen release to tissues by 10%.
e. In primary metabolic acidosis, the $PaCO_2$ in mm Hg should equal the 2 digits to the right of the decimal point of the pH if no other derangement exists. For example a pH of 7.22 corresponds to a $PaCO_2$ of 22 mm Hg in pure acute metabolic acidosis.

Table 15.3.1B3 Compensatory blood gas changes

DISORDER	INITIAL CHANGE	COMPENSATORY CHANGE
Respiratory Acidosis	10 mm Hg $PaCO_2$ increase	HCO_3 increases 1 mEq/L (acute), HCO_3 increases 3 to 4 mEq/L (chronic)
Respiratory Alkalosis	10 mm Hg $PaCO_2$ decrease	HCO_3 decreases 1 to 3 mEq/L (acute), HCO_3 decreases 2 to 5 mEq/L (chronic)
Metabolic Acidosis	1 mEq/L HCO_3 decrease	$PaCO_2$ decreases 1 to 1.5 mm Hg
Metabolic Alkalosis	1 mEq/L HCO_3 increase	$PaCO_2$ increases 0.5 to 1 mm Hg
$PaCO_2$ = partial alveolar pressure of carbon dioxide; HCO_3 = bicarbonate		

15.3.2 Causes of Metabolic Alkalosis

A. Chloride responsive causes (urine chloride <10 mEq/L) : gastrointestinal chloride loss (vomiting, gastric suction, chloride diarrhea), diuretics, rapid correction of hypercapnia, and cystic fibrosis.

B. Chloride resistant causes (urine chloride >20 mEq/L): excess mineralocorticoid activity, hyperaldosteronism, Cushing's syndrome, Bartter's syndrome, excess licorice, and severe K^+ depletion.

C. Variable chloride response: milk-alkali syndrome and alkali administration.

15.3.3 Causes of Metabolic Acidosis

A. Increased Loss of Bicarbonate or Chloride Addition (Normal Anion Gap)
   1. Associated with K^+ retention (hyperkalemia): early uremic acidosis, renal tubular acidosis type IV, hypoaldosteronism, K^+-sparing diuretics, resolving diabetic ketoacidosis, and early obstructive uropathy.
   2 Associated with K^+ depletion (hypokalemia): acute diarrhea with bicarbonate and chloride losses, renal tubular acidosis type I or II, and dilution acidosis.
   3. Increased Organic Acids (Increased Anion Gap). See section 21.1.2.

15.3.4 Causes of Respiratory Alkalosis (Relative Tachypnea)

A. Central nervous system pathology: infection, trauma, and tumors.

B. Respiratory: hypoxia, mild bronchospasm, pneumonia, pulmonary emboli, and respiratory center stimulating drugs (salicylates, catecholamines).

C. Others: congestive heart failure, severe anemia, anxiety with hyperventilation, pregnancy, pain, fever, sepsis, hepatic dysfunction, and hyperthyroidism.

15.3.5 Causes of Respiratory Acidosis

A. Central nervous system depression of the respiratory drive: drug overdose, central nervous system lesions, and infections.

B. Pulmonary diseases: obstructive pulmonary disease, severe bronchospasm, pneumonia, pulmonary edema, and smoke inhalation.

C. Mechanical abnormalities: airway obstruction, foreign body, croup, epiglottitis, retropharyngeal abscess, laryngeal edema, aspiration, pleural effusion, pneumothorax, flail chest, and scoliosis.

D. Neuromuscular abnormalities: Guillain-Barré syndrome, poliomyelitis, Werdnig-Hoffman disease, myasthenia gravis, botulism, tetanus, muscular dystrophy, severe hypokalemia, and myxedema.

319. If a newborn weighs 4.0 kg, what is the total body water weight — A 15.1.1

A. 3.0 kg
B. 2.0 kg
C. 1.0 kg
D. 0.5 kg

320. What percent of total body water is extracellular fluid — C 15.1.1

A. 11%
B. 22%
C. 33%
D. 44%
E. 66%

321. A patient's sodium is 140 mmol/L, glucose is 72 mg/dL, and blood urea nitrogen is 28 mg/dL. What is the calculated osmolality — B 15.1.2

A. 164 mOsm/kg
B. 294 mOsm/kg
C. 306 mOsm/kg
D. 330 mOsm/kg

322. A 3-month-old with a history of vomiting and diarrhea has been fed nothing except half-strength formula for 2 days. On arrival to your emergency department, he is having a seizure. Which of the following sodium values (in mmol/L) reflects this history — D 15.2.3

A. 146
B. 136
C. 126
D. 116

323. What is the most accurate way to determine whether or not total body water is decreased in an individual child — D 15.2.1

A. calculate the estimated percent of dehydration
B. measure the child's heart rate and compare it to norms for age
C. measure the child's urine output
D. compare recent weight measurements with the current weight

324. How quickly should the free water be replaced in children with hypertonic dehydration — A 15.2.3

A. 48 hours
B. 24 hours
C. 18 hours
D. 12 hours

325. How quickly should the fluid deficit be replaced in children with isotonic dehydration — C 15.2.3

A. 72 hours
B. 48 hours
C. 24 hours
D. 18 hours

326. At what point is maintenance potassium added to intravenous fluids when treating a child with severe dehydration — A 15.2.3

A. when urine output is assured
B. when intravenous fluids are started
C. when the serum potassium falls below 4.0 mmol/L
D. potassium should not be added to the intravenous fluid until the deficit fluids are replaced

327. Calculate the 24 hour maintenance fluid requirements for a 30 kg child C 15.2.2

A. 1000 ml
B. 1300 ml
C. 1700 ml
D. 1900 ml

328. How much sodium does a 30 kg child require a day B 15.2.2

A. 3 mEq
B. 9 mEq
C. 15 mEq
D. 20 mEq

329. What is the water deficit in a 16 kg child with hypernatremic dehydration, who normally weighs 20kg, and has a serum sodium of 160 mmol/L A 15.2.3

A. 1500 ml
B. 1200 ml
C. 1000 ml
D. 900 ml

330. A child with meningitis has a sodium level of 124 mmol/L and a blood urea nitrogen of 6 mg/dL. What is the recommended course of therapy if the hyponatremia is not symptomatic B 15.2.3

A. continue maintenance intravenous fluids with 0.45 normal saline
B. impose fluid restriction
C. replace fluid with hot salt (3% saline)
D. change fluid to normal saline and run it at 1.5-times maintenance

331. What is the anion gap with a sodium of 140 mmol/L, potassium of 4 mmol/L, chloride of 108 mmol/L, and bicarbonate of 20 mmol/L A 15.1.2

A. 16
B. 10
C. 18
D. 20

332. How many ml of 3% saline is required to raise the serum sodium from 110 to 120 mmol/L in a 20 kg patient C 15.2.3

A. 60 ml
B. 100 ml
C. 240 ml
D. 300 ml

333. A dehydrated child is inadvertently given intravenous fluids containing 60 mmol/L of potassium. An electrocardiogram is performed that reveals peaked T waves. The best next action is to D 15.2.3

A. administer calcium chloride
B. perform dialysis
C. administer insulin
D. administer calcium gluconate

334. A child presents with a history of vomiting. On exam, you note dry mucous membranes, reduced tearing, acrocyanosis, tachycardia, prolonged capillary refill time, lethargy, and a concentrated urine. What is the estimated level of dehydration. C 15.2.1

A. <5%
B. <7%
C. 10%

335. If a patient presents with a primary metabolic acidosis without other derangement and a pH of 7.24, the $PaCO_2$ (in mm Hg) should be E 15.3.1

A. 16
B. 18
C. 20
D. 22
E. 24

336. A patient presents with sepsis. His bicarbonate level is 14 mmol/L and his $PaCO_2$ is 47 mm Hg. What is his acid-base status C 15.3.1

A. combined metabolic and respiratory alkalosis
B. mixed metabolic acidosis and respiratory alkalosis
C. combined metabolic and respiratory acidosis
D. mixed metabolic alkalosis and respiratory acidosis

337. What condition is associated with clinical signs of dehydration at lower levels of fluid deficit B 15.2.1

A. hypernatremia
B. hyponatremia
C. isonatremia
D. acidosis
E. alkalosis

16 NEUROLOGIC DISORDERS

16.1 GENERAL CONCEPTS

16.1.1 Brain Growth

A. Optimal brain growth and development requires structural integrity, adequate nutritional substrates at the appropriate time, absence of toxic and traumatic insults, and environmental stimulation. Deficiencies in any of these areas can result in suboptimal neurological development.

B. The skull grows in response to developing brain tissue.
   1. Microcephaly is due to smaller than average brain volume. Lack of skull growth does not cause microcephaly.
   2. Macrocephaly results from a large brain or increased intracranial contents (hydrocephalus).

C. Physical brain growth continues until around 10 years of age.
   1. At birth the head is nearly 2/3 the adult size.
   2. More than 8/10 the adult size is reached by 1 year of age.

D. Myelinization of the spinal cord is not completed until 2 years after birth.

16.1.2 Diagnostic Modalities

A. Serum Electrolytes, Glucose, Magnesium, and Calcium
   1. A fingerstick glucose should be done early in evaluation of altered sensorium. Hypoglycemia can cause profound and, if not rapidly reversed, permanent central nervous system (CNS) changes.
   2. Determination of electrolytes and minerals may detect treatable causes of CNS dysfunction such as hyponatremia.

B. Toxicology Screens
   1. A toxicology screen should always be considered in cases which neurologic changes do not have an obvious explanation.
   2. In seizure patients with neurologic changes, anticonvulsant levels are indicated.

C. Lumbar Puncture (LP) and Cerebrospinal Fluid (CSF) Analysis
   1. The most common parameters assessed via an LP are opening pressure, CSF cell count, CSF protein, CSF glucose, counter current immune electrophoresis (CCIE), and Gram stain.
   2. In uncooperative infants and children, the opening pressure is of questionable validity.
   3. Before performing the LP, evaluate for evidence of significantly increased intracranial pressure by examining for papilledema or, if time permits, perform a computed tomography (CT) scan of the head.
   4. Focal neurologic deficits should raise the question of a significant intracranial mass effect.
   5. Normal CSF Values (Table 16.1.2)

D. Electroencephalography (EEG)
   1. The electroencephalogram is being replaced by magnetic resonance imaging (MRI), evoked potentials, CT scans, and regional blood flow studies as both a diagnostic and prognostic tool in many of the neurological conditions.
   2. It is still useful to confirm, classify, and monitor seizure activity and its response to anticonvulsant therapy.

E. Evoked Potentials. Computer enhanced averaging of responses to cortical auditory, visual, or somatosensory-evoked responses can be used by skilled interpreters to arrive at clinical interpretations of brain functional integrity with fairly reproducible results.

F. Computed Tomography (CT) Scan of the Head
   1. The CT scan can reveal structural abnormalities, midline shifts from mass lesions, acute and chronic bleeds, tumors, and cerebral edema.
   2. A CT scan without contrast media is indicated in suspected acute CNS bleeds. It may not detect chronic subdural hematomas if the clot has organized sufficiently to be of similar density to surrounding brain tissue.
   3. A CT scan with contrast media is needed to best delineate vascularized tumors, arteriovenous malformations, and chronic subdural clots. Contrast media should not be used if the patient has evidence of decreased glomerular filtration rate (elevated blood urea nitrogen/creatinine ratio) because its use in such as situation can result in acute renal failure.

G. Magnetic Resonance Imaging (MRI)
   1. The MRI is a noninvasive technique that provides detailed delineation of white and gray matter of the brain and can provide information about not only

Table 16.1.2 Normal cerebrospinal fluid values

Age	Opening Pressure (cm H_2O)	Glucose (mg/dl)	Protein (mg/dl)	Polymorpho-nuclearcytes	Lymphocytes	Red Blood Cells
Newborn	70 to 180	50-80	150	<8	<30	<50
3 months	70 to 180	(2/3 of blood glucose)	<65	<3	<15	<30
>6 months	70 to 150	(2/3 of blood glucose)	10 to 40	0	<5	<5

structural abnormalities, but histological and biochemical information as well.

2. MRI cannot detect calcified lesions and it requires much longer immobilization.
3. MRI usually requires sedation in children.

16.1.3 The Neurologic Exam

A. **Cranial Nerves** (CN) and Disease Manifestations.

1. Olfactory Nerve (CN I). Anosmia (loss of sense of smell) is most commonly due to upper respiratory tract infections, but may be seen with frontal lobe tumors or damage to the cribriform plate. Congenital lesions are very infrequent.
2. Optic Nerve (CN II)
   a. Examine by testing visual acuity and optic nerve disc visualization after pupillary dilatation, unless contraindicated (monitoring neurologic status by following pupil reaction).
   b. Cataract formation interferes with exam.
   c. Papilledema is present if the optic disc margins are blurred. Hyperemia, dilated veins, and constricted arterioles may be present. Visual acuity and color vision generally remain intact.
3. Oculomotor Nerve (CN III)
   a. Innervates the superior, inferior, and medial rectus, as well as the inferior oblique and superior levator muscles.
   b. Damage results in ptosis, dilated pupils, and deviation of the eye out and down.
4. Trochlear Nerve (CN IV). Innervates the superior oblique muscle. Damage results in paralysis of upward, outward gaze.
5. Trigeminal Nerve (CN V)
   a. This nerve provides sensory innervation to the face, part of the neck, and cornea.
   b. It provides motor innervation to the masseter, temporalis, and pterygoid muscles.
   c. It has three branches: ophthalmic, maxillary, and mandibular.
6. Abducens Nerve (CN VI). Innervates the lateral rectus muscle. Damage results in the inability to move the eye laterally past midline.
7. Facial Nerve (CN VII)
   a. Its motor function is innervation of the facial musculature and the stapedius muscle of the middle ear.
   b. Its sensory function is to provide taste to the anterior 2/3 of the tongue.
   c. Injury to the central portion of CN VII motor neurons results in decreased movement of the lower face with a flattened nasolabial fold on the same side as the lesion.
   d. Injury to the peripheral nerve affects the upper and lower face equally (Bell's palsy).
8. Auditory Nerve (CN VIII)
   a. CN VIII is responsible for hearing and vestibular function.
   b. Risk factors for injury include prematurity, ototoxic drugs, asphyxia, family history of deafness, severe hyperbilirubinemia, bacterial meningitis, congenital malformation, and TORCH infection. Children with these conditions should be screened for hearing loss in infancy.
   c. Vestibular function can be assessed by caloric testing. Five milliliters of ice water is instilled into the ear canal of a patient. If nerve function is intact, the eyes deviate toward the stimulus or nystagmus is demonstrated with the quick movement away from the stimulated labyrinth. Warm water has the reverse effect. These results can be recalled by the phrase "cold opposite, warm same" in reference to the quick component of nystagmus. If there is no response, the brainstem is not functioning.
9. Glossopharyngeal Nerve (CN IX). Innervates the stylopharyngeal muscle and provides taste to the posterior 1/3 of the tongue.
10. Vagus Nerve (CN X). Provides innervation to the vocal cords and muscles of the soft palate. Isolated vocal cord paralysis may occur after chest and neck surgery due to damage of the recurrent laryngeal nerve.
11. Accessory Nerve (CN XI). Innervates the sternocleidomastoid and trapezius muscles.
12. Hypoglossal Nerve (CN XII). Innervates the tongue. With damage, the tongue cannot be extended. If damage is unilateral, the tongue will curve towards the side of injury upon protrusion.

B. **Motor Testing**

1. Assess muscle bulk and tone.
2. Strength Testing
   a. Grade 0/5 is flaccidity.
   b. Grade 1/5 is flicker or fasciculation.
   c. Grade 2/5 is active movement if gravity is eliminated.
   d. Grade 3/5 is active movement against gravity.
   e. Grade 4/5 is movement against gravity and mild resistance.
   f. Grade 5/5 is normal strength.
3. Observe posture, gait, and motility for abnormality.
4. Muscle Stretch (Deep Tendon) Reflexes
   a. Grade 0/4 is no reflex elicited.
   b. Grade 1/4 is less than normal.
   c. Grade 2/4 is normal.
   d. Grade 3/4 is more brisk than normal.
   e. Grade 4/4 is hyperreflexic.
   f. Note if symmetry is present or absent.
   g. Deep tendon reflexes may be absent in peripheral neuropathy or myopathy.
   h. Deep tendon reflexes are increased in upper mo-

tor neuron disease.

5. Abnormalities on Motor Testing
   a. Common abnormalities include weakness, fasciculations, atrophy, hypotonicity, and hypertonicity.
   b. Clonus is a rhythmic cycle of contraction and relaxation in response to rapid forced movement of a muscle group.
   c. Tics may be transient or chronic and are nonrhythmic movements of a muscle group. If they are chronic and associated with a vocal component, the diagnosis is likely Tourette's syndrome.
   d. Rigidity is resistance to movement of a muscle group. It may be characterized as having a cogwheel sensation or a clasp-knife feel.
   e. Ataxia is incoordination of movement or a problem with balance.
   f. Romberg's sign is unsteadiness when standing with the eyes shut.
   g. Dysmetria is a cerebellar sign characterized by difficulty in measuring distance (past pointing).
   h. Decorticate posturing is characterized by extension of the lower extremities and flexion of the upper extremities.
   i. Decerebrate posturing is extension of the extremities signifying brainstem injury.
   j. Dystonia is a slow, twisting movement of proximal muscle groups.
   k. Opisthotonus is tonic arching of the back with the head and heels forced backwards.
   l. Chorea is rapid jerking movements of the head and extremities associated with basal ganglia lesions. A classic example is the "milkmaid" sign where the hand grasps and releases repetitively.
   m. Athetosis is slow writhing hand movements due to basal ganglia lesions.
   n. Babinski's sign is the abnormal extension of the great toe upon stroking of the sole of the foot. It is abnormal if present after one year of age and signifies an upper motor neuron lesion.

C. The Primitive Reflexes

1. These reflexes are present in normal infants and appear and disappear in sequence. Persistence beyond certain ages signifies abnormal neurologic function.
2. Palmar grasp begins at 28 weeks estimated gestational age and disappears about 3 months of age.
3. Moro reflex is symmetric abduction and extension of the arms followed by flexion and adduction when the head falls backwards. It is abnormal after 6 months of age.
4. Tonic neck reflex is extension of the arm in the direction which the head is manually rotated with flexion of the opposite arm. It is abnormal after 6 months of age.
5. Parachute sign is a protective reflex characterized by spontaneous extension of the upper extremities when the suspended child is flexed forward. It appears at 7 months of age and persists throughout life.

D. Gait Disturbance

1. Circumduction gait is a lateral circular motion about the hip in a patient with hemiparesis.
2. Waddling gait is associated with weakness of the hip girdle.

E. Sensory Testing

1. Address the presence of numbness, tingling, burning sensation, and pain.
2. Sensory function can be tested by two-point and sharp-dull discrimination.
3. Position sense, light touch, pain, and vibratory sensation should be assessed.
4. Infants and young children are unable to cooperate well with sensory exam. Impressions are based upon the child's response to a given stimulus.

16.1.4 Pathophysiologic Manifestations

A. Upper Motor Neuron Disease

1. This includes the corticospinal tract and its associated motor neurons.
2. All muscle groups below the level of the lesion are affected.
3. Muscle tone and reflexes are increased.
4. Atrophy is absent.
5. Posture is that of upper extremity flexion and lower extremity extension.
6. A common example of this type of lesion is cerebral palsy.

B. Lower Motor Unit Disease

1. This includes the anterior horn cells, motor nerves, peripheral motor nerves, neuromuscular junction, and muscles.
2. Individual units of muscles or muscle groups are affected.
3. Muscles are flaccid with decreased or absent reflexes.
4. Fasciculations may be present.
5. Atrophy is prominent.
6. Representative examples of this process include spinal muscular atrophy, poliomyelitis, Guillain-Barré syndrome, botulism, muscular dystrophy, thyroid disease, hyperkalemia, and glycogen storage disease.

16.2 DISEASE PROFILES

16.2.1 Neural Tube Defects

A. These are a group of conditions due to embryologic failure of the neural tube to close between 3 and 4-weeks estimated gestational age. There is a known association with folate deficiency.

1. Spina bifida occulta is a midline closure defect of the vertebral arch without protrusion of the spinal cord or meninges. Overlying skin may have a birthmark or hairy patch.
2. Meningocele is spina bifida with herniation of the meninges and an associated Arnold-Chiari malformation (Arnold-Chiari malformation is protrusion of the brainstem through the foramen magnum with associated hydrocephalus).
3. Myelomeningocele is a defect that involves herniation of the meninges and spinal cord elements.
   a. Arnold-Chiari malformation and hydrocephalus is present.
   b. The degree of deficit corresponds to the level of the lesion.
4. Encephalocele is dysraphism of the skull with herniation of the cranial vault contents. Nasal encephaloceles may be mistaken for polyps.
5. Anencephaly is absence of the cranial vault associated with severe brain malformation. The brainstem may be functional, but the condition is generally considered incompatible with life.
6. Diplomyelia is duplication of the spinal cord.
7. Diastematomyelia is a cleft in the spinal cord.
8. Syringomyelia is a fluid-filled cyst in the spinal cord.
9. Sacral dysgenesis is seen in 1% of infants of diabetic mothers.
10. Neurodermal sinus may be a site of entry for recurrent CNS infections. Consider this when evaluating sacral pits.

B. Treatment

1. Therapy depends upon the nature of the condition.
2. Surgical closure of spinal defects is accomplished with concomitant placement of a ventriculoperitoneal shunt for hydrocephalus.
3. Most children will require evaluation of their urinary tract and clean intermittent bladder catheterization.
4. A multidisciplinary approach involving primary care, neurosurgery, orthopedics, occupational therapy, physical therapy, urology, neurology, and social services is necessary for coordinated care.
5. Anencephaly is usually not treated.
6. Management of encephaloceles depends upon the extent of the lesion.

C. Complications of dysraphism and treatment include hydrocephalus, ventriculoperitoneal shunt malfunction or infection, renal disease, urinary tract infection, scoliosis, tethered cord, developmental and cognitive delay, constipation, and social adaptation problems.

16.2.2 Disorders of Cellular Proliferation and Migration

A. Agenesis of the Corpus Callosum

1. This condition is usually identified when a child undergoes an evaluation for developmental delay or new-onset seizures.
2. On neuroimaging, the ventricles are farther apart than normal.
3. Predisposing conditions include maternal ingestion of toxic substances and genetic abnormalities.
4. Symptoms range from none to seizures and severe mental retardation.
5. Prognosis depends on the severity of the malformation.

B. Microcephaly

1. Head circumference is more than 2 standard deviations below average.
2. Predisposing conditions include chromosomal anomalies, idiopathic causes, hypothyroidism, Hurler's syndrome, rickets, and craniosynostosis.

C. Macrocephaly

1. Head circumference is the more than 2 standard deviations above average.
2. Hydrocephalus is most common cause in infants. Inherited metabolic anomalies, chromosome anomalies, arachnoid cysts, and leukodystrophies are also associated.

D. Hydrencephaly

1. This condition results from necrosis of the cerebral cortex in utero.
2. Prognosis. Affected infants usually die within the first year of life.

E. Hydrocephalus

1. Noncommunicating hydrocephalus is ventricular enlargement due to obstruction of CSF flow.
   a. It may result in signs and symptoms of increased intracranial pressure.
   b. It generally requires placement of a ventriculoperitoneal or ventriculoatrial shunt.
2. Communicating hydrocephalus is due to abnormal absorption of CSF.
3. Hydrocephalus ex vacuo is the appearance of increased fluid-filled spaces on neuroimaging secondary to brain atrophy instead of obstruction.
4. Predisposing conditions include prenatal or perinatal intraventricular bleeds, infections, brain tumors, and malformations.
5. Symptoms include accelerated rate of head growth, irritability, headaches, and vomiting.

F. Dandy-Walker Malformation

1. This is cystic dilation of the fourth ventricle with resulting hydrocephalus.
2. Pathophysiology is atresia or blockage of the foramen of Magendie and foramen of Luschka.
3. Shunting is always required.
4. Prognosis depends upon the severity of associated brain malformations. Developmental delay may be mild or severe.

16.2.3 Craniosynostosis

A. This is premature closure of the cranial sutures.
   1. Primary craniosynostosis is closure of one or more sutures due to an abnormality of skull development.
   2. Secondary craniosynostosis is closure due to lack of brain growth.

B. Incidence in 1 in 2,000 infants.

C. **Abnormal Head Shapes**
   1. Scaphocephaly is a prominent forehead and occiput secondary to closure of the sagittal suture.
   2. Frontal plagiocephaly is unilateral flattening of the forehead with elevation of the orbit due to closure of the coronal and sphenofrontal sutures.
   3. Trigonocephaly is a triangular-shaped skull secondary to premature closure of the metopic (mid-frontal) suture.
   4. Occipital plagiocephaly is most often due to positioning in infancy rather than craniosynostosis of the lambdoid sutures. It is characterized by occipital flattening with bulging of the frontal bone.
   5. Turricephaly is a conical skull due to coronal suture closure.
   6. Kleeblattschädel deformity is a cloverleaf-shaped skull seen in association with Carpenter and Crouzon's syndromes.

D. Complications
   1. Premature closure of a single suture usually does not cause neurologic problems.
   2. There is risk of increased intracranial pressure and neurologic dysfunction if 2 or more sutures are involved.

16.2.4 Seizure Disorders

A. Seizures result from abnormal neuronal discharges in the cerebral cortex.

B. They have many causes that can be grouped by age of onset.
   1. Day of life #1: hypoxia, drugs, birth trauma, infection, hyperglycemia, hypoglycemia, and pyridoxine deficiency.
   2. Day of life #2 and #3: infection, drug withdrawal, hypoglycemia, hypocalcemia, developmental brain malformation, intracranial hemorrhage, inborn error of metabolism, infection, hyponatremia, and hypernatremia.
   3. One week to 6 months of life: infection, hypocalcemia, hyperphosphatemia, hyponatremia, developmental malformation, trauma, drug withdrawal, and inborn error of metabolism.
   4. Six months to 3 years of age: febrile seizure, birth injury, infection, toxin exposure, trauma, metabolic disorder, and cerebral degenerative disease.
   5. Over 3 years of age: idiopathic, infection, trauma, and cerebral degenerative disease.

C. Classification
   1. Partial seizures have a focal onset.
      a. Simple implies that consciousness is retained.
      b. Complex seizures are associated with impairment of consciousness.
      c. Motor seizures are most common. Sensory and autonomic seizures may also occur.
      d. Associated signs may be an aura or automatisms (lip smacking, chewing, picking motion, and pulling motion).
   2. Generalized Seizures
      a. Absence seizures are the sudden cessation of normal activity associated with a blank stare and no postictal period. The classic EEG pattern is 3 per second spike and wave discharges.
      b. Generalized tonic-clonic seizures may occur spontaneously or result from secondary generalization of a partial seizure. They are usually associated with a postictal phase. They can occur at any age with or without an aura.

D. Recognized Seizure Disorders
   1. **Benign Rolandic Epilepsy of Childhood**
      a. These seizures are transmitted as an autosomal dominant trait with a family history of seizures present in approximately 40% of affected children.
      b. Seizures are nocturnal in 70% of patients.
      c. The typical seizure is paresthesia followed by twitching of the face and mouth with associated drooling and loss of speech. Consciousness is preserved unless secondary generalization occurs. Duration is approximately 1 to 2 minutes.
      d. The epileptogenic focus is high-voltage spikes in the central or centrotemporal (Rolandic) area of the brain.
      e. MRI and CT studies of the brain are normal.
      f. Treatment is not needed if seizures are not frequent or if they only occur at night. Seizures respond well to phenobarbital or phenytoin.
      g. Prognosis is very good with seizures resolving with age whether or not the child was treated.
   2. **Rasmussen's Encephalitis**
      a. This condition is characterized by focal, partial seizures that do not stop spontaneously.
      b. Progressive neurologic deficits such as paralysis develop and may persist.
      c. EEG shows spike discharges that spread to adjacent areas and to the mirror focus in the opposite hemisphere.
      d. Aggressive drug therapy, including pentobarbital coma in refractory status epilepticus is indicated. Hemispherectomy may provide the best long-term control.
      e. Etiology is unknown, but is thought to be due to a low-grade encephalitis.

3. **Benign myoclonus of infancy** is myoclonic jerks without associated EEG change. Treatment is not indicated.
4. **Juvenile myoclonic epilepsy** presents in adolescents with myoclonic jerks on arising in the morning, abating later in the day. Over the course of years, the child may develop generalized tonic-clonic epilepsy.
5. **Progressive myoclonic epilepsy** is myoclonic jerking associated with progressive neurologic deterioration within 1 year of seizure onset.
6. **Infantile Spasm**
   a. Presents in infants at 4 to 8 months of age as brief, repetitive, symmetric contractions of the flexor neck, trunk, and extremity musculature.
   b. Hypsarrhythmia is the classic EEG finding.
   c. The prognosis depends upon the etiology. In infants with a preceding neurologic insult or genetic syndrome, the incidence of mental retardation is up to 90%.
   d. Treatment is with anticonvulsants or occasionally intramuscular adrenocorticotropic hormone has a varied success rate.
7. **Febrile Seizures**
   a. This is the most common seizure disorder of childhood occurring in children without underlying neurologic disorder.
   b. It has an excellent prognosis, but may be indicative of a serious underlying disease (meningitis, sepsis).
   c. Age of incidence is 6 months to 6 years with a peak at 18 months of age.
   d. There is a familial predisposition.
   e. Typically the seizure is generalized tonic-clonic activity less than 10 minutes in duration with only a brief postictal phase.
   f. Seizures are atypical if they last >15 minutes, occur repeatedly during the illness, or have a focal component.
   g. EEG and neuroimaging are not routinely indicated.
   h. The risk of maintenance antiepileptic drug therapy outweighs the benefit because only 30% of children who experience a first febrile seizure will have a subsequent episode.
   i. Prognosis is good with an incidence of progression to epilepsy of only 2% by 7 years of age. This incidence is slightly increased if the child has atypical febrile seizures.

E. Commonly Used Antiepileptic Drugs
1. Carbamazepine (Tegretol®): generalized tonic-clonic or partial epilepsy.
2. Ethosuximide (Zarontin®): absence seizures or myoclonic seizures.
3. Gabapentin (Neurontin®): adjunctive therapy for poorly controlled seizures.
4. Lamotrigine (Lamictal®): adjunctive therapy for poorly controlled seizures.
5. Phenobarbital: generalized tonic-clonic seizure maintenance and acute status epilepticus.
6. Phenytoin (Dilantin®): generalized tonic-clonic or partial complex epilepsy, and treatment of status epilepticus.
7. Valproic acid (Depakene®, Depakote®): generalized tonic-clonic, partial complex, akinetic, or absence epilepsy, and myoclonus.
8. Primidone (Mysoline®): generalized tonic-clonic and partial epilepsy.

F. Treatment side effects include dizziness, drowsiness, liver dysfunction, bone marrow dysfunction, weight gain, abdominal pain, gingival hyperplasia, developmental delay, skin rash (Stevens-Johnson syndrome), and birth defects.

G. Alternative Treatments
1. Adrenocorticotropic hormone has been used with some success in infantile spasm.
2. Epilepsy surgery to ablate the offending focus of activity or to implant automated vagal nerve stimulators (defibrillates the brain) decrease seizure frequency.
3. Ketogenic diets may work in some disorders to decrease seizure activity.

H. Differential diagnosis includes many episodic events that mimic seizure activity.
1. **Pseudoseizure** ("Hysterical" Seizure)
   a. Occur most often in adolescents, especially females.
   b. Forty percent of individuals have a true seizure disorder. The pseudoseizures begin when the true concurrent seizures are effectively controlled.
   c. They are attention-seeking behaviors with a great deal of secondary gain. Typically a history of psychosocial stressor can be obtained.
   d. "Seizures" are characterized by bilateral or unilateral, tonic posturing and tremulousness with thrashing or jerking instead of true tonic-clonic activity. Expressions of distress followed by semipurposeful activity or unresponsiveness may also occur.
   e. Diagnosis is by observation. Video EEG is very useful.
   f. Present the diagnosis to the patient and the family carefully. Reassure them that the child is not "faking" or "crazy." Determine the secondary gain and address this issue. Pseudoseizures generally cease when the diagnosis is made and explained.
2. Other episodic disorders confused with seizures include breath-holding spells, night terrors, sleep

walking, benign paroxysmal vertigo, pallid attacks, simple syncope, prolonged QT syndrome, cataplexy, narcolepsy, and shuddering attacks.

16.2.5 Neurocutaneous Syndromes

A. Neurofibromatosis (Von Recklinghausen's Disease)

1. Autosomal dominant disease characterized by skin, ocular, and neurologic findings.
2. Physical Findings
   - **a.** Six or more café au lait spots are diagnostic.
   - **b.** Lisch nodules (pigmented nodules) in the iris are present in 90% of patients.
   - **c.** Neurofibromas of the skin also occur.
3. Potential complications include seizure disorders, optic nerve gliomas, acoustic neuromas, meningiomas, and spinal cord tumors.
4. Genetic counseling is warranted.

B. Tuberous Sclerosis (Bourneville's Disease)

1. This autosomal dominant inherited disorder is a triad of skin lesions, seizures, and mental retardation.
2. Symptoms include epilepsy, mental retardation, and autistic features. Severity of symptoms varies among affected individuals.
3. Physical findings include ash-leaf spots seen with a Wood's lamp, shagreen patches, café au lait spots, and facial angiokeratomas seen during the second decade of life. Retinal hamartomas are present in 50% of patients.
4. Potential complications are periventricular tumors, cysts, and malignant tumors in the heart, kidneys, pancreas, and peritoneal cavity.
5. Treat the associated conditions and lesions. Provide genetic counseling.

C. Sturge-Weber Syndrome

1. These are capillary hemangiomas over the trigeminal nerve distribution on the face. The condition may be linked with certain kinds of brain damage.
2. Seizures may occur if the lesion involves the optic branch of the trigeminal nerve.
3. Physical findings include port-wine stain due to capillary hemangiomas on the face and glaucoma.
4. Seizures may be intractable to medications and require surgery to remove the inciting part of the brain.

D. Ataxia-Telangiectasia (Louis-Bar Syndrome)

1. This autosomal recessive condition affects the skin, cerebellum, and immune system.
2. Ataxia usually presents in first 5 years of life.
3. Telangiectasias are most prominent in the second 5 years of life and involve the conjunctivae and ears.
4. Potential complications include lung infections due to immunoglobulin A deficiency by 10 years of age and malignant lymphomas by 15 to 20 years of age.
5. Differential diagnosis includes cerebral palsy and Friedreich's ataxia.
6. Death usually occurs due to infection or malignancy.

16.2.6 Degenerative CNS diseases

A. Most diseases of this category are genetically transmitted and may involve metabolic derangements. While they are characterized by a deterioration of function, this deterioration may initially manifest as arrested neurologic development.

B. Table 16.2.6 Entities detectable by "metabolic screen"

DISEASE	DETECTED BY
Phenylketonuria	Ferric chloride
Maple syrup urine disease	Ferric chloride
Hypothyroidism	Thyroid-stimulating hormone, Thyroxine
Tyrosinosis	Ferric chloride
Galactosemia	Benedict's solution
Fructosemia	Benedict's solution
Homocystinuria	Nitroprusside
Hypermethionemia	Nitroprusside
Mucopolysaccharidosis	Cetrimonium bromide

C. Degenerative diseases of the basal ganglia are reflected primarily via movement disorders such as dystonia, chorea, athetosis, and tremor.

D. Wilson's Disease (Hepatolenticular Degeneration)

1. This autosomal recessive disorder is due to a defect in copper metabolism causing copper accumulation in tissue, including the brain, liver and cornea.
2. Physical findings include hepatomegaly, choreoathetoid movements, and Kayser-Fleischer rings in the corneas.
3. Laboratory Findings
   - **a.** Copper levels greater than 250 mcg/g of liver is diagnostic.
   - **b.** Decreased serum copper and decreased serum ceruloplasmin are also present.
4. Treatment is with lifelong chelation therapy using D-penicillamine.
5. Prognosis is poor with progressive neurologic deterioration if untreated.

E. Degenerative changes of the cerebellum, brainstem, and spinal cord are usually reflected in an ataxic gait.

1. **Friedreich's ataxia** is progressive ataxia, weakness and wasting of distal muscles with death usually due to cardiomyopathy by 30 years of age.
2. **Ramsay Hunt syndrome** is dentate cerebellar ataxia.
3. Hereditary cerebellar ataxias may occur as a familial condition.

F. Degenerative diseases of the cerebral cortex white matter manifest primarily by visual impairment and spasticity. Dementia and seizures may occur late in the course of disease.

1. **Metachromatic leukodystrophy** is due to defi-

ciency of the arylsulfatase A enzymes. The infantile form is fatal by 5 to 6 years of age.

2. **Adrenoleukodystrophy** has onset at 8 to 10 years of age with death 2 to 5 years later. It is characterized by adrenal insufficiency with dementia and spastic gait.
3. **Rett's syndrome** occurs in girls and presents with a peculiar wringing motion of the hands, progressive ataxia, and dementia.

G. Many degenerative diseases of gray matter are neuronal storage diseases.

1. **Tay-Sachs disease** is a gangliosidosis due to a deficiency of hexosaminidase A. Findings are cherry red macula, hyperacusis to noise, and death by 3 to 4 years of age.
2. **Niemann-Pick disease** is due to accumulation of sphingomyelin in the reticuloendothelial system resulting from a deficiency of sphingomyelinase. Findings include an enlarged liver and spleen.
3. **Gaucher's disease** is due to a deficiency of glucocerebrosidase characterized by hepatosplenomegaly.
4. **Menkes' kinky hair syndrome** is an X-linked defect in copper absorption. Profound neurologic deficits are present with death occurring before 2 years of age.

H. Miscellaneous Degenerative CNS Disease

1. **Dystonia musculorum deformans** is muscle spasms causing slow, twisting movements. The cause is unknown.
2. **Lesch-Nyhan syndrome** is characterized by self-mutilation, elevated uric acid due to a purine metabolism defect, mental retardation, and choreoathetosis.

I. Anterior Horn Cell Diseases

1. **Spinal muscular atrophy** is similar to amyotrophic lateral sclerosis in adults.
2. **Werdnig-Hoffman disease** is a progressive disease. It is often fatal by 2 years of age.

J. Degeneration of the Neuromuscular Junction – **Myasthenia Gravis**

1. Autoimmune disease with antibodies developing against acetylcholine receptors at the motor endplate.
2. Pathophysiology
   a. Neonatal myasthenia gravis is transient and is due to transplacental antibodies from the mother. It resolves within 2 months of birth.
   b. Congenital myasthenia gravis does not have detectable antibodies. Ptosis is noted by 2 years of life.
   c. Juvenile myasthenia gravis is similar to the adult form.
3. Physical findings include muscle weakness that returns to normal with an edrophonium test.
4. Treatment is with pyridostigmine. Immunosuppression with steroids may help.
5. Prognosis. If ocular muscle weakness alone is present for more than 2 years, progression of the disease tends to be limited.

K. Peripheral Neuropathies – **Guillain-Barré Syndrome**

1. Guillain-Barré syndrome is a demyelinating polyneuropathy that typically follows a viral infection or immunization.
2. Paresthesias may accompany the weakness.
3. Physical findings include an ascending muscle weakness with paralysis.
4. Laboratory findings include an elevated CSF protein with a normal CSF cell count.
5. Complications include respiratory failure and autonomic instability (hypertension).
6. Treatment is primarily supportive care. Prednisone, intravenous immune globulin, or plasmapheresis may help minimize disease progression.
7. Prognosis. Fatality is rare, but recovery may take up to a year. Up to 15% of affected individuals may have residual neuromuscular deficits.

L. Hereditary Sensory and Motor Neuropathy

1. This is a family of disorders. **Charcot-Marie-Tooth disease** (peroneal muscle weakness) is the most common disorder in this group.
2. Weakness begins in the feet during the first decade of life.
3. Physical findings include ataxia, retinitis, and deafness.
4. Delayed nerve conduction time is evident on electromyography.
5. The condition may progress to significant loss of muscle strength, but most often is of a mild course with normal life expectancy.

16.2.7 Encephalopathies

A. **Cerebral Palsy** (CP)

1. This is a static disorder of posture and movement that may have associated seizures, speech disorder, decreased visual acuity, and mental retardation.
2. Pathophysiology
   a. CP was originally felt to be primarily related to birth trauma, prematurity, and asphyxia. Despite advances in perinatal care, the incidence of CP is not declining.
   b. The Collaborative Perinatal Project found an incidence of CP of 4:1,000 live births. Birth asphyxia was an uncommon cause. Intrauterine infection and low birth weight were associated with the highest incidence of CP, however most causes were not identified.
3. Classification
   a. Spastic hemiplegia is decreased spontaneous movement on the affected side. Affected children may demonstrate an early hand preference

(Hand preference is normally not manifested until about 18 months of age).

b. Spastic diplegia is bilateral spasticity of the legs. Children usually have normal intellect and a low incidence of seizures.

c. Spastic quadriplegia is the most severe form of CP. Affected children have motor impairment of all extremities with a high incidence of mental retardation and seizures. They may be prone to aspiration pneumonia secondary to associated bulbar palsy.

d. Athetoid CP is a rare form of the disorder characterized by hypotonia, prominent tongue thrust, drooling, slurred speech, and athetoid movements. Seizures and deficient intellect are rare.

B. Reye's Syndrome

1. This is an acquired encephalopathy associated with fatty degeneration of the viscera and mitochondrial abnormalities.
2. The condition is sporadic.
   a. The association with salicylate ingestion in the presence of influenza B and varicella virus infection is well known.
   b. It occurs with valproic acid hepatotoxicity in the presence of a genetic disposition.
   c. It is seen in "Jamaican vomiting sickness" due to toxin exposure.
   d. It may be recurrent in disorders of fatty acid oxidation.

C. Acquired immunodeficiency syndrome's encephalopathy is an acute onset of brain growth arrest with developmental delay and progressive neurologic deterioration.

D. Other causes of encephalopathy include lead, renal hypertension, and radiation exposure.

16.2.8 Stroke Syndromes

A. Stroke in children occurs with a yearly incidence of 1 to 3/100,000.

B. Etiologies

1. **Arterial Thrombosis or Embolism**
   a. Blunt trauma to the posterior pharynx due to a fall on a Popsicle stick or pencil held in the mouth with subsequent damage to the carotid artery is relatively common.
   b. Retropharyngeal abscess causes inflammation of the internal carotid artery with intimal thrombus formation.
   c. Thromboembolic events also occur in association with congenital and acquired heart disease and vasoocclusive disorders.
2. **Venous Sinus Thrombosis**
   a. Sepsis (bacterial meningitis and encephalitis) are associated with thrombosis.
   b. Nonseptic causes include severe dehydration, hypercoagulable states (cyanotic congenital heart disease, protein C deficiency, protein S deficiency, antithrombin III deficiency), hyperviscosity syndromes (polycythemia, leukemia), and sickle cell disease.
3. Intracranial Hemorrhage
   a. Subarachnoid bleeding is associated with headache, nuchal rigidity, and altered consciousness.
   b. Intracerebral hemorrhage is associated with focal neurologic findings and may be seen with arteriovenous malformation, cerebral aneurysm, idiopathic thrombocytopenic purpura, and hemophilia.

C. Differential diagnosis includes migraine, alternating hemiplegia of childhood, metabolic disease, Todd's paralysis following seizure, tumor, encephalitis, and focal postviral encephalitis.

D. Treat the underlying condition and provide supportive care for the acute signs and symptoms of stroke.

16.2.9 Muscular Dystrophy (MD)

A. MD is a group of primary myopathies with a genetic basis associated with progressive degeneration of muscle fibers.

B. Representative Diseases

1. **Duchenne's MD**
   a. This is the most common form of MD and is an X-linked recessive disorder. Carrier females are not affected.
   b. Early motor development may be normal or associated with subtle signs of dysfunction.
   c. Signs and symptoms include a Trendelenburg gait (hip waddle), Gower's sign, primarily proximal muscle weakness, pseudohypertrophy of the calves with wasting of thigh muscles, and intellectual impairment.
   d. Complications include cardiomyopathy, joint contractures, scoliosis, and respiratory compromise.
   e. Laboratory evaluation shows elevated creatinine kinase even in asymptomatic individuals.
   f. Additional evaluation should include echocardiography, electromyography, and muscle biopsy.
   g. The disease is a painless process that results in death, usually by 18 years of age.
   h. Treatment is supportive with care for complications as they occur.
2. **Becker's MD** is the same as Duchenne's MD except patients remain ambulatory until late adolescence, with death occurring in their 20's.
3. **Emery-Dreifuss MD** (Scapuloperoneal or Scapulohumeral MD)
   a. This is an X-linked disorder with onset of slowly progressive symptoms in middle childhood.

b. Signs and symptoms include muscle wasting in a scapulohumeroperoneal distribution. Myotonia is not present.
c. Intelligence is not affected.
d. Creatinine kinase is only mildly elevated.
e. Death occurs in late adulthood, usually due to severe cardiomyopathy.

4. **Myotonic MD (Steinert's Disease)**
a. This is the second most common form of MD.
b. It is an autosomal dominant disorder characterized by multisystem involvement.
c. Signs and symptoms include a characteristic facial appearance (inverted V-shaped upper lip, thin cheeks, high arched palate), mild weakness with progressive wasting of distal muscles initially and proximal muscles later, myotonia (very slow relaxation of muscles after contraction), expressive speech disorder, slow gastric emptying, and heart block with arrhythmia.
d. Other associated conditions include hypothyroidism, adrenocortical insufficiency, diabetes mellitus, testicular atrophy, cataracts, and immunoglobulin G deficiency.
e. Infants born to mothers with myotonic dystrophy may have a severe form of the disorder with death occurring in the first year of life.

5. **Limb-Girdle MD**
a. This condition affects the muscles of the hips and shoulders. Facial muscles may be involved. Eventually, distal muscles are affected as well.
b. Symptoms begin in middle to late childhood with muscle weakness and decreased deep tendon reflexes, progressing to severe disability after 20 years of age.
c. Cardiac involvement is unusual and joint contractures rarely occur.
d. Affected children have normal intelligence.
e. Creatinine kinase is elevated but not to the extent seen in Duchenne's MD.
f. This form of MD is difficult to distinguish from Becker's MD.

6. **Facioscapulohumeral Syndrome**
a. This is a form of MD with histologic evidence of myopathy, neuropathy, and inflammation. It may be a different presentation of the same genetic abnormality that causes Emery-Dreifuss MD.
b. Symptom onset is insidious. Usually weakness begins in the shoulders and extends to the face in the second decade of life. It may be asymmetric.
c. The first noticed sign of the disease may be a change in facial expression (mouth is rounded and puckered, incomplete eyelid closure). Late in the course of the disease, speech may be affected and lower extremity weakness may occur, interfering with ambulation.
d. Creatinine kinase may be normal or elevated.
e. The course of disease is variable with severe disability seen in the infantile form and other patients with normal lifespans and no functional disability.
f. Retinal vascular disease occurs in almost all patients necessitating treatment to prevent blindness.

16.2.10 Metabolic Myopathy

A. **Potassium Related Periodic Paralysis**
1. This is an autosomal dominant condition associated with paralysis on awakening with gradual recovery over the course of the day.
2. Potassium may be high or low (most common).
3. Symptoms become more frequent as the child ages.
4. Eventually patients show evidence of a progressive myopathy.

B. **Malignant Hyperthermia**
1. This is an autosomal dominant inherited tendency toward life-threatening extreme fever, muscular rigidity, respiratory and metabolic acidosis, increased creatinine kinase, and myoglobinuria precipitated by exposure to general anesthetics.
2. Symptoms may be prevented by giving dantrolene sodium before administering anesthetics.

C. **Vitamin E Deficiency Myopathy**. Patients with chronic malabsorption, on dialysis, or premature infants, may develop progressive myopathy and neuropathy resembling MD. The condition can be prevented by consuming an adequate intake of vitamin E.

16.2.11 Neuropathy

A. **Familial Dysautonomia (Riley-Day Syndrome)**
1. This is an autosomal recessive disorder common in Eastern European Jews.
2. Patients have fewer unmyelinated nerve fibers for autonomic functions, pain, temperature, and taste sensation, as well as decreased myelinated afferent nerves.
3. Signs and symptoms include poor suck and swallow, increased sweating, breath-holding with syncope, insensitivity to pain, clumsy walking, absent deep tendon reflexes, seizures, prolongation of the QT interval, and poor body temperature control.
4. Complications include heat related syndromes, aspiration pneumonia, recurrent nonrecognized trauma, and cardiac arrhythmia.
5. Elevations of homovanillic acid and vanillylmandelic acid are noted on laboratory evaluation.
6. Treatment is symptomatic.

B. **Bell's Palsy**
1. This is acute facial nerve peripheral neuritis.
2. It most commonly occurs from infancy through adolescence.

3. Its typical presentation is occurrence of facial weakness and facial droop approximately 2 weeks after an infectious illness. The most common infections involved are Ebstein-Barr virus, herpes simplex virus, mumps, and Lyme disease.
4. Neonatal disease is usually due to facial nerve compression rather than infection with symptoms resolving in days to weeks.
5. Recovery is complete in 85% of individuals. The remaining patients have either mild (10%) or severe (5%) facial paralysis.
6. Treatment
   - **a.** Steroid use is controversial and generally not recommended.
   - **b.** If the etiology is not known, some authors recommend routine use of acyclovir for possible herpes simplex virus infection.
   - **c.** Surgical decompression is not useful.

16.2.12 Headaches. See Section 4.3.2.

338. A 6-year-old male presents with fever and new onset focal seizure. What test should be performed before proceeding with a lumbar puncture for cerebral spinal fluid collection — E 16.1.2

A. serum chemistry
B. complete blood count
C. urinalysis
D. liver function tests
E. computed tomography of the brain

339. The electroencephalogram is used primarily to — E 16.1.2

A. identify the location of brain tumors
B. classify seizure types
C. monitor response to antiepileptic drug therapy
D. all of the above
E. B and C

340. Which of the following is a contraindication to performing a computed tomography scan of the brain with contrast enhancement — C 16.1.2

A. acute cerebral hemorrhage
B. chronic subdural hematoma
C. elevated serum creatinine
D. the presence of a central nervous system vascular tumor

341. Which cranial nerve is responsible for lateral gaze — D 16.1.3

A. II
B. III
C. IV
D. VI
E. IX

342. Which cranial nerves are responsible for the sensation of taste — B 16.1.3

A. VII, X
B. VII, IX
C. V, IX
D. V, VII

343. Which cranial nerve can be damaged with severe hyperbilirubinemia — A 16.1.3

A. VIII
B. VII
C. VI
D. V

344. A child has a surgical repair of a tracheoesophageal fistula. After surgery. he has mild inspiratory stridor and vocal hoarseness that fails to resolve. What is the probable etiology of his hoarseness — B 16.1.3

A. irritation from the endotracheal tube
B. recurrent laryngeal nerve injury
C. cranial nerve IX injury
D. vocal cord polyp

345. What differentiates upper motor neuron disease from lower motor neuron disease — A 16.1.4

A. absence of atrophy
B. presence of atrophy
C. absent reflexes
D. muscle fasciculations

346. A child, with a history of stroke, has muscle weakness. He is able to flex his right arm at the elbow if gravity is eliminated. What is his strength rating for the tested muscle group — B 16.1.3

A. 1 out of 5
B. 2 out of 5
C. 3 out of 5
D. 4 out of 5
E. 5 out of 5

347. A child is noted on an physician's report to have "normal" reflexes. On a rating scale, what is considered to be a "normal" reflex — B 16.1.3

A. 1 out of 4
B. 2 out of 4
C. 3 out of 4
D. 4 out of 4

348. A 7-year-old has cerebral palsy. Which of the following would be closest to his deep tendon reflex rating — A 16.1.3

A. 4 out of 4
B. 2 out of 4
C. 1 out of 4
D. 0 out of 4

349. A 10-year-old boy presents for an attention deficit hyperactivity disorder evaluation. He is referred by his teacher, who states, "He is so disruptive. He is constantly shouting and making rude noises during our lessons." During your interview with the family, you note that the child frequently grimaces and has blepharospasm. What is your diagnosis — D 16.1.3

A. poor child-teacher match
B. attention deficit hyperactivity disorder
C. learning disability
D. Tourette's disease
E. lead poisoning

350. In which of the following children would the presence of a Babinski sign be considered abnormal — A 16.1.3

A. 18-month-old
B. 12-month-old
C. 6-month-old
D. 1-month-old

351. When does the parachute sign disappear in normal individuals — E 16.1.3

A. 7 months of age
B. 12 months of age
C. 2 years of age
D. 4 years of age
E. it does not disappear

352. A 15-year-old is scheduled for surgery. His father is concerned because he had an episode of malignant hyperthermia during general anesthesia. What drug should you administer to this child prior to giving anesthetic agents — D 16.2.10

A. midazolam
B. ibuprofen
C. acetaminophen
D. dantrolene sodium
E. diazepam

353. Which vitamin deficiency is associated with neural tube defects — C 16.2.1

A. niacin
B. thiamine
C. folate
D. riboflavin

354. A 4-year-old is referred to an otolaryngologist for removal of a persistent nasal polyp. What is your advice to the family regarding the surgery — D 16.2.1

A. "He is a healthy child. Surgery should be no problem."
B. continue intranasal steroids and forego surgery at present
C. "Have them take his tonsils out at the same time."
D. get magnetic resonance imaging study of the brain to assess anatomy before attempting surgery

355. A child presents to your office for evaluation of a possible immune deficiency. She has had 3 distinct episodes of culture proven bacterial meningitis. Her history is otherwise unremarkable. You decide that she is not immune deficient. Why? — A 16.2.1

A. she has a draining sacral pit
B. she has a normal total white blood cell count
C. she has never had the chicken pox
D. she has never had recurrent candidal skin infections

356. What is the most common cause of macrocephaly in infants — B 16.2.2

A. benign megalencephaly
B. obstructive hydrocephalus
C. hydrocephalus *ex vacuo*
D. toxoplasmosis
E. Hurler's syndrome

357. A child with craniosynostosis has scaphocephaly. Which suture is prematurely fused — C 16.2.3

A. lambdoid
B. metopic
C. sagittal
D. coronal

358. A child with craniosynostosis has trigonocephaly. What suture is prematurely fused — B 16.2.3

A. lambdoid
B. metopic
C. sagittal
D. coronal

359. Which of the following etiologies for neonatal seizure is more likely to cause seizure on day of life 3, as opposed to day of life 1 — D 16.2.4

A. hypoglycemia
B. hypoxia
C. infection
D. inborn error of metabolism

360. What is the life expectancy of a patient with Becker's muscular dystrophy — B 16.2.9

A. death occurs before 18 years of age
B. death occurs in the 20's
C. death occurs in the 30's
D. death occurs in the 40's

361. What is the recommended course of treatment for benign rolandic epilepsy when the seizures only occur at night — D 16.2.4

A. carbamazepine
B. phenytoin
C. phenobarbital
D. no treatment

362. A 6-month-old infant presents with paroxysms of seizure activity characterized by flexion of the neck, trunk, and extremities. What is the classic electroencephalogram finding seen with this seizure type. — C 16.2.4

A. 3 per second spike and wave
B. diffuse slowing
C. hypsarrhythmia
D. delta waves

363. What is the peak age of onset of febrile seizures — D 16.2.4

A. 3 months of age
B. 6 months of age
C. 12 months of age
D. 18 months of age
E. 3 years of age

364. A 2-year-old has his first simple febrile seizure. What is his risk of developing epilepsy by 7 years of age — A 16.2.4

A. 2%
B. 4%
C. 10%
D. 20%
E. 30%

365. Which of the following is used to treat absence seizures — E 16.2.4

A. gabapentin
B. carbamazepine
C. phenobarbital
D. lamotrigine
E. ethosuximide

366. A 14-year-old is referred from another hospital for status epilepticus. He failed to respond to standard doses of antiseizure medications. His seizures are characterized by rapid head turning and thrashing movements. Of note, the seizures only occur when his family is present. What is your diagnosis — C 16.2.4

A. malingering
B. atypical seizures
C. pseudoseizure
D. schizophrenia

367. A previously normal 12-month-old presents with fever and new onset seizures. A computed tomography scan of his brain reveals diffuse calcifications. He has several faint hypopigmented macules on his trunk. What is your diagnosis — A 16.2.4

A. tuberous sclerosis
B. Neurofibromatosis
C. toxoplasmosis
D. febrile seizure
E. familial seizure disorder

368. What is the treatment of choice for pseudoseizure — E 16.2.4

A. identify stressors
B. benzodiazepines
C. address secondary gain
D. all of the above
E. A and C

369. A partial complex seizure is one that — C 16.2.4

A. consciousness is maintained
B. activity is generalized
C. is focal in onset
D. is not controlled with antiepileptic drugs

370. A 9-year-old presents with hepatomegaly, choreoathetoid movements, and Kayser-Fleischer rings on the corneas. What is the chelating agent of choice — A 16.2.6

A. D-penicillamine
B. 2.3-dimercaptosuccinic acid (DMSA)
C. edetate calcium disodium (EDTA)
D. deferoxamine
E. dimercaprol (BAL)

371. A 4-year-old girl was developmentally normal at birth. As she grew, her parents noted that she did not gain new milestones as easily as her peers, and for the past 2 years, is actually regressing. When you are conducting your interview, you note that the child does not communicate. She just sits and wrings her hands. You diagnose — B 16.2.6

A. Lennox-Gastaut syndrome
B. Rett's syndrome
C. spinocerebellar ataxia
D. spinal muscular atrophy

372. A 2-year-old child of Jewish descent is noted to have severe mental retardation, hyperacusis, and a cherry red macula on eye exam. You diagnose Tay-Sach disease. What is the enzyme deficiency — C 16.2.6

A. glucocerebrosidase
B. sphingomyelinase
C. hexosaminidase A
D. arylsulfatase A

373. You see a 12-year-old boy with severe mental retardation in the neurology clinic. He is restrained in his wheelchair. When his hands are released, you see that he has choreoathetosis and that he constantly tries to hit and bite himself. His serum uric acid is elevated. What is your diagnosis — D 16.2.6

A. Tay-Sach disease
B. Gaucher's disease
C. adrenoleukodystrophy
D. Lesch-Nyhan syndrome

374. A 10-year-old had a recent upper respiratory tract infection. He now presents with a 4 day history of weakness, beginning in the legs. His speech is slurred and he cannot swallow well. You note generalized weakness and hyporeflexia. What will his cerebral spinal fluid studies show — B 16.2.6

A. Gram-positive cocci on staining
B. normal cerebrospinal fluid cell count with elevated protein level
C. high cerebrospinal fluid cell count with elevated protein level
D. increased red blood cell count in the cerebrospinal fluid
E. normal cerebrospinal fluid cell count and normal protein level

375. A child with cerebral palsy has bilateral lower extremity spasticity without other symptoms. His intelligence quotient is likely to be — C 16.2.7

A. less than his peers
B. less than his siblings
C. normal
D. none of the above

376. A 17-year-old presents in January with an acute encephalopathy. His parents report, he had been self-medicating with aspirin for muscle aches, fever, and headache. He had been previously healthy. What is your diagnosis — B 16.2.7

A. congenital fatty acid oxidation defect
B. Reye's syndrome
C. drug overdose
D. malingering

377. A 16-year-old female presents with bilateral facial nerve palsy, 1 week after returning from a bicycling trip through Connecticut. What infection should you be especially concerned about — A 16.2.11

A. Lyme disease
B. group A β-hemolytic streptococcus
C. cat-scratch disease
D. Epstein-Barr virus
E. mumps

378. What is the most favorable prognostic indicator in patients with myasthenia gravis — C 16.2.6

A. stable isolated ocular weakness
B. impaired respiratory function
C. neonatal myasthenia gravis with transplacental antibodies
D. muscle weakness responding to edrophonium

17 MUSCULOSKELETAL DISORDERS

17.1 DEVELOPMENTAL CONSIDERATIONS

17.1.1 The Fetus and the Newborn

A. Many skeletal deformities in infancy are due to positional pressures and force *in utero* and will resolve spontaneously.

B. Normal Musculoskeletal Deformation

1. After a breech or cephalic delivery, the hips will lie in flexion of 30 to 60 degrees.
2. Knee contracture of 20 to 40 degrees is present.
3. There is10 to 30 degrees of internal tibial torsion.

C. Intrauterine postural deformities that can be manipulated back to normal position will generally spontaneously resolve by 3 months in over 90% of infants.

17.1.2 Developmental Variation

A. Terminology

1. Varum. Angulation of a bone toward the midline.
2. Valgum. Angulation of the bone distal to a joint away from the midline.

B. "Bowlegs" and "Knock-Knees'"

1. **Genu Varum**; "bowlegs." The leg distal to the knee bends toward the midline.
2. **Genu Valgum**; "knock-knee." The bone distal to the knee angles away from the midline.
3. Progression
   a. From birth to about 18 months of age, there is a normal stage of development in which genus varum persists. Early walking is associated with valgus deformity.
   b. After 24 months of age, children develop increasing valgus until, in adolescence, they finally have knees which are straight or with a minor degree of varus or valgus.
4. Follow up and reassurance to parents are generally the only needed treatment for genus varum or genus valgum.
5. Either entity may have a positive family history.

C. Intoeing

1. Developmental Femoral Anteversion (Hip Intoeing)
   a. This condition presents between 2 and 6 years of age and is the most common cause of intoeing.
   b. Treatment usually is not needed and this will resolve with age.
2. Internal Tibial Torsion
   a. Present between 3 months and 2 years of age, it is the second most common cause of intoeing.
   b. It is a result of intrauterine positioning and is common in normal children, especially neonates.
   c. No treatment is required.

D. Flat feet (Flexible Pronated Feet)

1. This condition commonly presents at ages 3 to 7 years of age, almost always without symptoms. The primary concern is cosmetic.
2. Therapy
   a. For many years various forms of treatment have been used to correct this "problem," including surgery.
   b. Two things to remember: the foot is not mature until around 12 years of age and no treatment (except surgery) has any permanent effect. Research suggests, even in severe cases, the flexible pronated adult is not disabled by the condition.

17.2 DISEASE PROFILES

17.2.1 Trauma

A. General Fracture Information

1. Fractures are common accidental injuries in children that usually heal without sequelae.
2. A careful exam to assure that no neurological or vascular injury has occurred is needed.
   a. Neurologic injury results in loss or altered sensation and loss of function.
   b. Vascular changes manifest as decreased blood flow and a cool, pale extremity.
   c. Both are emergencies and will likely need orthopedic consultation.
3. Fractures in children less than 2 years of age without a reasonable, consistent explanation, and any fracture in a child less than 1 year of age is suspicious for abuse.
4. Clavicle fractures are common and heal without problems. Splint for comfort.
5. Generally fractures that do not have neurovascular injuries and are not open can be splinted and treated definitively with casting in a few days when the swelling subsides. A few types of fractures will need surgical pinning to stabilize. Consult orthopedic surgery if this occurs.

B. Physis Fractures

1. The physis or growth plate is the main difference between young and mature bone.
2. The physis lies between the epiphysis and the metaphysis.
3. Because fractures that involve growth plates can have long lasting consequences, there is a separate fracture classification for immature bone.
4. **Salter-Harris Physis Fracture Classification (Figure 17.2.1)**
   a. Type I: the fracture extends through the physeal plate.
   b. Type II: the fracture includes a triangular piece of the metaphysis.
   c. Type III: the fracture extends from the joint surface to the epiphyseal plate.
   d. Type IV: this is a type III fracture that involves

the metaphysis as well.

e. Type V: this is a crush injury of the growth plate.

C. **Sprains**

1. Sprain, strains, and contusions all involve some degree of tissue injury and inflammation.
2. Ankle injury is usually associated with a sprain.
   a. If the patient can support weight within 30 minutes of injury, the joint is probably sprained and not fractured.
   b. Sprains are more common as the child's age increases.
3. Ligaments around joints are stronger than epiphyseal plates in children. Be wary of diagnosing sprains in joints that still have growth plates. Usually, the epiphysis gives way before the ligament.
4. Treatment
   a. The involved limb can be splinted for comfort, elevated, and periodically iced down for the first 48 hours.
   b. Nonsteroidal anti-inflammatory drugs are usually adequate for pain control.

D. Puncture wounds of the soles of the feet (especially through dirty tennis shoes) are prone to osteomyelitis (organism commonly *Pseudomonas aeruginosa*).

E. Lacerations of the feet often need splinting to maintain sutures in active children.

17.2.2 Infection

A. **The Limping Child**

1. In the child who refuses to bear weight, after exam and interview have lowered the suspicion for fracture, septic joint must be considered.
2. Painless limps may present as changes in muscle tone, strength, or joint function. These may be caused by neurologic disease, muscle disease, bone and joint disorders, or hysteria.
3. Painful limps may be caused by trauma or infection, either of the legs, hips, back, or intra-abdominal processes (appendicitis).
4. Laboratory study is dictated by findings, but usually includes a blood culture, complete blood count, and erythrocyte sedimentation rate or C-reactive protein at a minimum.
   a. Erythrocyte sedimentation rate is a sensitive but not very specific test. However, if it is normal, it moves osteomyelitis and septic joint down on the list of the differential diagnose.
   b. An elevated white blood cell count or a shift to immature cells is more concerning for an infectious process.

B. **Transient (Toxic) Synovitis**

1. This is a common condition in children from ages 4 to 10 years. Toddlers are affected as well.
2. Boys are affected 2:1 over girls.
3. It presents as acute onset of a painful limp. The child suddenly refuses to walk and may have a slightly elevated temperature. Often there is a history of viral illness in the recent past.
4. Diagnostic Testing
   a. An erythrocyte sedimentation rate may be only slightly elevated.
   b. An x-ray may be normal or show widening of the joint space.
   c. Toxic synovitis is a diagnosis of exclusion. If clinically indicated (ill appearance, significant fever, increased white blood cell count, increased erythrocyte sedimentation rate, joint effusion) septic arthritis has to be considered and a joint aspiration performed.
5. Conservative treatment with bed rest is needed and the prognosis is very good.

C. **Septic Arthritis**. See section 7.3.10A.

D. **Osteomyelitis**. See section 73.10B.

1. Osteomyelitis occurs most frequently in younger children but can be seen at any age.
2. Boys are affected 3:1 over girls.
3. Spread is most commonly hematogenous, but can be by direct extension from soft tissue or direct external introduction (puncture wound).
4. In children less than 18 months of age, where the physis has not yet formed, the infection can reach across the nonexistent growth plate to the epiphysis, leading to septic arthritis.
5. Pain is the most common symptom. Patients may

Figure 17.2.1 Salter-Harris physis fracture classification

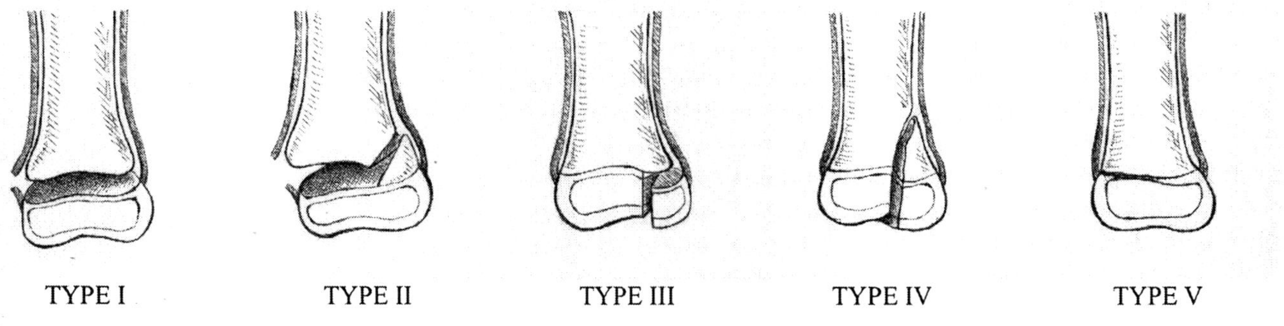

also have fever, localized erythema, and swelling.

6. Treatment with early diagnosis may be parenteral antibiotics alone. Surgical debridement and drainage may be necessary in some cases.
7. Common Organisms (Septic Arthritis and Osteomyelitis)
   a. Neonatal: group B streptococcus, Gram-negative enteric bacilli, and *Staphylococcus aureus*.
   b. Toddlers and children: *Staphylococcus aureus* (most common), streptococci, and *Haemophilus influenzae*.
   c. Adolescence: the causative agents are the same as children plus *Neisseria gonorrhoeae*.
   d. Sickle cell disease: *Streptococcus pneumoniae*, *Salmonella species*, and *Staphylococcus aureus*.

17.2.3 Arthritis and Joint Pain in Children

A. Rheumatoid arthritis can occur at any age in childhood, but the greatest prevalence is from 5 to 8 years of age. See section 8.2.1.

B. Hemophiliacs may have hemarthrosis causing synovial inflammation which, with reoccurrence, can lead to osteoarthritis. This generally occurs in a weightbearing joint. Treatment is early diagnosis and intravenous transfusion of the missing factor. See section 11.3.5.

C. Sickle cell disease may first present as dactylitis in infants. There are radiographic changes secondary to the red marrow expansion. Also, bony infarcts lead to increased bony trabeculation and sclerosis. The infarcted areas have a high risk of infection. See section 11.3.3B.

D. Neoplastic disorders can also present as bone or joint pain. Leukemia with neoplastic growth within the bone marrow may first present as bone pain. See section 12.2.1.

17.2.4 General Musculoskeletal Disorders

A. **Rickets** occurs when growing bone is inadequately mineralized and softens. See section 5.2.12B.

B. **Congenital amputations** may be due to amniotic bands, teratogens, or rarely, hereditary defects. Most are spontaneous and are not expected to recur in future offspring.

C. **Achondroplasia** (Classic Chondrodystrophy)
   1. This is a heritable condition characterized by short limbs, with the humerus and femur proportionately shorter than the radius and tibia, and varum deformities.
   2. Moderate hydrocephalus, lumbar lordosis, short, stubby digits, and motion restriction of major joints are common.
   3. Cognitive and sexual functions are normal.

D. **Osteopetrosis** (Albers-Schönberg Disease, Marble Bone Disease)
   1. This is an inherited disorder characterized by pathologic fractures, myelophthisic anemia, splenomegaly, dwarfing, pigeon breast, square head, facial paralysis, and auditory and visual disturbances.
   2. Calcification of soft tissues may occur.
   3. It can present at any age.

E. **Osteochondrodystrophy** (Morquio's Disease)
   1. This condition is a result of abnormal deposition of mucopolysaccharides.
   2. It is characterized by shortening of the spine, scoliosis, kyphosis, pigeon breast, hepatosplenomegaly, and corneal clouding.
   3. The child appears normal at birth and develops the deformities between 1 and 4 years of age.
   4. The condition is autosomal recessive when familial.

F. **Chondroectodermal Dysplasia** (Ellis-van Creveld Syndrome)
   1. This familial condition occurs more frequently in the Amish people of Pennsylvania.
   2. Mental retardation, ectodermal dysplasia, poor dentition, congenital heart disease, polydactyly, and syndactyly are major components of this syndrome.

G. **Marfan's syndrome** is characterized by unusually long digits (arachnodactyly) and hypermobility of the joints. Other associations include ectopia lentis and intrathoracic aneurysms.

H. **Arthrogryposis Multiplex Congenita**
   1. This condition involves fibrous ankylosis of most of the joints of the body with poor muscular development.
   2. Physical activity can be severely restricted.
   3. Affected patients usually have normal mentation.

I. **Osteogenesis Imperfecta**
   1. Inheritance is usually autosomal dominant.
   2. In the severe fetal type (osteogenous imperfecta congenita), fractures may occur *in utero* and are common during the birth process.
   3. Growth retardation occurs because of recurrent fractures.
   4. Mentation is normal.
   5. Blue sclera are the characteristic associated finding in addition to bony deformity.

17.2.5 Regional Musculoskeletal Disorders

A. Foot Problems
   1. **Posturing** is the habitual position in which one holds the foot. It can be manipulated into a normal position. A deformity is present if the foot cannot be manually manipulated into normal position.
   2. **Pes Planus (Flatfoot).** If a longitudinal arch is present when the child is not weight bearing, the arch will develop normally and no treatment is needed.
   3. **Cavovarus Foot.** A unusually high longitudinal arch of the foot. Neurologic abnormalities such as Charcot-Marie-Tooth disease, Friedreich's ataxia, and diastematomyelia should be ruled out.

4. **Intoeing**. See section 17.1.2.
5. **Metatarsus Adductus**. A positional deviation of the forefoot that can be corrected by manipulation. Serial castings may be needed to prevent development of a high arch with medial inclination of the heel.
6. **Metatarsus Varus** A medical deformity of the forefoot that cannot be corrected by manipulation.
   a. It is due to an intrauterine subluxation of tarsometatarsal joints with adduction and inversion of the metatarsal bones.
   b. Serial casting or surgery may be needed to prevent development of a high arch with medial inclination of the heel.
7. **Talipes Equinovarus (Clubfoot)**
   a. The foot is pointed downward like a horse (equinus = horse), with medial deviation of the forefoot, and medial inversion of the heel.
   b. Spontaneous correction does not occur. Aggressive treatment is indicated.
   c. Those not responding to serial casting will require surgical correction.
8. **Talipes Calcaneovalgus**. The reverse of clubfoot.
   a. It is a benign condition due to intrauterine molding pressures.
   b. The foot is averted and dorsiflexed at the ankle. Passive stretching usually results in correction.

B. Lower Leg Problems
1. **Tibial Torsion**. The tibia is normally internally rotated and bowed until about 9 years of age.
2. **Blount's Disease**
   a. This is a disturbance of the growth plate at the proximal tibia.
   b. It is more common in those with precocious walking and African ancestry.
   c. If not corrected with braces and/or surgery, it can leave permanent deformities.
   d. It may follow fractures involving the growth plates.
3. **Osgood-Schlatter Disease**
   a. Tenderness and swelling over the tibial tuberosity due to fibrocartilage microfractures at the insertion of the patellar tendon.
   b. It occurs in late childhood and early adolescence, and is more common in males.
   c. The condition is generally benign, but pain may persist with activity for up to a year after skeletal maturity.

C. **Osteochondritis Desiccans**
1. This is the result of necrosis and separation of bone adjacent to articular cartilage.
2. The knee is a common site for this to occur, though it can also be found in the talus, femoral head, or lateral humeral condyle.
3. The area is at risk for fractures.

D. Leg Length Discrepancies
1. Shortening of a femur is a common cause of discrepancies in leg length.
2. Orthopedic evaluation is indicated if the difference in leg lengths is >2.5 cm.

E. Hip Problems
1. **Developmental Dysplasia of the Hip** (DDH)
   a. This condition is characterized by a hip that can be dislocated in a normal newborn or a newborn with neuromuscular disease.
   b. This tendency can be demonstrated on exam by a Barlow test (a click of dislocation is felt as the hip is adducted toward midline in a flexed position) or an Ortolani test (the hip is abducted away from midline, producing a clunk as the dislocated femoral head slips into the acetabulum).
   c. Asymmetric gluteal folds and apparent shortening of the affected leg are also clues to the presence of this condition.
   d. DDH is more common in girls.
   e. Whether the hip is dislocatable or dislocated, it needs to be detected and treated before the child walks, otherwise permanent deformity will ensue.
   f. A major complication is aseptic necrosis of the femoral head caused by reduction of the dislocation under pressure. It too results in permanent hip deformity.
   g. Treatment is with a Pavlik harness (holds the hips in flexion and abduction) or, in older children, surgical reduction.
2. **Slipped Capital Femoral Epiphysis** (SCFE)
   a. A fracture through the physis of the femoral head can occur during the pubescent growth spurt.
   b. Shortening of the thigh and loss of internal rotation of the hip are characteristic findings of this condition, as well as anterior thigh and knee pain.
   c. The vulnerable age groups are males 10 to 17 years and females 8 to 15 years of age.
   d. This condition is associated with African Americans, males, obesity with delayed skeletal maturation, tall stature, thin body habitus, and hypothyroidism (prepubertal SCFE).
   e. Hip necrosis is the feared complication.
   f. Treatment is surgical repair.
3. **Legg-Calvé-Perthes Disease** (LCP)
   a. LCP is avascular necrosis of the femoral head.
   b. The highest incidence is between 4 and 8 years of age, during the period of rapid growth of the epiphysis.
   c. LCP occurs in males 6-times more often than in females.

d. Most children have a painful thigh and a limp. Persistent pain is common, yet some affected children have only mild intermittent pain.
e. Radiography reveals, in order of appearance in the disease process, decreased growth of the capital femoral epiphysis, fracture, reabsorption of bone with collapse, reossification, and residual chronic change.
f. Treatment is with observation, bedrest, physical therapy, and pain control. Surgical treatment or casting may be considered in certain cases in an effort to improve tissue structure and function.

F. Spine Problems

1. **Scoliosis**
   a. Adolescent idiopathic scoliosis has its onset after 10 years of age and can progress rapidly during the pubescent growth spurt.
   b. Females are at high risk for progressive deformity.
   c. A history of pain should initiate search for lesions of the spinal cord or neoplasms since the idiopathic condition is generally painless.
   d. Patients with curves more than 20 degrees should have an orthopedic evaluation for consideration of surgical repair.
   e. If untreated, and the condition is progressive, severe restrictive lung disease, gross cosmetic deformity, and joint disease may occur.
2. **Torticollis**
   a. This condition is common in the neonatal period and is associated with a contracture of the sternocleidomastoid muscle.
   b. Torticollis may also be seen from gastroesophageal reflux (Sandifer's syndrome) and with subluxation of cervical spine facets. Hint: muscle spasm occurs on the side of shortening of the sternocleidomastoid in spastic torticollis and the opposite side in subluxation.
3. **Klippel-Feil Anomaly**. The result of segmentation failure in the cervical spine. This has a high association with other abnormalities, including cardiac lesions, urinary tract problems, and auditory apparatus anomalies.
4. **Diastematomyelia**
   a. The spinal cord is split and anchored in the spinal canal by bony or fibrous spicules.
   b. The result can be dysfunction of the bladder or lower extremity muscles.
   c. A hairy patch is often present over the affected area of the spine.
   d. The differential diagnosis includes a tethered spinal cord which can produce similar symptoms.
   e. Down's Syndrome. Subluxation of C1 can occur in children with Down's syndrome due to ligamentous laxity.

G. Elbow Problems

1. **Subluxation of the Radial Head**
   a. Referred to as **nursemaid's elbow**, this condition occurs when the toddler is picked up by the wrist.
   b. The child typically holds the arm by his side with the palm down (pronated) and refuses to use it until it is reduced by supination of the palm while flexing the elbow. Distal traction is applied during the reduction maneuver.
2. **Elbow Fracture**. Supracondylar fractures of the elbow are at high risk for development of compartment syndrome (Volkmann's contracture) and neurologic deficit if not adequately treated. Needs orthopedic consultation.

379. A child sustains a fracture of his distal tibia. The fracture line passes through the growth plate and includes a piece of the metaphysis. What is the fractures Salter-Harris classification B 17.2.1

A. I
B. II
C. III
D. IV
E. V

380. A 3-year-old presents to your office because of a 1 day history of refusal to bear weight on his left leg. He has no history suggestive of recent injury. His initial evaluation should include all of the following except B 17.2.2

A. complete blood count
B. bone scan
C. C-reactive protein
D. blood culture
E. a careful physical exam

381. A 15-year-old twists her ankle while playing basketball. Thirty minutes after the injury occurs, she is able to support her own weight and walk, albeit, with pain. What is the recommended course of treatment for this injury E 17.2.1

A. place a splint while she is in the emergency department
B. keep the limb elevated
C. apply an ice pack several times a day for a couple of days
D. take ibuprofen for pain control
E. all of the above

382. A 3-week-old infant presents with a stiff right knee. The parents report that she cries when they try to straighten it out. Her white blood cell count is 28,000 cells/mm^3 with an erythrocyte sedimentation rate of 80 mm/hr. A blood culture is pending. What is the best next step in evaluation and treatment D 17.2.2

A. place an intravenous catheter and start parenteral antibiotics
B. reassure her parents that the stiffness is from intrauterine positioning and treatment other than passive stretching is not indicated
C. refer her to physical therapy
D. perform a joint aspiration for fluid analysis and culture
E. perform a lumbar puncture

383. A 2-year-old presents with acute refusal to bear weight on his right leg. His examination reveals no fever, mild pain on manipulation of the right hip, normal plain x-rays, normal complete blood count, and normal erythrocyte sedimentation rate. Further history is significant for recent recovery from a viral upper respiratory infection. What is the most likely diagnosis C 17.2.2

A. osteomyelitis
B. septic hip
C. toxic synovitis
D. muscle strain
E. occult hip fracture

384. A 2-year-old child presents with scoliosis, kyphosis, pigeon breast, hepatosplenomegaly, and corneal clouding. By history, he appeared normal at birth. He had a great uncle who had the same deformities. What is his diagnosis C 17.2.4

A. arthrogryposis
B. achondroplasia
C. osteochondrodystrophy
D. osteogenesis imperfecta
E. rickets

385. A 5-year-old presents with a 4 day history of worsening limp and thigh pain. The white blood cell count and erythrocyte sedimentation rate are elevated, plain x-rays of the limb are normal, and a blood culture is pending. There is no evidence of joint infection. If osteomyelitis is a concern, the next step in evaluation is — A 17.2.2

A. nuclear medicine bone scan
B. magnetic resonance imaging
C. wait 5 days and repeat the x-ray
D. perform a percutaneous bone biopsy

386. Which of the following organisms is the most likely etiology for osteomyelitis in a 2-week-old infant — A 17.2.2

A. group B streptococcus
B. group A β-hemolytic streptococcus
C. *Neisseria* species
D. *Salmonella* species
E. pneumococcus

387. What is the mode of inheritance for most congenital amputations — E 17.2.4

A. multifactorial
B. autosomal dominant
C. autosomal recessive
D. X-linked recessive
E. they are not inherited

388. A mother voices concern that her 18-month-old child intoes when she walks. Your advice to her is — D 17.1.2

A. she should see an orthopedic surgeon
B. she needs to wear leg braces
C. she should wear high topped shoes
D. reassure her that this condition will resolve with age
E. this condition is genetic and will persist throughout life

389. A parent asks about her toddler's feet. She has noticed that since he started walking, he seems flat footed. Your response is — B 17.2.5

A. you examine the child's feet and note that an arch is present when he does not bear weight. You recommend inserts for his shoes
B. you note that the arch is present when the child is not weight bearing. You reassure the mother that this is normal
C. you recommend physical therapy
D. you recommend referral to an orthopedic surgeon
E. you recommend that the child not be placed in shoes

390. When doing newborn nursery rounds, you identify a child fixed with a plantar flexed foot with medial deviation of the forefoot and medial inversion of the heel. When addressing the problem with the parents of the infant you recommend — E 17.2.5

A. home stretching exercises and careful follow-up in your office
B. physical therapy
C. no treatment until the child is older
D. application of flexible splints
E. referral to an orthopedic surgeon for casting or surgery

391. Knock-knees' are an example of what kind of deformity — A 17.1.2

A. valgus
B. varus
C. torsion
D. anteversion

392. A 13-year-old boy presents to your office complaining of knee pain. You discover he has been participating in rigorous basketball practices for the past 2 weeks. On exam he is acutely tender with palpation of the tibial tuberosity. What is your diagnosis D 17.2.5

A. osteochondritis desiccans
B. arthritis
C. ligament injury
D. Osgood-Schlatter disease
E. Legg-Calvé-Perthes disease

393. What is the minimum degree of leg length discrepancy necessitating orthopedic evaluation A 17.2.5

A. 3 cm
B. 2 cm
C. 1.5 cm
D. 1 cm
E. 0.5 cm

394. When examining an infant's hip, a palpable clunk is felt as the flexed hip is abducted away from midline. You diagnose developmental hip dysplasia. The maneuver you used is called B 17.2.5

A. Barlow maneuver
B. Ortolani maneuver
C. Murphy's sign
D. Moro reflex
E. Thompson test

395. Treatment for developmental hip dysplasia is A 17.2.5

A. a Pavlik harness
B. surgical reduction in early infancy
C. no treatment is necessary
D. physical therapy
E. passive stretching exercises

396. A 12-year-old presents for evaluation of scoliosis. She has an angle of curvature of 23 degrees. She also reports that she has chronic, activity limiting back pain. What should you do next C 17.2.5

A. refer to an orthopedic surgeon for repair
B. evaluate for spinal cord abnormalities
C. both
D. neither

397. A 6-year-old presents with radicular low back pain, overflow urinary incontinence, and constipation. On examination you note a hairy patch over her lower spine. Which of the following is the most likely diagnosis B 17.2.5

A. musculoskeletal strain
B. diastematomyelia
C. herniated intervertebral disk
D. scoliosis
E. vertebral fracture

398. A child is born with severe respiratory distress. On exam, you note multiple fractures of the ribs, skull, and extremities. What color are his sclera B 17.2.4

A. white
B. blue
C. red
D. yellow

399. An overweight African American 14-year-old male presents for evaluation of acute onset of anterior thigh and knee pain. On exam, you notice thigh shortening and internal rotation of the leg at the hip. Based on this history, the appropriate treatment is D 17.2.5

A. provide analgesics for pain and discharge the patient to home
B. refer for physical therapy
C. recommend bedrest
D. immediately refer to an orthopedic surgeon for repair
E. do not treat

400. A 2-year-old is brought to the emergency department by his parents due to refusal to use his left arm. He holds his arm pronated by his side. His symptoms started shortly after his father grabbed his wrist to prevent a fall. What is your diagnosis A 17.2.5

A. subluxation of the radial head
B. elbow fracture
C. elbow sprain
D. wrist sprain
E. child abuse

401. A 6-year-old boy presents with a 9 day history of anterior thigh and knee pain associated with a limp. He is afebrile. His pain worsens with passive movement of his hip. His x-rays are remarkable only for flattening of the femoral epiphysis on the painful side. What is your course of treatment for his condition D 17.2.5

A. ibuprofen for pain
B. immediate referral for surgical correction
C. bedrest
D. A and C
E. none of the above

18 DERMATOLOGY

18.1 GENERAL CONCEPTS

18.1.1 Anatomy

A. Epidermis consists of stratified epithelial tissue composed of keratinocytes. Cells at the basal layer move upward during development providing constant renewal for upper cell layers.

B. Dermis is the fibrous supporting layer between the epidermis and subcutaneous fat tissue.

C. The adnexal structures include apocrine glands, eccrine sweat glands, hair follicles, sebaceous glands, and nails.

18.1.2 Patient Management

A. Evaluation

1. History and physical examination, as always, may provide clues to the diagnosis.
2. Woods lamp examination (fungal infection, neurocutaneous syndrome skin lesions), potassium hydroxide exam (fungal infection), Tzank's smear (viral infections), skin biopsy (rarely required for diagnosis), and serum testing for circulating antibodies are some of the ancillary examinations performed when investigating cutaneous disease.

B. Treatment

1. Weeping skin lesions respond better to wet dressings followed by lotions or creams.
2. Dry skin lesions respond better to ointments.
3. Avoid soap on acutely inflamed skin.
4. Shampoos containing tar and sulfur are useful in conditions with significant scalp scaling.
5. Fine powders are useful in preventing maceration in areas of excessive moisture.
6. Keratolytic agents dissolve keratin, making them beneficial in the treatment of conditions characterized by thickened, scaling skin.
7. Topical corticosteroids are excellent in reducing inflammation associated with certain skin conditions (eczema, contact dermatitis).
8. Other treatment is geared to the underlying diagnosis.

18.2 VASCULAR MALFORMATIONS

18.2.1 Port Wine Stain

A. Sharply circumscribed, usually unilateral, pink to purple patches that are present at birth.

B. The lesions are composed of mature dermal capillaries.

C. As affected children age, the lesions may become darker or develop a cobblestoned surface.

D. Representative Syndromes

1. **Sturge-Weber Syndrome**. Trigeminal port wine stain associated with glaucoma, leptomeningeal venous angioma, seizures, and intracranial calcifications.
2. **Klippel-Trenaunay-Weber Syndrome**. Port wine stain with bone and soft tissue hypertrophy, and venous varicosities.
3. **Cobb's Syndrome**. Port wine stain with spinal arteriovenous malformation.

E. Treatment, in an effort to minimize the cosmetic impact of the lesion, is pulse dye laser therapy beginning in infancy.

18.2.2 Capillary Hemangioma (Strawberry Nevus)

A. These lesions are bright red, well-demarcated, raised, compressible vascular malformations.

B. They usually appear within the first 2 months of life as solitary or multiple skin lesions.

C. They are characterized by a phase of rapid growth, followed by a stationary phase, with ultimate involution in 95% of cases by 10 years of age.

D. Complications include ulceration, infection, bleeding, interference with vital functions (vision, breathing).

E. Treatment is observation. Steroids and interferon are reserved for more serious lesions.

18.2.3 Cavernous Hemangioma

A. These are cystic, firm, compressible, deeply placed vascular lesions.

B. Their natural history and treatment is the same as with capillary hemangiomas.

C. **Maffucci's Syndrome**. Cavernous hemangioma with lymphangiomas and nodular chondromas.

D. Complications of Hemangiomas

1. **Kasabach-Merritt Syndrome**. This syndrome is characterized by rapidly enlarging hemangiomas with thrombocytopenia, consumptive coagulopathy, and microangiopathic anemia. It is discussed in section 113.6C.
2. **Disseminated Hemangiomatosis**. Extensive skin and visceral lesions associated with high output heart failure, visceral hemorrhage, or respiratory distress.

18.2.4 Pyogenic Granuloma

A. This is an overgrowth of granulation tissue (fibroblasts, capillaries) resulting in a red, moist papule that is easily injured with resultant bleeding.

B. It is usually located at sites of previous injury.

C. Treatment is removal.

18.2.5 Hereditary Hemorrhagic Telangiectasia (Osler-Weber-Rendu Disease)

A. This is an autosomal dominant condition characterized by the development of skin and mucous membrane telangiectasias at the onset of puberty.

B. Skin lesions are 1 to 4 mm papules and macules with spider-like projections of blood vessels.

C. The lesions may bleed. Sometimes the hemorrhage is

severe. Clotting mechanisms are normal.

18.2.6 Ataxia-Telangiectasia (Louis-Bar) Syndrome

A. This is an autosomal recessive condition that affects the cerebellum, skin, and immune system.

B. Signs and symptoms are age-related.

1. Telangiectasias on the face, conjunctiva, and ears enlarge as the child ages.
2. Ataxia is also present early and must be distinguished from other causes of neurologic symptoms.
3. Pulmonary infections secondary to immunoglobulin A deficiency develop in the first decade.
4. Lymphomas are seen in the teen years.

C. Treatment is symptomatic, with death resulting from infection or malignancy.

18.2.7 Angiokeratoma Corporis (Fabry's Disease)

A. This is an X-linked recessive disorder involving an error of glycolipid metabolism (decreased α-galactosidase with accumulation of ceramide trihexoside).

B. Affected children develop small, red to blue papules, with hyperkeratotic surfaces over the genitalia, hips, buttocks, and thighs.

C. Other symptoms include recurrent fever, pain, parathesias, corneal opacities, and hypohidrosis.

D. Death occurs secondary to renal disease and cardiac involvement.

18.3 CUTANEOUS NEVI

18.3.1 Acquired Melanocytic Nevus

A. This lesion is a benign proliferation of melanocytes at the epidermal-dermal junction.

B. Natural History

1. The numbers of nevi increase during childhood, reaching a plateau in the third to fourth decade, then begin to decrease.
2. The average adult has 25 to 35 acquired nevi.

C. The nevus' location in the skin may be junctional, dermal, or compound.

D. Malignant transformation, if it occurs, is characterized by rapid increase in size, development of satellite lesions, color variegation (red, gray, black, blue), irregular borders, or a change in texture.

18.3.2 Congenital Melanocytic Nevus

A. This skin lesion is due to the presence of nevus cells in the lower dermis between collagen bundles and around appendages, extending into subcutaneous tissue.

B. It is present in 1% of newborns.

C. Categories (Grouped by Size)

1. Small: <2cm.
2. Intermediate: 2 to 20 cm.
3. Giant: >20 cm.

D. Complications

1. Giant nevi on the head are associated with leptomeningeal melanocytosis which leads to increased intracranial pressure, seizures, developmental delay, and mental retardation.
2. Giant nevi also may develop areas of malignant melanoma (10%).

E. Treatment is controversial (observation versus excision).

18.3.3 Melanoma

A. Melanoma accounts for 1 to 3% of pediatric cancers.

B. Risk factors include familial atypical mole-melanoma syndrome, xeroderma pigmentosa, excessive numbers of melanocytic nevi, giant nevi, fair complexion, excessive sun exposure, first degree relative with melanoma, and immunosuppression.

C. Mortality from melanoma is approximately 40%.

D. Treatment

1. Prevention by avoidance of sun exposure from 10 AM to 3 PM, protective clothing, and use of sunscreen.
2. Complete surgical excision of the lesion is performed when possible.

18.3.4 Halo Nevus

A. A halo will occasionally form around a melanocytic nevus. It forms as melanocytes disappear.

B. The halo is formed as a result of inflammation directed against the nevus cells.

C. Individuals with halo nevi have antibodies in their serum against malignant melanoma cells.

D. Although specific treatment is not needed, careful observation of the lesion for evidence of malignant transformation is warranted.

18.3.5 Nevus' of Ota and Ito

A. Nevus of Ota

1. This lesion is a speckled patch of blue, black, and brown coalescing macules resembling Mongolian spots.
2. It is unilateral and occurs in areas supplied by the first and second branches of the trigeminal nerve.
3. Malignant transformation is rare.

B. The **nevus of Ito** is less mottled than the nevus of Ota, and is localized to the supraclavicular, scapular, and deltoid regions.

18.3.6 Epidermal Nevi

A. Hamartomas are areas of hyperplasia of epidermal and adnexal structures, occasionally associated with other abnormalities of skin, soft tissue, eyes, central nervous system, heart, and urogenital system.

B. Nevus Sebaceous of Jadassohn

1. This is a linear, yellow, hairless plaque that is due to an abundance of sebaceous gland structures.
2. Nevus sebaceous most commonly occurs on the

head and neck.
3. The lesion becomes verrucous in adolescence.
4. Excision prior to adolescence is recommended due to the high rate of malignant transformation.

18.4 HYPERPIGMENTED LESIONS

18.4.1 Freckles (Ephelides)

A. Development of freckles is controlled by an autosomal dominant gene.

B. Most freckles are <3 mm in diameter with poorly defined margins occurring in sun exposed skin.

C. They are more common in fair skinned individuals.

D. They are a risk factor for development of melanoma independent of the presence of nevi (very likely because of the association with sun exposure.)

18.4.2 Lentigines

A. These are <3 cm benign, round, dark brown macules occurring anywhere on the skin.

B. Associated Syndromes
1. LAMB syndrome is characterized by *l*entigines on the face and vulva, *a*trial and mucocutaneous *m*yxoma, and *b*lue nevi.
2. LEOPARD syndrome is an autosomal dominant syndrome of symmetric *l*entigines associated with *e*lectrocardiogram abnormalities, *o*cular hypertelorism, pulmonic stenosis, *a*bnormal genitalia, growth *r*etardation, and sensorineural *d*eafness.
3. Peutz-Jeghers syndrome is an autosomal dominant disease associated with melanotic macules on the lips and mucous membranes, gastrointestinal polyposis, and both gastrointestinal tract and nongastrointestinal tract tumors.

18.4.3 Café au Lait (CAL)

A. These are sharply demarcated, hyperpigmented macules found on any area of skin.

B. Associated Syndromes
1. McCune-Albright syndrome has precocious puberty, large CAL, fibrous bony dysplasia, and endocrinopathy.
2. Neurofibromatosis type 1 (von Recklinghausen's disease) is an autosomal dominant disease with multiple CAL (>5 lesions of >5 mm in diameter prepuberty or >6 lesions of >15 mm in diameter postpuberty) and tissue neurofibromas.

18.4.4 Incontinentia Pigmenti

A. This is a disorder caused by random inactivation of an X chromosome that affects dermatologic, dental, and ocular structures.

B. Stages of Disease (Phases may Overlap)
1. First phase is erythematous linear streaks and plaques of vesicles.
2. Second phase includes formation of verrucous plaques at the site of previous vesicles.
3. Third phase is characterized by hyperpigmentation in whorls, patches, flecks, and streaks at sites not necessarily associated with preceding phases.
4. Fourth phase consists of hypopigmented, hairless, anhidrotic patches.

C. Associated defects include alopecia, late dentition, hypodontia, conical teeth, developmental delay, seizures, spasticity, microphthalmos, strabismus, optic atrophy, cataracts, and nail dysplasia.

18.4.5 Postinflammatory Skin Findings

A. Hyper- or hypopigmentation may occur after even minor skin inflammation.

B. The skin change may be persistent for weeks to months.

C. Treatment is not required except as directed toward the cause of the inflammation.

18.5 HYPOPIGMENTED LESIONS

18.5.1 Albinism

A. Partial or complete failure of melanin production in the skin, hair, and eyes.

B. Types
1. **Ocular Albinism**. An X-linked, autosomal dominant, or autosomal recessive condition associated with pigmentary defects of the eyes alone. It may also be associated with deafness.
2. **Tyrosinase Negative Type I Oculocutaneous Albinism**
   a. This condition is characterized by lack of visible pigment in the skin, hair, and eyes.
   b. Photophobia, decreased visual acuity, blue gray irises, white hair, and white skin are associated physical findings.
3. **Tyrosinase Positive Type II Oculocutaneous Albinism**
   a. This is the most common etiology of albinism
   b. Affected children have some pigment to their skin, hair, and eyes. Pigment continues to darken throughout life.
   c. Patients may have decreased visual acuity and nystagmus that also improves with age.
   d. Patients with Angelman's syndrome or Prader-Willi syndrome who have deletions on chromosome 15 may have this form of albinism.
4. **Hermansky-Pudlak Syndrome**. A tyrosinase positive albinism associated with variable pigmentation, defective platelets, hemorrhagic diathesis, pulmonary fibrosis, granulomatous colitis, cardiomyopathy, and renal failure.
5. **Partial Albinism** (Piebaldism). An autosomal dominant condition with amelanotic patches found most frequently on the forehead, scalp (producing a white forelock), anterior trunk, and extensor extremities.
6. **Waardenburg's syndrome**. An autosomal dominant form of albinism associated with a white fore-

lock, wide nasal bridge, heterochromia of the iris, and sensorineural deafness.

18.5.2 Tuberous Sclerosis

A. This is an autosomal dominant condition, mapped to chromosome 9 that is comprised of skin lesions, epilepsy, and mental retardation.

B. Associated skin findings include ash-leaf lesions (hypopigmented macules), adenoma sebaceum (reddish-brown angiofibromatous papules), shagreen patch (skin colored plaques with orange-peel texture), and periungual fibromas.

18.5.3 Hypomelanosis of Ito

A. The skin lesions in this condition are a negative image of those seen in incontinentia pigmenti.

B. The areas of hypopigmentation fade in adulthood.

C. Associated abnormalities include mental retardation, seizures, hypotonia, microcephaly, scoliosis, strabismus, nystagmus, and heart defects.

18.5.4 Vitiligo

A. This condition appears as sharply circumscribed, depigmented macules.

B. The etiology is unclear.

C. Risk factors include a family history of vitiligo, thyroid disease, adrenal insufficiency, pernicious anemia, and diabetes mellitus.

D. Treatment is with psoralen compounds with exposure to sunlight or ultraviolet light.

18.6 VESICULOBULLOUS DISORDERS

18.6.1 Erythema Multiforme

A. This condition occurs in children and young adults.

B. The skin lesions are erythematous macules, papules, vesicles, bullae, and urticaria. The center of the lesion may become purpuric or necrotic.

C. Types

1. Erythema multiforme minor occurs with crops of skin lcsions primarily on the extremities with sparing of the mucous membranes. Management is supportive.
2. Erythema multiforme major (Stevens-Johnson syndrome) is skin involvement with mucous membrane involvement.
   a. The affected skin may slough leading to fluid loss, anemia, and bacterial superinfection.
   b. Vision may be impaired secondary to corneal involvement.

D. The potential etiologies include infection, neoplasm, drug reaction (antibiotics, anticonvulsants), and idiopathic causes.

E. Toxic epidermal necrolysis has the same predisposing factors and is likely a more severe form of erythema multiforme major.

18.6.2 Epidermolysis Bullosa

A. This is a hereditary, congenital blistering disorder characterized by the sudden occurrence of blisters after even minor trauma to the skin due to cytolysis of the basal layer.

B. The disease exacerbates in warm weather.

C. Types

1. Epidermolysis bullosa simplex is autosomal dominant, nonscarring epidermolysis bullosa that improves with age.
2. Epidermolysis bullosa junctional is an autosomal recessive disorder with severe skin and mucosal involvement. It carries the risk of serious disfigurement and death within the first 3 years of life secondary to sepsis, organ failure, or cachexia.
3. Dystrophic EB is the autosomal recessive form and the most disabling. It is characterized by extensive blister formation with scarring, cutaneous carcinomas, digital fusion, esophageal strictures, and joint contracture. Autosomal dominant forms do occur.

18.6.3 Pemphigus Vulgaris

A. Skin findings in pemphigus vulgaris are large, flaccid bullae on the skin and painful oral ulcers.

B. Nikolsky's sign is positive.

C. Ruptured bullae heal poorly with residual hyperpigmentation.

18.7 ECZEMA

18.7.1 Contact Dermatitis

A. Eczematous skin lesions are characterized by erythematous oozing lesions acutely, and thickened, dry, scaling lesions with increased pigmentation and lichenification in the chronic state.

B. Contact dermatitis is an eczematous skin reaction caused by prolonged or recurrent contact with an irritative substance.

C. Examples of this condition include diaper dermatitis, allergic contact dermatitis, rhus dermatitis (poison ivy, poison oak, poison sumac), juvenile plantar dermatosis (skin lesions arising because of cycles of excessive hydration followed by rapid drying), and nicked dermatitis (characteristically seen at sites of clothing snap closures).

D. Treatment is by removal of the offending agent, cool compresses, topical steroids, and antihistamine for sedation when itching is severe.

18.7.2 Nummular Eczema

A. These are coin shaped, eczematous plaques on the extensor extremities, buttocks, and shoulders.

B. It is often confused with tinea corporis.

C. Treatment is similar to atopic eczema including topical corticosteroids for flares and aggressive skin moisturizing.

18.7.3 Pityriasis Alba

A. These lesions are hypopigmented, round or oval, nonpruritic macules with a fine scales and irregular borders.

B. Distribution is on the face, neck, trunk, and proximal arms.

C. The condition is exacerbated by skin dryness.

D. It is self-limiting, but skin changes may last for weeks to months.

E. The differential diagnosis includes tinea versicolor and tinea corporis.

18.7.4 Seborrheic Dermatitis

A. This common cause of the neonatal condition, cradle cap, is a focal, scaling, crusting, greasy, erythematous dermatitis.

B. Distribution is on the face, neck, scalp, retroauricular area, axillae, and diaper area (distribution of the sebaceous glands).

C. Etiology is unknown.

D. Treatment is with antiseborrheic shampoo and topical corticosteroids.

18.8 DISORDERS OF THE EPIDERMIS

18.8.1 Psoriasis

A. Psoriasis is characterized by erythematous papules that coalesce into plaques with sharply demarcated borders.
   1. Removal of the superficial, silvery scale results in pinpoint bleeding (Auspitz's sign).
   2. Köbner's phenomenon is the formation of new lesions at sites of trauma.
   3. Distribution is on the scalp, knees, elbows, and genitalia.
   4. Pitting of the nails is common.

B. Guttate psoriasis predominates in children.
   1. It is characterized by multiple, small, oval lesions that look like the larger plaques of psoriasis.
   2. It can follow a group A β-hemolytic streptococcus infection, a viral infection, sunburn, or withdrawal from systemic steroid therapy.

C. Psoriasis has a pattern of remission and exacerbation.

D. Psoriatic arthritis is a well recognized disease complication.

E. Treatment
   1. Avoid trauma to the skin.
   2. Tar preparations are beneficial if prolonged sun exposure is not anticipated.
   3. Topical corticosteroids may provide early transient improvement in individual lesions.
   4. Treatment with a phenol and saline solution followed by a tar shampoo is useful for scalp psoriasis.
   5. Psoralen and ultraviolet light treatment or oral retinoids and methotrexate are used in severe psoriasis.
   6. Infantile and guttate psoriasis should be treated conservatively because aggressive therapy may worsen the condition.
   7. Consultation with a dermatologist is appropriate.

18.8.2 Pityriasis Rosea

A. This is a benign skin reaction of unknown etiology.
   1. Pityriasis rosea begins with a herald patch (solitary, oval, dry skin lesion) with occurrence of a symmetric eruption of oval, pink, scaling lesions following skin cleavage planes on the trunk and proximal extremities approximately 5 to 10 days later.
   2. The classic rash distribution is of a "Christmas tree" pattern on the posterior trunk.
   3. The skin lesions may be pruritic and last up to 12 weeks.

B. Differential diagnosis is tinea corporis, guttate psoriasis, eczema, and in sexually active individuals, secondary syphilis.

C. Pityriasis rosea is self-limiting so treatment is not necessary. It may resolve faster with ultraviolet light exposure. Itching may be treated with antihistamines or topical steroids.

18.8.3 Lichen Striatus

A. This is a linear band of papules along a skin dermatome.

B. The condition evolves over days to weeks and resolves slowly over months without sequelae.

C. Treatment is not necessary.

18.8.4 Papular Acrodermatitis of Childhood (Gianotti-Crosti Syndrome)

A. The rash is this disease is a coppery colored, flat-topped papule 1 to 5 mm in diameter.
   1. Distribution in symmetric over the face, buttocks, and limbs.
   2. Köbner phenomenon occurs.

B. Associated symptoms include fever and malaise.

C. In Italy, this condition used to be associated with hepatitis B virus infection.

18.8.5 Acanthosis Nigricans

A. This condition presents as hyperpigmented, velvety plaques most often located on the neck and skin folds.

B. It is associated with obesity, drugs, and illnesses such as diabetes mellitus, thyroid disease and Cushing's syndrome. When present in a child with obesity, it is known as pseudoacanthosis migricans.

C. It usually improves over time following appropriate treatment of the underlying disorder.

18.8.6 Disorders of Keratin Formation

A. **Ichthyosis**. This is a group of dermatoses characterized by hyperkeratosis and scaling.

1. **Harlequin Fetus**
   a. These infants are noted to have markedly thickened, cracked skin over the entire body at the time of birth.
   b. They have a poor suck, respiratory distress, and are prone to severe cutaneous infection.
   c. Prognosis is poor. Most infants die within weeks.
2. **Collodion Baby**
   a. At birth, these infants are covered by a thick, leathery membrane that soughs over a period of weeks, rarely revealing normal skin, usually revealing the thick skin scales of ichthyosis.
   b. Features include flattening of the facies and an O-shaped lip configuration.
   c. Hair is sparse.
   d. Prognosis is guarded because these infants are at high risk for death by cutaneous fluid loss, infection, or aspiration.
3. **Lamellar Ichthyosis**
   a. Autosomal recessive condition presenting usually as a collodion infant.
   b. Affected children have erythroderma and thickened skin scales.
   c. Biopsy reveals marked thickening of the stratum corneum.
   d. Complications. Itching is a distressing symptom that does not respond well to antihistamines. Cutaneous superinfection is common.
   e. Treatment is aggressive moisturization with long, oil laden baths, high humidity environment, keratinolytic agents, and emollient creams.
4. **Ichthyosis Vulgaris**
   a. This is a very common autosomal dominant condition that presents during the first year of life with scaling that is not as debilitating as in lamellar ichthyosis.
   b. Disease flares in the winter months and may resolve completely in the summertime.
   c. Treatment is with an emollient.
5. **X-linked Ichthyosis**
   a. In this ichthyosis, skin changes are present at birth. It occurs predominantly in males, but female carriers may show some scaling.
   b. This condition worsens as the child ages.
   c. Deep corneal opacities are a hallmark complication. They do not interfere with visual development.
   d. Like other forms, an emollient is the mainstay of treatment.

18.8.7 Mucous Membrane Findings

A. **Cheilitis** is inflammation of the lips at the angles of the mouth usually due to chapping, excessive salivation, or lip licking.

B. **Fordyce spots** are ectopic sebaceous glands on the vermillion border of the lips.

C. **Mucoceles** are painless, bluish, fluctuant, papules on the lips, tongue, and palate due to traumatic damage to minor salivary gland ducts.

D. **Ranulas** are mucoceles arising as a result of damage to the submaxillary and sublingual salivary ducts.

E. **Aphthous stomatitis** (canker sores) are painful, shallow ulcers of the oral mucosa with varied causes. Contrary to popular belief, they are not a manifestation of herpes simplex virus infection.

F. **Geographic tongue** (benign migratory glossitis) is a condition with sharply demarcated, irregular, smooth, red plaques on the tongue due to atrophy of the filiform papillae. No treatment is needed.

G. **Black hairy tongue** is a dark coating of the tongue caused by hyperplasia of filiform papillae, overgrowth of chromogenic bacteria and fungus, and entrapped food particles. Poor hygiene and smoking are risk factors.

18.9 DISORDERS OF THE DERMIS

18.9.1 Keloid

A. Keloids are overgrowth of connective tissue after trauma.

B. The lesions are raised, red, rubbery, tender or pruritic lesions distinct from hypertrophic scars. Both lesions are due to collagen formation over longer periods of time than in normal wound healing. Hypertrophic scars remain confined to the site of injury. Keloid overgrows the area of original injury.

18.9.2 Granuloma Annulare

A. These are skin colored to mildly erythematous, firm, smooth papules that form annular plaques with a raised border and atrophic central area.

B. Lesions can occur anywhere on the body.

C. It is commonly mistaken for tinea corporis (ringworm), but is not scaly.

18.9.3 Ehlers-Danlos Syndrome

A. This is a genetic connective tissue disorder which predominantly effects skin and ligament elasticity.

B. Types
   1. Type I (Gravis Type). Autosomal dominant condition with skin hyperelasticity and fragility, easy bruising, joint hypermobility, scoliosis, mitral valve prolapse, and premature birth.
   2. Type II (Mitis Type). Autosomal dominant disease with mild skin and joint (hands and feet) manifestations.
   3. Type III (Benign Hypermobile Type). Autosomal dominant disease with minimal skin changes, but severe, generalized joint hypermobility.
   4. Type IV (Ecchymotic Type). Autosomal dominant or recessive disease with marked dermal thinning,

ecchymosis, keloid formation, bowel rupture, aortic aneurysm, and stroke.

5. Type V (X-linked Type). Minimal joint and skin laxity, moderate bruising, skin fragility, and scarring.
6. Type VI (Autosomal Recessive Ocular Type). Joint hypermobility, kyphoscoliosis, fragile cornea, keratoconus, fragile bones, and skin hyperelasticity.
7. Type VII (Arthrochalasis Multiplex Congenita). Autosomal recessive condition with short stature, joint hypermobility and dislocation, hyperelastic skin, and easy bruising.
8. Type VIII (Periodontitis Type). Autosomal dominant disease with mild skin hyperelasticity, small joint hypermobility, bruising, skin fragility with scarring, and periodontitis leading to permanent tooth loss.
9. Type IX (X-linked Recessive Skeletal Type). Occipital exostosis, widening and bowing of long bones, bladder diverticula, inguinal hernia, chronic diarrhea, and mild skin hyperelasticity.
10. Type X (Dysfibronectinemic Type). Autosomal recessive failure of platelet aggregation, easy bruising, joint hypermobility, and hyperelasticity.

18.9.4 Mastocytosis

A. Collection of disorders characterized by clusters of mast cells in the dermis.

B. Urticaria pigmentosa is single or multiple skin lesions that, upon stroking, develop a wheal and flare. It is self-limiting with resolution by adulthood (75%).

18.10 DISORDERS OF SWEAT GLANDS

18.10.1 Miliaria

A. This is retention of sweat in blocked eccrine sweat ducts.

B. Types
1. Miliaria crystallina are noninflammatory pinpoint, clear vesicles. It is a very superficial process.
2. Miliaria rubra (prickly heat) are erythematous, papules and vesicles localized to skin folds or areas of occlusion.

18.10.2 Hidradenitis Suppurativa

A. Chronic inflammation of apocrine glands with onset at puberty.

B. The disease presents as solitary or multiple, painful nodules and deep abscesses with subsequent scarring.

C. The most severe complications are formation of chronically draining sinus tracts or fistulas.

D. Treatment
1. Avoid tight fitting clothing.
2. Topical and systemic antibiotics for treatment of infection.
3. Incision and drainage of abscesses.
4. Other useful medications include intralesional or oral steroids and oral contraceptive pills.

18.11 DISORDERS OF THE HAIR

18.11.1 Excessive Growth

A. Hypertrichosis is defined as excessive hair growth at inappropriate locations. It has many causes including familial tendency, drugs, local trauma, nevi, and both endocrine and congenital disorders.

B. Hirsutism is male pattern hair growth in women.

18.11.2 Deficient Hair Growth

A. **Hypotrichosis** and **alopecia** are deficient or absent hair growth.

B. **Telogen effluvium** is the sudden loss of hair in large amounts, caused by premature conversion of anagen (growing) hairs to telogen (resting) hairs. It usually occurs 1 to 3 months after a physiologically stressful event (illness, injury, surgery).

C. **Anagen effluvium** (toxic alopecia) is severe, diffuse growth inhibition of anagen follicles with >80% loss of scalp hair. Causes include radiation, chemotherapy, and hypervitaminosis A.

D. **Traction alopecia** is due to trauma to hair follicles by tight braids, rubber bands, headbands, or rollers. If the practice leading to the alopecia persists, it can result in permanent scarring of the hair follicles.

E. **Trichotillomania** is compulsive pulling and twisting of hairs resulting in breakage. The hairs remaining in the area and are of varying lengths. Treatment is interruption of the behavior.

F. **Alopecia**
1. Alopecia areata is complete loss of hair in well-circumscribed patches.
2. Alopecia totalis is loss of all scalp hair.
3. Alopecia universalis is complete loss of all body hair.
4. The cause is unknown.
5. It can be confused with tinea capitis, however with alopecia, the underlying skin is normal as compared to the scaling plaque seen with tinea.
6. Alopecia areata resolves within 6 to 12 months without treatment and recurrences are common. Alopecia universalis and totalis are less likely to resolve.

18.12 SKIN INFECTIONS

18.12.1 Impetigo

A. Nonbullous impetigo is a localized skin infection at the site of preceding trauma characterized by golden crusts on an erythematous base.
1. The most common causative agent is *Staphylococcus aureus* followed by group A β-hemolytic streptococcus.
2. Spread is by fomites or autoinoculation.
3. The condition is most often confused with cutaneous herpes simplex virus.

B. Bullous impetigo is the development of transparent, thin-walled bullae on the skin of the face, buttocks, trunk, perineum, and extremities.

1. The bullae rupture easily leaving a collarette of scales at the margin of a shallow erosion. These typically heal without scarring.
2. This form of impetigo is always caused by *Staphylococcus aureus.*

C. Treatment for impetigo is topical or systemic antistaphylococcal antibiotics.

18.12.2 Staphylococcal Scalded Skin Syndrome (SSSS)

A. SSSS is a generalized cutaneous disease secondary to epidermolytic and exfoliative toxin elaboration from localized *Staphylococcus aureus* infection.

1. SSSS is associated with a prodrome of malaise, fever, and tenderness of the skin.
2. A scarlatiniform erythema is usually present.
3. As the disease progresses, areas of epidermis will separate with light lateral pressure (Nikolsky's sign).
4. The lesions usually heal without scarring because the skin separation occurs in the granular layer of the epidermis.

B. Complications of the disease include secondary bacterial infection and fluid and electrolyte disturbance due to loss of substances from denuded skin.

C. Treatment is with antistaphylococcal antibiotics and supportive care.

18.12.3 Other Bacterial Infections

A. **Blistering distal dactylitis** in a blistering infection of the fingertips and toes caused most commonly by group A β-hemolytic streptococcus. Treatment is with penicillin.

B. **Ecthyma** resembles impetigo, but involves deeper skin structures. Group A β-hemolytic streptococcus is the usual pathogen followed closely by *Staphylococcus aureus.*

C. **Ecthyma gangrenosum** is necrotic ulcer formation with an eschar associated with *Pseudomonas aeruginosa* infection. It is seen most commonly in patients with immune deficiency.

D. **Folliculitis** is a superficial infection of the hair follicles most often caused by *Staphylococcus aureus.*

18.12.4 Fungal Infections

A. **Tinea versicolor**

1. These are reddish-brown, scaling macules that merge to form confluent patches.
2. The etiology is *Malassezia furfur.*
3. Potassium hydroxide preparation reveals a classic "spaghetti and meatballs" appearance of fungal elements.

B. **Dermatophytosis**

1. **Tinea capitis** is a scalp infection caused usually by *Trichophyton tonsurans* growth in the hair shaft.
   a. The skin lesion is a scaling, red eruption with a raised margin associated with hair breakage.
   b. Treatment is with oral griseofulvin. Topical preparations are not useful because the fungus is located within the hair shaft (endothrix).
   c. **Kerion formation** is a complication of tinea capitis due to a severe inflammatory response to the fungus. It is a boggy mass studded with pustules. Treatment is with oral antifungals with or without oral steroids and oral antibiotics.
2. **Tinea corporis** is a fungal infection of nonscalp skin, excluding the palms and soles, acquired by direct contact with contaminated skin, hair, or surfaces.
   a. The lesions are annular, dry, red, raised, scaling skin lesions with raised margins and central clearing.
   b. Treatment is with topical antifungal medications.
3. **Tinea cruris** (jock itch) is a scaling red patch on the inner thigh with vesicle formation at the well-demarcated, advancing margin. Treatment is with topical antifungals.
4. **Tinea pedis** (athlete's foot) presents as fissured, malodorous, erythematous skin with maceration, peeling, itching, and tenderness of the involved area.
5. A **dermatophytid ("id") reaction** is a papular and vesicular grouped skin eruption seen in individuals with fungal infections and a hypersensitivity to the offending pathogen.

C. **Candidal Infection**

1. **Thrush** is an overgrowth of *Candida albicans* forming thick, white, adherent, pruritic plaques on the buccal mucosa. It can be effectively treated with nystatin or fluconazole.
2. **Fungal diaper dermatitis** is an erythematous, confluent plaque with defined margins and satellite lesions distinct from the main area of involvement. Treatment is with topical antifungal medications.

18.12.5 Viral Infections

A. **Human papilloma virus** infection (warts) presents as well circumscribed papules with irregular (verrucous), hyperkeratotic surfaces.

1. Warts occur in 5 to 10% of all children.
2. They are spread primarily by direct contact and autoinoculation.
3. Treatment is with ablation by liquid nitrogen, cantharidin, curettage, lactic acid, or salicylic acid.

B. **Molluscum contagiosum** are flesh-colored, pearly papules with a central umbilication that occur anywhere on the body.

1. Lesions are caused by a poxvirus spread via direct contact, autoinoculation, or fomite.
2. The condition is self-limited with resolution within 9 months of onset in most cases. Some children will have lesions that persist for years.

3. They may be treated with curettage, liquid nitrogen, or topical cantharidin.

18.12.6 Infestations

A. **Scabies**
   1. The manifestations of scabies are caused by a delayed sensitivity reaction to the burrowing female mite, *Sarcoptes scabei*, her eggs, and her feces.
   2. The rash is red papules and threadlike burrows associated with intense itching and subsequent excoriations from scratching.
   3. Treatment is with topical permethrin cream.

B. ***Pediculosis capitis*** (head lice), ***corporis*** (body lice), and ***pubis*** (pubic lice).
   1. These parasites survive on the host by feeding on human blood.
   2. They are spread by direct contact and fomites.
   3. Treatment is with permethrin, lindane (carefully), or oral sulfamethoxazole (interferes with louse's gut bacteria), nit removal, and environmental cleansing.
   4. The primary complication of infestation is secondary bacterial infection from scratching.

C. **Seabather's eruption** consists of inflammatory papules developing within 12 hours of swimming in salt water, usually in sites covered by the swimsuit.
   1. In addition to the pustular, vesicular, or urticarial rash, patients may experience fever, malaise, chills, and gastrointestinal upset.
   2. It is a hypersensitivity reaction to the venom from the larvae of the thimble jellyfish.

18.13 MISCELLANEOUS SKIN DISEASE

18.13.1 Common Neonatal Skin Lesions

A. **Milia** are superficial epidermal inclusion cysts. They are 1 to 2 mm in diameter, white papules, occurring primarily on the face and gingiva. When located on the palate, they are referred to as Epstein's pearls.

B. **Sebaceous hyperplasia** are numerous, small, yellow-white papules on the forehead, nose, lips, and cheeks. They resolve spontaneously within a few weeks.

C. **Sucking blisters** are bullae on the limbs of infants caused by in utero sucking on the affected part.

D. **Cutis marmorata** is a lacy, red to blue, reticular, vascular pattern in the skin, caused by environmental exposure to cool temperatures.

E. **Harlequin color change** is skin color change related to poor autonomic control of the vasculature. Dependent areas become deep red while nondependent areas become pale.

F. **Nevus simplex** are flat, pink, vascular lesions occurring on the glabella, eyelids, upper lip, posterior neck, and occiput. The facial lesions fade with age. The nuchal lesion ("stork bite") often persists.

G. **Mongolian spots** are blue, flat, macular areas usually found on the thighs, back, shoulders, and sacrum. They are seen primarily in dark-skinned infants.

H. **Erythema Toxicum**
   1. Erythema toxicum is a condition seen in 50% of all newborns.
   2. It consists of 1 to 2 mm erythematous papules with a yellow, central pustule.
   3. Wright staining of material from the pustule reveals eosinophils.
   4. No treatment is needed.

I. **Transient Neonatal Pustular Melanosis**
   1. This dermatosis presents as superficial pustules noted at delivery that rupture, leaving a hyperpigmented macule surrounded by a collarette of scale.
   2. The hyperpigmentation may persist for several months.
   3. Wright staining of pustule contents reveal polymorphonuclear leukocytes, however this is not an infectious condition.
   4. No treatment is necessary.

J. **Infantile Acropustulosis**
   1. This condition begins at 2 to 10 months of age and has erythematous papules that become vesicopustular, followed by crusting.
   2. The lesions are intensely pruritic.
   3. Episodes of the dermatosis last 7 to 14 days with lesions appearing in crops.
   4. Infants may experience cyclic recurrence every 2 to 4 weeks for up to 2 years from onset.

K. **Supernumerary nipples** are single or multiple, unilateral or bilateral, residual, rudimentary nipples occurring along a line from the anterior axilla to the inguinal area. They are commonly mistaken for nevi.

L. **Aplasia Cutis Congenita** (Cutis Aplasia)
   1. Cutis aplasia is the absence of skin, usually on the scalp, due to developmental failure of the skin structures.
   2. The lesions are oval, well-demarcated, noninflammatory ulcerations or fibrotic scars.
   3. Complications include bleeding, local infection, and meningitis.
   4. Cutis aplasia may be associated with intrauterine toxin exposure or infection, or may be seen as part of a syndrome of malformations.

18.13.2 Acne Vulgaris

A. Acne vulgaris is an inflammatory process involving the sebaceous glands, occurring in up to 80% of adolescents.

B. Pathophysiology
   1. Androgens produced during puberty cause increased sebum production that causes plugging of the sebaceous gland follicles, forming comedones.
   2. The material trapped in the follicle ruptures into

the surrounding tissue. Bacteria present in the follicles attract leukocytes. The leukocytes release hydrolytic enzymes causing a local inflammatory reaction.

3. The lesion will eventually heal, but may do so with scarring.

C. Types of lesions
1. Closed comedones (whiteheads) are the result of hyperkeratosis of the follicular epithelium resulting in an elevated skin papule.
2. Open comedones (blackheads) are a later stage of enlarged comedones containing melanin.
3. Pustules are the typical "zit" that results when comedones rupture into the surrounding tissue and the inflammatory response results.
4. Nodulocystic lesions are not truly cysts. They are deep skin nodules resulting from rupture of glandular contents into surrounding tissues.

D. Treatment is usually effective in 1 to 2 months.
1. Benzyl peroxide is an organic peroxide and oxidizing agent that peels superficial skin layers. It is bacteriostatic for *Propionibacterium acne.*
2. Topical antibiotics (clindamycin, erythromycin) and oral antibiotics (tetracyclines) inhibit the growth of *Propionibacterium acne*. Be aware that oral antibiotics may decrease the effectiveness of oral contraceptive pills.
3. Tretinoin causes increased turnover of epithelial cells and decreased cohesiveness of epidermal cells resulting in decreased comedone formation.
4. Isotretinoin is used in treatment of moderate to severe nodulocystic acne. It reduces sebum formation, decreases the population of *Propionibacterium acne,* and decreases ductal cornification. Use with caution because of teratogenic effects.

18.13.3 Nutritional Dermatoses

A. **Acrodermatitis enteropathica** is an autosomal recessive skin disorder caused by an inability to absorb dietary zinc in the gastrointestinal tract.
1. Affected patients develop vesicles and bullae in the perioral, perineal, and acral areas.
2. Other symptoms include photophobia, conjunctivitis, diarrhea, stomatitis, irritability, and growth retardation.
3. Therapy with oral zinc supplementation produces dramatic improvement in symptoms.

B. **Kwashiorkor**
1. This is severe protein and essential amino acid malnutrition in the presence of adequate caloric intake.
2. Patients have cutaneous erythema progressing to desquamation, circumoral pallor, skin depigmentation, and purple skin patches that progress to waxy lesions and erosions. They may also have the skin lesions of acrodermatitis enteropathica secondary to dietary zinc deficiency.
3. Skin appendage effects include thin nails and sparse hair with a flag sign (linear depigmentation with alternating light and dark bands).

C. Cystic fibrosis patients may experience similar skin findings as seen in kwashiorkor due to protein calorie malnutrition.

D. **Pellagra** is due to inadequate dietary intake of niacin and/or tryptophan.
1. Patients present with edema, erythema, and sunburn of exposed skin. Local trauma to the skin can also cause lesions.
2. Skin may become lichenified (thickened, hyperpigmented, cracked).
3. When the rash is present on the neck, it is called "Casal's necklace."
4. Skin infections may be a significant complication.

E. **Scurvy** is caused by a deficiency of vitamin C or ascorbic acid.
1. The classic dermatologic finding is follicular hyperkeratosis with perifollicular petechiae and coiling of hairs on the extremities and buttocks.
2. Other symptoms include gingivitis and subperiosteal hematomas.
3. Treatment is with oral vitamin C supplementation.

F. Vitamin A deficiency is associated with nightblindness, xerosis, hyperkeratosis, and desquamation.

G. Fatty acid deficiency may be seen in individuals with gastrointestinal malabsorption, consumers of fat free diets, or those receiving total parenteral nutrition without lipid supplementation. These children may have thickened red skin with desquamation and alopecia in addition to failure to thrive and thrombocytopenia.

402. All of the following are adnexal skin structures except — A 18.1.1

A. keratinocytes
B. apocrine glands
C. eccrine glands
D. hair follicles
E. sebaceous glands

403. An infant is born with a port wine stain of the skin supplied by the ophthalmic branch of the trigeminal nerve. At 4 months old, he begins having seizures. Evaluation reveals intracranial calcifications. What is his diagnosis — B 18.2.1

A. congenital cytomegalovirus
B. Sturge-Weber syndrome
C. congenital toxoplasmosis
D. infantile spasm

404. An infant is noted at birth to have hypertrophy of his right upper extremity and blotchy skin discoloration. Subsequently, the discoloration is noted to be diffuse areas of port wine stain. What is his diagnosis — C 18.2.1

A. Cobb syndrome
B. Sturge-Weber syndrome
C. Klippel-Trenaunay-Weber syndrome
D. harlequin baby syndrome

405. A 4-month-old infant is brought in for a well child check. His parents are concerned about a bright red, raised, soft "mole" on his head that seems to be growing faster than he is. What is your diagnosis — D 18.2.2

A. cavernous hemangioma
B. port wine stain
C. nevus simplex
D. strawberry nevus
E. pyogenic granuloma

406. An infant is brought to your office to establish care. In his history you find that he has a cavernous hemangioma, lymphangiomas, and nodular chondromas. What is his diagnosis — B 18.2.3

A. Kasabach-Merritt syndrome
B. Maffucci's syndrome
C. Cobb's syndrome
D. Klippel-Trenaunay-Weber syndrome
E. Osler-Weber-Rendu syndrome

407. A child is noted on physical exam to have sharply demarcated, irregular, smooth, red plaques on the tongue. What is the etiology of these lesions — C 18.8.7

A. herpes simplex virus infection
B. sucking on too many popsicles
C. atrophy of filiform papillae
D. overgrowth of bacteria
E. fungal growth

408. A 17-year-old female presents with lesions consistent with pityriasis rosea. She reports that she is sexually active. What condition should you rule out — C 18.8.2

A. group A β-hemolytic streptococcus
B. group B streptococcus
C. syphilis
D. chlamydia
E. gonorrhea

409. A teenager presents with a new diagnosis of lymphoma. Her past history is significant for facial and conjunctival telangiectasias, ataxia, and immunoglobulin A deficiency with recurrent pulmonary infection. What is her diagnosis — B 18.2.6

A. Osler-Weber-Rendu disease
B. Louis-Bar syndrome
C. Klippel-Trenaunay-Weber syndrome
D. Fabry's disease

410. All of the following are indicators of malignant transformation of a nevus except — A 18.3.1

A. slow increase in size
B. variegation in color
C. irregular margins
D. changes in texture

411. Leptomeningeal melanocytosis is associated with what overlying skin lesion — C 18.3.2

A. small congenital melanocytic nevus on the head
B. intermediate congenital melanocytic nevus
C. giant congenital melanocytic nevus on the scalp
D. bathing suit nevus

412. What is the incidence of malignant transformation in areas of giant nevi — A 18.3.2

A. 10%
B. 20%
C. 30%
D. 40%
E. 50%

413. What is the mortality rate from malignant melanoma — B 18.3.3

A. 30%
B. 40%
C. 50%
D. 60%
E. 70%

414. What is the recommended management of nevus sebaceous — A 18.3.6

A. excision prior to adolescence
B. excision in infancy
C. observation for malignant change
D. no treatment is necessary

415. Where is the nevus of Ota located — B 18.3.5

A. scapular region
B. face
C. deltoid region
D. back
E. supraclavicular region

416. An obese 15-year-old African American female presents with acanthosis nigricans on her neck and polydipsia and weight loss. Which of the following laboratory tests would be indicated — D 18.8.5

A. hemoglobin A_{1C}
B. thyroid stimulating hormone
C. insulin level
D. all of the above
E. A and B

417. Incontinentia pigmenti demonstrates what form of inheritance — A 18.4.4

- **A.** random inactivation of an X chromosome
- **B.** X-linked recessive
- **C.** autosomal dominant
- **D.** autosomal recessive
- **E.** it is not a genetic disorder

418. Which phase of incontinentia pigmenti are hyperpigmented whorls present — C 18.4.4

- **A.** phase I
- **B.** phase II
- **C.** phase III
- **D.** phase IV

419. A child with Prader-Willi syndrome has pale skin, hair and eyes, decreased visual acuity, and nystagmus. What kind of albinism is this — B 18.5.1

- **A.** ocular albinism
- **B.** tyrosinase-positive oculocutaneous albinism
- **C.** tyrosinase-negative oculocutaneous albinism
- **D.** partial albinism

420. A child is noted to have hypertelorism, deafness, and a white forelock, just like his mother. What is their diagnosis — A 18.5.1

- **A.** Waardenburg's syndrome
- **B.** piebaldism
- **C.** Prader-Willi syndrome
- **D.** type I oculocutaneous albinism

421. A child who has been taking a sulfa based antibiotic, presents with raised, red, urticarial lesions and target lesions with central purpura. He has no mucosal lesions. What is his diagnosis — A 18.6.1

- **A.** erythema multiforme minor
- **B.** erythema multiforme major
- **C.** toxic epidermal necrolysis
- **D.** staphylococcal scalded skin syndrome

422. Separation of the superficial layers of the skin with slight lateral pressure is called — D 18.12.2

- **A.** Koebner's phenomenon
- **B.** dermatographism
- **C.** Auspitz's sign
- **D.** Nikolsky's sign

423. A child presents with multiple, oval, sharply demarcated, red plaques with silvery scale. Auspitz's sign is positive. What illness may have preceded the development of this child's guttate psoriasis — B 18.8.1

- **A.** group B streptococcus
- **B.** group A β-hemolytic streptococcus
- **C.** shigellosis
- **D.** hemolytic-uremic syndrome

424. A 4-month-old Hispanic child is referred to your office for evaluation of bruising without a known history of trauma. You note blue macules over the sacrum and buttocks. What is your diagnosis — A 18.13.1

- A. Mongolian spots
- **B.** accidental bruising
- **C.** nonaccidental trauma
- **D.** idiopathic thrombocytopenic purpura

425. What is the treatment of choice for pyogenic granuloma — A 18.2.4

A. removal
B. intralesional steroid injections
C. benign neglect
D. topical retinoids

426. At what stage of life do the manifestations of Osler-Weber-Rendu disease present — D 18.2.5

A. infancy
B. preschool years
C. elementary school years
D. adolescence
E. young adulthood

427. What distinguishes granuloma annulare from tinea corporis — A 18.9.2

A. lack of scale
B. location
C. shape
D. central clearing

428. Chemotherapy results in which of the following disorders — B 18.11.2

A. telogen effluvium
B. anagen effluvium
C. traction alopecia
D. trichotillomania

429. Which of the following is characterized by excessive hair growth in inappropriate locations — A 18.11.1

A. hypertrichosis
B. hirsutism
C. telogen effluvium
D. trichotillomania

430. What is the most common causative agent of nonbullous impetigo — D 18.12.1

A. group B streptococcus
B. group A β-hemolytic streptococcus
C. *Staphylococcus epidermidis*
D. *Staphylococcus aureus*

431. Which of the following statements about staphylococcal scalded skin syndrome is false — D 18.12.2

A. the skin lesions usually heal without scarring
B. complications of the disease include secondary infection and fluid loss
C. it is caused by *Staphylococcus aureus*
D. Köbner phenomenon is present

432. Which of the following acne medications is teratogenic — D 18.13.2

A. benzoyl peroxide
B. erythromycin
C. topical retinoids
D. isotretinoin

433. Which fungus looks like "spaghetti and meatballs" on potassium hydroxide preparation — B 18.12.4

A. *Trichophyton tonsurans*
B. *Malassezia furfur*
C. *Candida albicans*
D. all of the above

434. What is the most common etiologic agent of blistering dactylitis — C 18.12.3

- **A.** *Staphylococcus aureus*
- **B.** *Staphylococcus epidermidis*
- **C.** group A β-hemolytic streptococcus
- **D.** *Pseudomonas aeruginosa*
- **E.** *Candida albicans*

435. What is the treatment of choice for tinea capitis — C 18.12.4

- **A.** topical antifungal preparations
- **B.** intralesional steroids
- **C.** oral griseofulvin
- **D.** topical antibiotics

436. What is definitive treatment for scabies infestation — D 18.12.6

- **A.** topical antibiotics
- **B.** oral antihistamines
- **C.** oral sulfamethoxazole-trimethoprim for resistant cases
- **D.** topical permethrin
- **E.** topical antihistamines

437. A 6-month-old black female with a history of eczema has hypopigmentation of the skin in the diaper area. They are concerned about this finding. What is your recommendation — C 18.4.5

- **A.** apply topical steroids
- **B.** apply skin lotions
- **C.** reassure them that the change will resolve when the eczema clears
- **D.** refer the family to a dermatologist

438. What is the dietary deficiency in pellagra — D 18.13.3

- **A.** vitamin C
- **B.** vitamin D
- **C.** vitamin E
- **D.** niacin

19 EYE DISORDERS

19.1 GENERAL CONCEPTS

19.1.1 Neonatal Eye Development

A. At birth, the eye is 2/3 the size of the adult globe. Rapid growth occurs during the first year of life.

B. Eye color is light blue to gray at birth. Pigmentary change of the iris occurs during the first 6 months of life.

C. Acuity
   1. Infants are hyperopic with vision measuring approximately 20/400 at birth.
   2. By 3 years of age, vision may have improved to 20/30.

D. Gaze
   1. Infants intermittently have disconjugate gaze during the early weeks of life.
   2. Conjugate gaze is developed by 3 to 6 months of age.
   3. Fixed gaze deviations should prompt early referral to an ophthalmologist.

E. The ability to produce tears is present by 1 to 3 months of age.

19.1.2 Test Methods

A. Visual Acuity
   1. The testing method employed depends on the child's age.
   2. Infants
      a. A crude assessment of vision can be made by evaluating the infant's ability to fixate on and follow an object held by the examiner.
      b. Historical information regarding parental observations may also be useful.
      c. A subtle clue to unilateral vision disturbance is irritability displayed by the young child when the eye with better acuity is occluded.
   3. Toddlers 2.5 to 3.5 years of age can usually perform well on picture tests.
   4. The tumbling E test is useful for the preschool-aged child.
   5. Standard Snellen charts can be used on children who can recognize and read individual letters.

B. Optic pathways and cortical function may be assessed through the use of visual evoked response testing.

C. Formal visual field testing can be performed on any child who can understand and follow examiner instructions.

D. Color vision testing can be performed on children who can follow instructions. Even if they cannot read letters or numbers, they may be able to trace the figures with a finger.

19.2 DISEASE PROFILES

19.2.1 Refractive Error

A. Hyperopia (Farsightedness)
   1. Hyperopia occurs when parallel rays of light strike a focal point posterior to the retina.
   2. This occurs when either the anteroposterior diameter of the eye is too short, the cornea or lens refraction is less than normal, or the lens is dislocated posteriorly.
   3. Symptoms include blurred vision with near objects, eye strain, headache, fatigue, squinting, eye rubbing, lack of interest in reading, and poor school performance.
   4. Accommodative esotropia is a result of hyperopia in toddlers.
   5. Treatment in children is with corrective lenses.

B. Myopia (Nearsightedness)
   1. Myopia occurs when parallel rays of light focus anterior to the retina.
   2. The condition is caused when either the anteroposterior diameter of the globe is too long, the cornea or lens refraction is greater than normal, or the lens is dislocated anteriorly.
   3. Predisposing factors include prematurity and heredity.
   4. Symptoms include blurred vision when observing distant objects, lack of interest in distant activities, reading material held close to the face, frowning, squinting, and poor school performance.
   5. Treatment in children is with corrective lenses.

C. Astigmatism
   1. Astigmatism is differences in the refractive power of varying areas in the same eye.
   2. It is due to irregular corneal curvature.
   3. Symptoms include squinting, eye strain, headache, fatigue, and poor school performance.

D. Anisometropia
   1. The refractive ability of one eye differs from the other eye.
   2. This places patients at risk for amblyopia.
   3. Treatment is achieved by correction of the refractive error.

19.2.2 Errors in Vision With Normal or Corrected Refraction

A. Amblyopia
   1. This is abnormal vision in one or both eyes persisting despite correction for refractive error.
   2. Etiologies include trauma, intrinsic eye disease, impairment of visual pathways, or sensory deprivation amblyopia. Sensory deprivation amblyopia occurs when vision is occluded, interfering with formation of a clear retinal image during a developmental period (cataracts, strabismus with suppression of the deviated eye).
   3. Treatment is by providing the clearest retinal image possible. This is accomplished by patching the better seeing eye, or instilling cycloplegic drops that

blur vision in the good eye, forcing use of the amblyopic eye. The risk of treatment is development of sensory deprivation amblyopia in the better eye.

B. **Amaurosis**
1. Amaurosis is partial or total loss of vision.
2. Etiology
   a. Chronic symptoms may be due to congenital infection, hypoxia, trauma, genetic disease, congenital defects, retinal disease, or central nervous system disease.
   b. Acquired amaurosis may be due to retinal detachment or acute central nervous system disease such as encephalitis, encephalopathy, tumors, hydrocephalus, toxins, or trauma.
3. Symptoms include poor school performance or behavior problems, nystagmus, strabismus, and behavioral change.

C. **Nyctalopia** (Night Blindness)
1. Nyctalopia is decreased vision in poor light conditions.
2. It is usually due to poor rod function.
3. Causes include genetic predisposition, myopia, disk abnormalities, stationary congenital night blindness or progressive night blindness, vitamin A deficiency, or quinine use.

D. **Diplopia** (Double Vision)
1. Double vision is caused by malalignment of the visual axis.
2. It is common in disorders of conjugate gaze and proptosis.
3. Causes include increased intracranial pressure, brain tumor, orbital mass, strabismus, and myasthenia gravis.
4. Symptoms include intentional covering of one eye and abnormal head position (head tilt).

19.2.3 Disorders of the Pupil and Iris

A. **Aniridia** (AN)
1. Congenital absence of the iris tissue.
2. Types
   a. AN 1 is an autosomal dominant defect of the eye.
   b. AN 2 is an autosomal dominant defect (deletion on the short arm of chromosome 11) associated with Wilms' tumor, genitourinary abnormalities, and mental retardation.
   c. AN 3 is an autosomal recessive condition associated with cerebellar ataxia, congenital cataracts, and mental retardation.
   d. One third of cases are sporadic. Up to 25% of cases develop Wilms' tumor.
3. Cataracts occur in 50 to 85% of patients. Lens dislocation also occurs.

B. **Coloboma**
1. This is a developmental defect. It is a hole or notch in the iris tissue.
2. The defect may be simple (isolated to the iris) or extensive, involving the fundus and the optic nerve.

C. Microcoria is absence or malformation of the dilator pupillae muscle associated with a small pupil.

D. Congenital mydriasis is a large pupil.

E. Dyscoria is abnormal pupil shape.

F. Corectopia is abnormal pupil position.

G. Anisocoria is inequality of pupil size.

H. Tonic pupil is a large pupil that reacts poorly to light or accommodation. When seen in association with decreased deep tendon reflexes in women, it is known as Adie's syndrome.

I. **Marcus Gunn Pupil**
1. This pupil finding is an abnormal response to light due to an afferent conduction defect.
2. Examination Findings
   a. Direct and consensual response is diminished when light is shined into the affected eye.
   b. Shining light in the normal eye causes bilateral pupil constriction. Swinging the light back to the abnormal eye causes some bilateral pupil dilation.

J. **Horner's Syndrome** (Oculosympathetic Paresis)
1. This syndrome is characterized by miosis, mild ptosis, apparent enophthalmos (due to elevation of the lower eyelid), and anhidrosis. Very young children (<2 years of age) may also have decreased pigmentation of the pupil on the affected side.
2. It is caused by pathology in the midbrain, brainstem, upper cervical spinal cord, neck, orbit, or may be familial. Another common cause is Klumpke's brachial palsy secondary to birth trauma.

K. Heterochromia is irises of different colors or when a portion of the irides differs in color.

L. Lisch nodules are elevated ,pigmented areas in the iris associated with neurofibromatosis.

M. Hypopyon is an accumulation of white blood cells in the anterior chamber. It is seen in leukemia.

N. Nevoxanthoendothelioma is a yellow plaque on the iris seen in juvenile xanthogranuloma.

O. Hyphema is the presence of blood in the anterior chamber. It is usually due to ocular trauma.

P. Leukocoria is the "cat's eye" reflex previously discussed in association with retinoblastoma (see section 12.2.5D). It is also seen with retinopathy of prematurity, retinal detachment, cataract, and hypoplastic primary vitreus.

19.2.4 Disorders of Eye Movement

A. **Strabismus** is disconjugate gaze caused by deviation of one or both eyes.
1. Strabismus affects 5% of children <6 years of age. Half of these children have amblyopia.

2. Unless it is repaired early, strabismus results in a permanent loss of binocular vision. Surgical repair is indicated prior to 2 years of age.
3. Descriptive Terms
   a. Orthophoria is normal ocular alignment.
   b. Heterophoria (phoria = intermittent) is when the eye deviates when fatigued (during illness or testing), interfering with normal binocular fusion. Symptoms include double vision, headache, and eye strain. It can be elicited with the cover test.
   c. Heterotropia (tropia = persistent) is malalignment that is persistently present. It may involve one or both eyes or be alternating. Unilateral involvement is more serious because the affected eye develops amblyopia. In alternating tropia, both eyes are used so amblyopia occurs less frequently.
   d. Exo- is the prefix describing outward deviation of the eye ("walleye").
   e. Eso- is the prefix describing inward deviation ("cross-eye"). It is the most common form of strabismus.
   f. Hyper- is the reflex describing upward deviation.
   g. Hypo- is the reflex describing downward deviation.
4. Diagnostic Testing
   a. Corneal Light Reflex (Hirschberg's) Test. Shine a light source into the corneas of both eyes simultaneously. The light reflex should be symmetric in the pupils. Asymmetry implies disconjugate gaze.
   b. Cover-Uncover Test. As the child fixates vision on a distant object, one eye is covered while the other is observed. If the eye remains stable, there is no malalignment. If the eye moves, disconjugate gaze is present. The procedure is repeated on the other eye.
   c. Alternating Cover Test. The examiner rapidly covers and uncovers one eye then the other moving back and forth. The abnormal eye rapidly moves as the cover is shifted to the other eye.

B. Pseudostrabismus

1. This is the false appearance of esotropia secondary to a widened nasal bridge, prominent epicanthal folds, or narrow interpupillary distances.
2. Light reflex testing and cover tests are normal.

C. Accommodative Esotropia

1. This condition results when children with hyperopia are able to sharpen the image in the affected eye by accommodation. The eyes cross because accommodation is closely linked to convergence.
2. It occurs between 6 months and 7 years of age with a peak around 2 to 3 years of age.
3. The esotropia resolves with treatment of the refractive error.

D. Duane's Syndrome. A congenital disorder characterized by retraction of the globe on adduction secondary to abnormal innervation of the ocular muscles.

E. Möbius' Syndrome. Bilateral facial nerve palsy or absence with resultant facial paresis and abduction weakness.

F. Brown's Syndrome. When the eye is in the adducted position, upward gaze is restricted.

G. Parinaud's Syndrome A vertical gaze palsy due to a disorder affecting the midbrain.

H. Nystagmus. Rhythmic oscillations of one or both eyes.

I. Congenital Oculomotor Apraxia. An abnormality of voluntary horizontal gaze with compensatory jerking motion of the head.

J. Opsoclonus. Nonrhythmic, multidirectional movement of the eyes.

19.2.5 Eyelid Abnormalities

A. Ptosis

1. Drooping of the eyelid caused either by underdevelopment of the levator muscle or an abnormality of the oculomotor nerve.
2. It may lead to amblyopia.
3. Etiologies include myasthenia gravis, botulism, central nervous system lesions (tumor, stroke, nerve damage), or inflammatory conditions of the eyelid or orbit.

B. **Epicanthal folds** are redundant folds of skin covering the inner canthi. They are common in several genetic syndromes.

C. Lagophthalmos is difficulty in closing or incomplete closure of the eyelids over the globe. Exposure leads to drying, infection, ulceration, and vision loss.

D. Abnormal Eyelid Retraction
1. Dalrymple's sign is staring.
2. Stellwag's sign is infrequent blinking.
3. Von Graefe's sign is lag of the upper eyelid on downward gaze.

E. Entropion is inversion of the eyelid margin that leads to corneal abrasions due to trauma from the inverted eyelashes.

F. Ectropion is eversion of the eyelid margin associated with epiphora (tearing) and maceration of the eyelid secondary to chronic moisture.

G. **Blepharospasm** is spasmodic closure of the eyelids.

H. **Blepharitis** is inflammation of the eyelid margins with crusting, redness, and swelling. It may be secondary to bacterial infection with *Staphylococcus aureus* or due to seborrheic dermatitis.

I. **Hordeolum** is infection of the glands of the eyelids usually caused by *Staphylococcus aureus*.

J. Chalazion is a granulomatous inflammation of the meibomian glands resulting in a firm nodule in the eyelid.

19.2.6 Disorders of the Lacrimal System

A. **Dacryostenosis**
   1. This is a congenital nasolacrimal duct obstruction secondary to incomplete canalization of the duct.
   2. It occurs in approximately 5% of normal newborns and usually resolves by one year of age.
   3. Symptoms are tearing, eye matting, and maceration of the eyelid skin.
   4. Treatment is with nasolacrimal massage (questionable benefit) and time.

B. **Dacryoadenitis** is inflammation of the lacrimal gland. It may be infectious or due to connective tissue disease.

C. **Alacrima** is a unilateral or bilateral congenital deficiency of tearing.

19.2.7 Disorders of Conjunctival Tissues

A. **Subconjunctival hemorrhages** are blood-filled patches in the bulbar conjunctiva secondary to injury, infection, or other inflammatory process.

B. **Pterygium** is an elevated, thickened area of conjunctival tissue that requires treatment if it encroaches on the cornea.

C. **Dermoid cysts** are yellow to pink, smooth, raised, oval conjunctival tumors that may contain glandular tissue, hair follicles, or adipose tissue. Treatment is by removal of the dermoid cyst.

D. **Conjunctivitis**
   1. Inflammation of the conjunctiva caused by irritant exposure (toxins, allergens), systemic disease, viral (adenovirus, enterovirus), or bacterial agents (most often *Haemophilus influenzae,* staphylococcus, streptococcus, pneumococcus).
   2. Treatment is based on the suspected etiology and may include observation, cool compresses, topical antihistamines, or ocular antibiotics.

E. **Ophthalmia Neonatorum**
   1. This is conjunctivitis in infants <4 weeks of age.
   2. It is usually acquired during vaginal delivery.
   3. It may lead to corneal damage and blindness if untreated.
   4. The most common causative agent in the United States is *Chlamydia trachomatis*. Gonococcal infection has decreased since the institution of newborn antibiotic eye prophylaxis.

F. Chemical Injury
   1. Alkaline chemicals penetrate deeply into ocular tissue causing damage over hours to days if not removed.
   2. Acid coagulates tissue proteins, causing immediate injury that tends to be less extensive than alkali burns.
   3. Treatment is by flushing with copious amounts of water or saline immediately after exposure.

G. **Pseudomembranes** are superficial, adherent exudates that form on the conjunctiva during an inflammatory process. They usually can be easily stripped away. Therapy is by treatment of the underlying condition.

H. **Vernal conjunctivitis**
   1. Inflammation characterized by formation of large cobblestone-like lesions on the palpebral conjunctiva with pseudomembrane formation and exudates.
   2. Symptoms include tearing, redness, and itching.
   3. Smear of the exudates may reveal large numbers of eosinophils.

19.2.8 Corneal Disorders

A. Keratoconus is a condition that begins in adolescence, with progressive thinning and bulging of the cornea into a cone shape.

B. **Dendritic Keratitis**
   1. Branching treelike pattern of corneal epithelial destruction caused by herpes simplex virus infection.
   2. It can lead to corneal scarring and permanent vision loss.
   3. Symptoms include pain, photophobia, and redness.
   4. Treatment is with topical antiviral drops. Avoid topical steroids because they may exacerbate the condition.

C. **Corneal Ulcers**
   1. Ulcers form as a result of infections (bacterial, fungal).
   2. Symptoms include blurred vision, pain, red conjunctiva, photophobia, and blepharospasm.
   3. May cause permanent corneal damage and blindness if the underlying etiology is not treated.

D. Interstitial keratitis is inflammation of the corneal stroma most often caused by syphilis.

19.2.9 Lens Disorders

A. **Cataract**
   1. Cataracts are lens opacities.
   2. They may be developmental variants or related to congenital infection (TORCH), metabolic disease (galactosemia), genetic syndromes, drugs (corticosteroids), or trauma.
   3. Management is by removal if the density interferes with vision.

B. **Ectopia lentis** is abnormal lens placement.
   1. Luxation is complete displacement. Subluxation is partial displacement.
   2. Symptoms include blurred vision and diplopia.
   3. The most common cause is ocular trauma. Other causes are uveitis, tumor, glaucoma, and cataract.

19.2.10 Disorders of the Retina

A. **Retinopathy of Prematurity** (ROP)
   1. Retinal angiogenesis starts at the optic disk at approximately 16 weeks of age and proceeds peripherally until vascularization of the retina is complete at full-term.
   2. Interruption of the process results in pathologic vessel growth.
   3. Stages of ROP
      a. Stage 1 shows a flat demarcation line between vascular and avascular retina.
      b. Stage 2 has a ridged demarcation line extending out of the plane of the retina.
      c. Stage 3 has the aforementioned ridge with extra fibrovascular tissue.
      d. Stage 4 shows subtotal retinal detachment.
      e. Stage 5 is total retinal detachment.
   4. Up to 90% of infants have resolution of the abnormal vascularization with minimal to no effect on vision.
   5. Treatment, when needed, is with cryotherapy.

B. **Retinoblastoma** (See Section 12.2.5D)

C. **Retinitis Pigmentosa**
   1. Retinitis pigmentosa is a progressive retinal degeneration with optic atrophy, impaired vision, and decreased numbers of arterioles.
   2. Symptoms include nightblindness and loss of peripheral vision.
   3. It is inherited as an autosomal dominant, recessive, or X-linked condition.

D. **Stargardt's Disease**. An autosomal recessive disorder characterized by bilateral retinal degeneration starting as early as 8 years of age.

E. **Best Vitelliform Degeneration**. An autosomal dominant disease that presents at approximately 6 years of age with yellow, discoid, subretinal, macular lesions. It is usually bilateral and is associated with progressive vision deterioration.

F. **Cherry Red Spot**
   1. It is a red spot found on the central macula surrounded by a light colored halo.
   2. It occurs most frequently in congenital metabolic disease such as Tay-Sachs disease and metachromatic leukodystrophy.
   3. Occlusion of the central retinal artery is in the differential diagnosis.

G. **Diabetic Retinopathy**
   1. Nonproliferative diabetic retinopathy is aneurysms of the retinal vessels with hemorrhages and exudates noted around the disk and macula.
   2. Proliferative diabetic retinopathy is neovascularization and proliferation of tissue on the retina with blood vessels extending into the vitreous. It is associated with hemorrhage into the vitreous and retinal detachment.
   3. Presence depends upon the duration of the diabetes. The incidence is low in the first 5 years of the disease and increases dramatically after 10 years of the disease onset.
   4. Close ophthalmologic follow-up is a key part of multidisciplinary diabetes mellitus care.

H. Subacute Bacterial Endocarditis. Associated with hemorrhage, Roth's spots, papilledema, and central retinal artery occlusion.

19.2.11 Optic Nerve Disorders

A. **Optic Nerve Hypoplasia or Aplasia**
   1. This is a developmental defect of optic nerve fibers.
   2. Affected patients have poor visual acuity or blindness, strabismus, and nystagmus.
   3. It may occur as an isolated defect or with other ocular and central nervous system malformations.
   4. The condition may also result from acquired degeneration of optic nerve axons.

B. **Papilledema**
   1. Papilledema is swelling of the optic nerve head felt to be indicative of increased intracranial pressure.
   2. Examination reveals blurring of the disk margin, elevation of the nerve head (decreased cup to disk ratio), and engorgement of veins with loss of pulsations.
   3. Associated findings may include abducent palsy, esotropia, eyelid retraction, tonic downward deviation of the eyes with paresis of upward gaze (setting sun sign), and both nausea and vomiting.
   4. If the condition is not relieved, it leads to permanent nerve damage.

C. **Optic Glioma**
   1. This is the most frequent benign tumor of the optic nerve in childhood.
   2. The effect of the tumor is based on location, either intraorbital, intracranial, or intracanalicular.
   3. The usual symptoms are unilateral or bilateral loss of vision, increased intracranial pressure, pituitary dysfunction, nystagmus, or strabismus. Chiasmal lesions produce bitemporal hemianopsia.
   4. It occurs with increased frequency in children with neurofibromatosis.

D. **Glaucoma** causes damage to the optic nerve by increasing pressure within the globe.
   1. More than half of all cases are caused by an isolated abnormality of the trabecular network (drainage apparatus).
   2. Secondary glaucoma is due to associated ocular abnormalities such as cataracts, ectopia lentis, ROP, trauma, inflammation, or tumor.
   3. Symptoms are epiphora, photophobia, and blepharospasm.

4. Examination may reveal corneal enlargement, edema, conjunctival injection, and blurred vision.
5. Avoid mydriatic drugs to prevent an acute increase in ocular pressure.

19.2.12 Orbital Abnormalities

A. Developmental Defects
   1. Hypertelorism is widely-spaced eyes.
   2. Hypotelorism is close-set eyes.
   3. Exophthalmos is protrusion of the eyes.
   4. Enophthalmos is intrusion of the eyes.

B. Orbital and Preseptal Cellulitis (See Section 7.3.5)

C. Eye Injury
   1. Blunt Trauma
      a. Hemorrhage occurs into the periorbital tissues resulting in a "black eye" with a benign course. Examine thoroughly for other injury.
      b. Lacerations of the eyelids have a high risk of complications including ptosis, eversion, inversion, epiphora, and nasolacrimal duct obstruction. Examine the orbit carefully.
      c. Blunt trauma may result in a "blowout" fracture of the orbital floor with entrapment of the extraocular muscles. Exam reveals limitation of upward gaze. Ophthalmologic consultation is required.
   2. Corneal abrasions are traumatic disruptions of superficial corneal epithelium resulting in pain, tearing, photophobia, and decreased vision. Diagnosis is made by identifying fluorescein staining of the epithelial defect using a Wood's lamp. Therapy is geared toward pain control. Patching is not necessary.
   3. Foreign Body
      a. Foreign bodies can be removed by irrigation or gently wiping the object away.
      b. Metallic foreign bodies may result in rust rings which require curettage.
      c. If injury was secondary to a high velocity contact, perform an x-ray to rule out intraocular foreign body.
   4. Globe laceration or penetration requires emergent evaluation by an ophthalmologist.

439. A child presents with periorbital herpes simplex virus eruption. On examination of the cornea, you identify dendritic keratitis. Which of the following substances is contraindicated in this condition — A 19.2.8

A. topical steroid drops
B. topical antiviral drops
C. artificial tears
D. oral antihistamine
E. oral antivirals

440. What is the average visual acuity of a newborn infant — A 19.1.1

A. 20/400
B. 20/200
C. 20/100
D. 20/40
E. 20/20

441. Which of the following statements regarding amblyopia is false — D 19.2.2

A. amblyopia is abnormal vision in an eye despite correction for refractive error
B. sensory deprivation amblyopia results when vision is occluded in an eye
C. strabismus is a known cause of amblyopia
D. there are no risks associated with patching therapy for amblyopia
E. treatment is enhanced by providing the clearest retinal image possible

442. A child has been seen covering an eye with his hand when he is reading from the blackboard at school. On exam, he is noted to have esotropia. What vision disturbance has he been attempting to compensate for with the noted behaviors — C 19.2.2

A. amblyopia
B. myopia
C. diplopia
D. hyperopia
E. amaurosis

443. Anisocoria refers to — D 19.2.3

A. a large pupil
B. abnormal pupil shape
C. abnormal pupil position
D. unequal pupil size
E. a small pupil

444. When light is shined into the affected eye both the direct and consensual response are decreased. Shining light into the normal eye causes bilateral pupillary constriction. This is characteristic of what abnormality — A 19.2.3

A. Marcus Gunn pupil
B. Horner's syndrome
C. retinoblastoma
D. aniridia

445. An infant born 24 weeks premature is being examined for retinopathy of prematurity. The findings are consistent with subtotal retinal detachment. This corresponds to which stage — D 19.2.10

A. 1
B. 2
C. 3
D. 4
E. 5

446. All of the following conditions may be associated with leukocoria except — B 19.2.3

A. retinoblastoma
B. optic atrophy
C. retinopathy of prematurity
D. retinal detachment
E. cataract

447. Which of the following is the most common form of strabismus — A 19.2.4

A. esotropia
B. exotropia
C. hypertropia
D. hypotropia

448. Which of the following statements regarding pseudostrabismus is false — C 19.2.4

A. the child appears to have esotropia because of a wide nasal bridge
B. the child appears to have esotropia because of prominent epicanthal folds
C. the Hirschberg test is not normal
D. the child may have a narrow interpupillary distance
E. the child's vision is not affected

449. Which organism is commonly associated with blepharitis — B 19.2.5

A. group A β-hemolytic streptococcus
B. *Stphylococcus aureus*
C. Adenovirus
D. *Haemophilus influenzae*

450. What is the treatment of choice for congenital nasolacrimal duct obstruction — D 19.2.6

A. topical antibiotics
B. surgical exploration of the tear duct
C. saline eye drops
D. nasolacrimal massage

451. A child presents with a yellow, smooth, raised, oval conjunctival mass. The best treatment for this lesion is — C 19.2.7

A. topical antibiotics
B. topical antihistamines
C. surgical removal
D. benign neglect

452. What is the most common cause of ophthalmia neonatorum — B 19.2.7

A. *Neisseria gonorrhea*
B. *Chlamydia trachomatis*
C. *Haemophilus influenzae*
D. *Staphylococcus epidermidis*
E. Syphilis

453. A cherry red spot on the macula is seen most commonly in what condition — A 19.2.10

A. congenital metabolic disease
B. central retinal artery occlusion
C. retinal detachment
D. optic atrophy
E. increased intracranial pressure

454. What is the incidence of Wilms' tumor in sporadic aniridia — B 19.2.3

A. 15%
B. 25%
C. 40%
D. 60%

455. When parallel rays of light strike a focal point posterior to the retina, the condition is known as — D 19.2.1

A. myopia
B. amblyopia
C. presbyopia
D. hyperopia

456. Which of the following are causative agents for cataracts — D 19.2.9

A. "TORCH" infections
B. corticosteroids
C. trauma
D. all of the above
E. A and B

457. What is the mode of inheritance for retinitis pigmentosa — D 19.2.10

A. autosomal dominant
B. autosomal recessive
C. X-linked
D. all of the above
E. none of the above

458. Diabetic retinopathy dramatically increases in frequency how many years after disease onset — B 19.2.10

A. 5
B. 10
C. 20
D. 30

459. All of the following are associated with papilledema except — C 19.2.11

A. increased intracranial pressure
B. blurring of the disc margin
C. accentuated venous pulsations
D. elevation of the nerve head

460. A 15-year-old boy is hit in the eye with a baseball. On exam, you note that his upward gaze on the injured side is limited. What injury is present — C 19.2.12

A. hyphema
B. globe rupture
C. blow out fracture
D. corneal abrasion

461. What is the treatment of choice for rust rings in the cornea that have resulted from metallic foreign bodies — B 19.2.12

A. remove by irrigation
B. curettage of the ring
C. topical antibiotics
D. patch the eye

20 PEDIATRIC EMERGENCIES

20.1 GENERAL CONCEPTS

20.1.1 Evaluation of the Critically Ill Child

A. Effective evaluation requires a systematic approach.

B. The approach must include a plan to identify and begin emergent treatment for stabilization of the patient even before a complete history and physical examination are obtainable.

C. A timely, directed evaluation of each body area must be performed in order to identify potentially serious additional illnesses or injuries.

20.1.2 The Primary Survey (A,B,C,D,E)

A. The primary survey is an initial assessment of the status of the patient's airway, oxygenation, ventilation, circulation and neurologic state.

1. During this phase life-threatening problems are identified.
2. Because it is not uncommon to encounter serious physiologic alterations in the course of the primary survey, it is frequently necessary to interrupt the order of the survey to perform resuscitative measures.

B. ***A*irway Management**

1. Goals include recognition and relief of obstruction, promotion of adequate gas exchange, prevention of gastric content aspiration, and attention to protection of the cervical spine.
2. Therapeutic Modalities
   - **a.** The triple airway maneuver involves tipping the head back (if cervical spine injury is not a concern), displacing the mandible forward (jaw thrust alone if neck injury is possible), and opening the mouth.
   - **b.** Use oral suction cautiously.
   - **c.** Maintain the airway with an oropharyngeal airway in the obtunded patient because the tongue is the most common obstruction to the pediatric airway. (Do not use an oropharyngeal airway in an awake patient.)
   - **d.** Definitive airway modalities such as endotracheal intubation and cricothyroidotomy may be necessary.

C. ***B*reathing and Ventilation**

1. Assessment of Breathing
   - **a.** Look for chest wall rise.
   - **b.** Listen for breath sounds.
   - **c.** Feel for air movement.
2. Deficient air exchange must be rapidly diagnosed and treated.
3. Etiologies of poor air exchange and appropriate interventions include:
   - **a.** Airway obstruction: jaw thrust.
   - **b.** Tension pneumothorax: aspiration and chest tube.
   - **c.** Open pneumothorax: aspiration and chest tube.
   - **d.** Massive pneumothorax: aspiration and chest tube.
   - **e.** Flail chest: positive pressure ventilation.
   - **f.** Cardiac tamponade: pericardiocentesis.
   - **g.** Gastric distension: nasogastric tube.
4. Methods to augment ventilation include mouth-to-mask breathing, bag-valve-mask ventilation, endotracheal intubation with mechanical ventilation, and cricothyrotomy (needle or surgical).
5. Children will electively place themselves in a position of maximal airway comfort when allowed to do so. Do not change this position unnecessarily until more definitive airway or breathing measures are available.
6. Generous use of oxygen (100%) is warranted initially in almost all emergency settings. NOTE: Oxygen should be supplied by a means that meets the patient's needs and by a delivery device that is acceptable to the patient.
7. Place an nasogastric or orogastric tube to allow for gastric decompression. If facial trauma is present do not place an nasogastric. Always confirm placement by auscultation.

D. ***C*irculation**

1. Assessment.
   - **a.** Determine the quality, rate, and regularity of the pulses (central and peripheral).
   - **b.** Determine capillary refill time at room temperature. Cool ambient temperature can delay capillary refill in an otherwise normal child.
   - **c.** Determine blood pressure but be aware that blood pressure is an insensitive measure of adequate circulation in children until profound deficiencies exist. Children have excellent compensatory mechanisms for maintaining blood pressure so compromised circulation can exist despite a normal blood pressure.
   - **d.** Note the mental status of the child.
   - **e.** Note the color of the skin.
   - **f.** Place a Foley catheter. Urine output is a good indicator of renal and other vital organ perfusion. Do not place the catheter if blood is present at the urethral meatus or if the prostate is high riding on rectal exam.
2. Circulatory Support
   - **a.** Identify both external and internal hemorrhage.
   - **b.** Control active hemorrhage by the application of direct pressure.
   - **c.** Provide external cardiac massage (cardiopulmonary resuscitation).
   - **d.** Defibrillate potentially responsive abnormal rhythms.
   - **e.** Drug administration (epinephrine, dopamine,

lidocaine, bicarbonate, dobutamine, amiodarone, norepinephrine, magnesium) to support normal heart rate, rhythm, and blood pressure.

f. Obtain reliable venous access (intravenous or intraosseous). Blood for laboratory studies (complete blood count, blood type and crossmatch, chemistries, coagulation studies) can be obtained as the intravenous catheter is placed.

g. Provide isotonic fluid boluses for shock. Colloids and blood may be required.

h. Medical anti-shock trousers (MAST) suit application for blood pressure support is rarely appropriate for a child.

D. *D*isability ("*D*e-Brain")

1. Rapid screening of the neurological system is essential.
2. Obtain "neuro vital signs."
   a. Observe the pupillary response.
   b. Assess the level of consciousness: *a*lert, *v*erbal response, *p*ain response, *u*nresponsive (AVUP) or Glasgow Coma Scale (best motor, verbal, and eye opening response).
   c. Note localizing signs.

E. *E*xposure/*E*nvironment

1. A complete physical exam requires the removal of all clothing.
2. Body Temperature
   a. Children cool rapidly because of their large surface-to-body ratio.
   b. Maintain temperature by radiant warmer or warming blanket at 36 to 37°C.
   c. Address hypo- or hyperthermia as needed.

F. Rapid Trauma History (**AMPLE History**)

1. *A*llergies.
2. *M*edication.
3. *P*ast medical illness.
4. *L*ast meal.
5. *E*vents surrounding illness and injury.

20.1.3 The Secondary Survey

A. The secondary survey includes a detailed, timely, complete physical examination.

1. It surveys each body area in a head-to-toe fashion.
2. Included here are a directed history, a brief past medical history, indicated lab and radiographic studies which may lead to a specific diagnosis or a list of problems which may require further attention.

B. Detailed Physical Exam

1. Maxillofacial trauma.
   a. Palpate bony prominences.
   b. Look for evidence of bloody or cerebrospinal fluid discharge from the nose, mouth, and ears.
   c. Evaluate for nasal septal hematoma.
   d. Check dentition.
   e. Check ocular muscle function.
   f. Suspect basilar skull fracture if Battle's sign, raccoon eyes, or hemotympanum are present.
2. Other head, eyes, ears, nose, and throat findings include sunken fontanelle and eyes (dehydration), hyphema, irregular pupil, retinal hemorrhage, decreased acuity (eye trauma), scalp lacerations, scalp hematomas, and bulging fontanel (increased intracranial pressure, meningitis, sepsis).
3. Neck.
   a. Palpate for obvious signs of fracture or dislocation and midline position of the trachea.
   b. Examine for subcutaneous emphysema, hematoma, localized pain, and the presence of jugular venous distension.
   c. Consider neck and cervical spine x-rays if indicated.
4. Chest
   a. Evaluate visually for adequacy of respiratory excursion, asymmetry of the chest wall motion, or presence of a flail segment.
   b. Carefully palpate chest wall and auscultate lung fields and the heart.
   c. Rule out pulmonary or myocardial contusion, and aortic, tracheobronchial, or esophageal disruption. chest x-ray is indicated.
   d. Assess respiratory adequacy by skin color, nasal flaring, use of accessory muscles, grunting, stridor, wheezing, and positioning of the child.
5. Abdomen
   a. On initial exam, inspect for ease of abdominal wall movement with respiration, gentle palpation for pain, and auscultation of bowel sounds.
   b. Observe and palpate flanks.
   c. Serial examinations are often needed to establish a definitive diagnosis.
   d. Investigate possible pregnancy and its related problems in female patients.
6. Pelvis
   a. Palpate bony prominences for tenderness or instability.
   b. Examine perineum for laceration, hematoma, acute bleeding, or discharge.
   c. Check the urethral meatus for blood.
   d. Observe for changes consistent with child sexual abuse.
7. Rectum. Evaluate the integrity of the vault wall, prostate, and muscle tone. Guaiac for occult gastrointestinal hemorrhage. Record evidence of child abuse if present.
8. Extremities
   a. Examine for signs of abrasion, contusion, hematoma, and soft tissue injuries.
   b. Examine for bony instability and neurovascular function.
   c. Examine for fractures and dislocations.
9. The back should be examined with neck and spine

immobilization maintained if spinal injury is a concern. This is accomplished if no obvious spinal cord injury or paralysis is present.

10. Skin
    a. Examine for bruises and petechiae. The color, size, shape, and "age" may be suggestive of trauma, coagulopathy, or physical abuse.
    b. Rashes that are hemorrhagic, stellate, or rapidly expanding may indicate a life-threatening illnesses (meningococcemia, septic shock, anaphylaxis).
    c. Look for burn and bite marks.
11. Neurologic
    a. In-depth neurologic exam should include motor, sensory, cranial nerve and level of consciousness determinations.
    b. Exam tympanic membranes, mastoid area, eyes, and nose for evidence of basilar skull fracture.
    c. Perform an examination of the optic fundi.
    d. Evaluate for the presence of spinal cord trauma and identify the suspected level.

C. A detailed history should be obtained when available.

D. Radiographic and Laboratory Studies. Additional evaluations should be based on the physical findings in the primary and secondary survey and history. Serial examinations may be necessary.

E. Monitoring. Continuous monitoring and frequent reevaluations are a must.

F. Definitive Care. Determine the need for hospitalization, operative intervention, and/or intensive care admission.

20.1.4 Useful Information

A. **Cardiopulmonary Resuscitation** (CPR)

1. Children >8 years of age can have CPR performed as in adults.
2. Airway
    a. Determine unresponsiveness.
    b. Call for help.
    c. Position the patient supine.
    d. Support the head and the neck.
    e. Perform a head tilt with chin lift or jaw thrust to open the airway.
    f. Do not perform blind finger sweeps of the child's mouth.
3. Breathing. Provide 2 rescue breaths, then support breathing at approximately 20 breaths per minute in the older child. The rate is 40 breaths per minute in the infant and young child.
4. Assess circulation by palpating the brachial or femoral pulse. The carotid pulse can be palpated in children >1 year of age.
5. Compressions should be provided at a rate of 80 to 100 per minute. The compression to ventilation ratio is 5:1 (3:1 in neonates).

B. Indications for intubation of the comatose child include:

1. Inability to maintain a patent airway.
2. Glasgow coma score <8.
3. Absent cough reflex.
4. Absent gag reflex.
5. Hypoxemia with adequate supplemental oxygen.
6. Hypoventilation.
7. Impending brainstem herniation with need for hyperventilation.

C. **Endotracheal Intubation**

1. Ensure that all equipment is at the bedside and is functional.
2. Equipment includes:
    a. A mask of the appropriate size with a bag and an oxygen source.

Table 20.1.4E Classification stages of the severity of shock in children

	I	II	III	IV
Estimated Blood Volume Deficit (%)	10 to 15	15 to 30	30 to 40	>40
Pulse (bpm)	>100	>120	>150	>150
Respirations	normal	increased	marked increase	tachypnea or apnea
Capillary Refill (sec)	<4	>4	6-8	>10
Blood Pressure	normal	narrowed pulse pressure	hypotensive	hypotensive to absent
Mentation	normal	anxious	confused	unconscious
Orthostatic Hypotension	+	++	+++	++++
Urine Output (ml/kg)	1 to 3	0.5 to 1	<0.5	none

b. Suction catheters, tonsil tip suction handle, tubing, reservoir, and suction unit.
c. Laryngoscope blades and endotracheal tubes of multiple sizes.
d. Equipment for venous access.
e. Drugs and syringes for intubation and resuscitation.
f. A ventilator appropriate for the patient's age and size.

3. Always check and recheck breath sounds following intubation.
4. Check a postintubation chest x-ray (anteroposterior and possibly the lateral view) for endotracheal tube placement.
5. Colorimetric end-tidal carbon dioxide monitors are useful to demonstrate the endotracheal location of the endotracheal tube.

D. Guidelines for Initiating Mechanical Ventilation

1. Choose a method of ventilation (volume or pressure controlled). Generally, the type of ventilator chosen is based on the patient's age, weight, reason for support, and the pathophysiology of the disease process.
2. Initial Ventilator Settings – No Pulmonary Disease
   a. Pressure ventilators are usually set up with a peak pressure of 16 to 24 mm Hg, a positive end-expiratory pressure (PEEP) of 0 to 5 mm Hg, a rate based on age, inspiratory:expiratory ratio of 1:1 or 1:2 (never >1 second), and an inspiratory oxygen fraction (FiO_2) of $\geq$30%, increased depending upon patient need.
   b. Volume ventilator settings are often initially adjusted to a tidal volume of 8 to 15 ml/kg, a PEEP of 0 to 5 mm Hg, an age-dependent rate, an inspiratory time of 25 to 33% of the respiratory cycle, and oxygen (FiO_2) based on need.
3. Initial Ventilator Settings – With Pulmonary Disease
   a. Begin with the ventilator set as noted above except raise the FiO_2 to 100%.
   b. Adjust settings based on the physical examination, noninvasive monitoring (pulse oximeter, capnography), and blood gas determinations.

E. Classification Stages of the Severity of Shock in Children (Table 20.1.4E)

F. Common Causes of Coma in Infants and Children (TIPS on the Vowels)

1. *A*—*A*lcohol. The adolescent patient is not the only pediatric group at risk for depressed levels of consciousness from alcohol. Infants may absorb enough alcohol through the skin from alcohol baths or from alcohol-containing medications to cause coma.
2. *E*—*E*pilepsy (and other causes of seizures). Both postictal states and continued subtle seizure activity without overt motor manifestations can cause the appearance of coma in the infant and child.
3. *I*—*I*nsulin (hypo- or hyperglycemia). Infants without adequate hepatic glycogen stores or depressed gluconeogenesis may succumb to hypoglycemia as the result of various disease processes. Hyperglycemia can also cause coma. A fingerstick glucose is indicated in all comatose children.
4. *I*—*I*ntussusception. A vacant, blank stare is often seen in the child with intussusception.
5. *O*—*O*verdose. Drug overdose may be intentional, accidental, or the result of misguided attempts at

Table 20.1.4G Glasgow Coma Scale

RESPONSE	ADULTS & CHILDREN	INFANTS	POINTS
Eye Opening	no response to pain to voice spontaneous	no response to pain to voice spontaneous	1 2 3 4
Verbal	no response incomprehensible inappropriate words disoriented conversation oriented and appropriate	no response moans to pain cries to pain irritable coos, babbles	1 2 3 4 5
Motor	no response decerebrate posturing decorticate posturing withdraws to pain localizes pain obeys command	no response decerebrate posturing decorticate posturing withdraws to pain withdraws to touch normal spontaneous movements	1 2 3 4 5 6
TOTAL SCORE			3 to 15

recreational use. They can even be acquired at birth. A toxic drug screen is indicated in all cases of coma without clear etiology.

6. *U*—*U*remia (and other metabolic causes). A serum ammonia and serum electrolytes are often helpful in providing clues to metabolic causes of coma.
7. *T* —*T*rauma. In comatose infants, retinal hemorrhages should alert the examiner to the possibility of intracranial trauma due to a "shaken baby" or other form of abuse. Intracranial bleeds or cerebral edema resulting from trauma that caused hypoxia or shock may be assessed by a computed tomography scan of the head.
8. *I*—*I*nfection. Infection is more common as a cause of altered sensorium in children than in adults. A high index of suspicion should lead to a lumbar puncture as soon as the probability of increased intracranial pressure is excluded.
9. *P* —*P*sychiatric. Factitious altered sensorium is exceedingly rare in children. It should be diagnosed by positive supporting evidence, not by lack of any other explanation for the altered level of consciousness.
10. *S*—*S*troke, shock, and other cardiovascular causes. An altered level of consciousness can be caused by shock resulting in inadequate brain perfusion or by local cerebrovascular accidents. Hypertensive encephalopathy can cause a stroke-like picture.

G. Glasgow Coma Scale (Table 20.1.4G)

20.2 SELECTED PEDIATRIC EMERGENCIES

20.2.1 Acute Respiratory Failure

A. This is a clinical condition marked by inadequate oxygen elimination and/or inadequate oxygenation of blood.

B. Criteria for diagnosis are: a respiratory rate >90 per minute (<12 months of age), a respiratory rate >70 per minute (≥12 months of age), apnea, a partial alveolar pressure of oxygen (P_aO_2) <40 mm Hg (without cyanotic heart disease), and a partial pressure of carbon dioxide (PCO_2) >65 mm Hg.

C. Etiologic Classification

1. Lung failure is due to diseases affecting airways, alveoli, capillary membranes, and pulmonary circulation such as croup, epiglottitis, tracheitis, bronchiolitis, asthma, pneumonia, bronchopulmonary dysplasia, and adult respiratory distress syndrome.
2. Respiratory pump failure results from disease along the pathway from brainstem, to the respiratory center, the spinal cord and phrenic nerves, and finally to chest wall muscles. Some examples include drug overdose, central nervous system disease, and neuromuscular disorders.

D. Evaluation

1. Physical examination is the most important tool.
2. Pulse oximetry (continuous or intermittent) gives information regarding oxygen saturation (oxygen saturation <90% = partial pressure of oxygen [PO_2] <60 mm Hg).
3. Lab tests may include arterial blood gases and a chest x-ray.

E. Signs and symptoms of respiratory failure include tachypnea, dyspnea, cyanosis, altered sensorium, diminished breath sounds, and retractions.

F. Management is by mechanical ventilation.

20.2.2 Shock

A. This is a syndrome of acute homeostatic derangement involving multiple organ systems which ultimately causes failure of cellular metabolism. Circulation is inadequate to provide oxygenation to the tissues and to carry away the byproducts of metabolism.

B. Classification

1. Hypovolemia is usually secondary to fluid (vomiting, diarrhea) or blood (trauma, surgery) loss.
2. Cardiogenic shock is hypoperfusion caused by heart failure (either inadequate filling or ejection).
3. Neurogenic shock occurs when diminished or absent central nervous system activity leads to loss of vascular tone.
4. Septic shock arises from overwhelming bacteremia or septicemia.

C. Signs and symptoms include vasoconstriction, acrocyanosis, poor peripheral pulses, altered consciousness, pallor, sweating, ileus, and oliguria. Peripheral vasodilatation can be seen in neurogenic and septic shock.

D. Differential Diagnosis

1. Infections include meningitis, bacterial sepsis, viral infection, and urinary tract infection.
2. Cardiac causes include dysrhythmias (sinus ventricular tachycardia, ventricular tachycardia, ventricular fibrillation, atrioventricular block), congestive heart failure, pulmonary hypertension, cardiomyopathies, myocarditis, pericardial effusion, and infiltrative disease.
3. Metabolic derangements such as electrolyte disturbances, hypo- or hyperglycemia, and inborn errors of metabolism can cause a shock state.
4. Gastrointestinal obstruction or ischemia, gastroenteritis with dehydration, and vomiting may lead to shock.
5. Miscellaneous etiologies include child abuse, anemia, hepatic failure, and intracranial bleeding.

E. Treatment

1. Hypovolemic shock requires vigorous fluid resuscitation.
2. Cardiogenic shock responds to vasopressors if intravascular volume is adequate.
3. Neurogenic shock is aided by a Trendelenburg position, fluids, and vasopressors.

4. Septic shock requires fluid resuscitation, vasopressors, and antimicrobial agents.

20.2.3 Congestive Heart Failure

A. Congestive heart failure is the inability of the heart to pump adequate blood volume for the circulatory and metabolic needs of the body.

B. Common Etiologies
   1. Volume overload: increased preload or excessive intravascular volume.
   2. Pressure overload: increased afterload or increased vascular resistance.
   3. Myocardial dysfunction: congenital lesions, acquired cardiomyopathy, myocarditis, and dysrhythmias. Ninety percent of children who develop congestive heart failure do so in the 1st year of life as a result of congenital heart disease.
   4. Other etiologies: cor pulmonale from chronic lung disease, cardiomyopathy, electrolyte abnormalities, endocarditis, rheumatic carditis, renal failure, systemic hypertension, anemia, hyperthyroidism, and overhydration.

C. Signs and symptoms include decreased exercise tolerance, altered behavior, weight loss, change in eating habits, tachycardia, gallop rhythm, cardiomegaly, venous congestion (hepatomegaly, jugular venous distension, edema), tachypnea with crackles, rhonchi, wheezing, orthopnea, and exercise intolerance.

D. Diagnosis is made by history and examination supported by chest x-ray, electrocardiogram, arterial blood gas analysis, and echocardiography.

E. Management focuses on improving contractility while reducing afterload.
Interventions include inotropic agents (digoxin, dopamine, dobutamine), reduction of volume overload (fluid restriction, diuretics), and reduction of afterload (vasodilators, antihypertensive agents).

20.2.5 Altered Mental Status

A. Altered levels of consciousness, stupor, and coma are signs of "brain failure" and should be treated emergently in an effort to minimize irreversible central nervous system injury.

B. Definitions
   1. Stupor is a state of unresponsiveness where the patient can be aroused by vigorous stimulation.
   2. Coma is a state of unresponsiveness where the patient cannot be aroused by vigorous stimulation.

C. Criteria for central nervous system failure include a Glasgow Coma Scale <5, fixed and dilated pupils, and an intracranial pressure >20 mm Hg for >20 minutes.

D. Management Goals
   1. Prevent secondary hypoxic-ischemic brain injury.
   2. Prevent herniation.
   3. Diagnosis and treatment (if possible) of the underlying cause of coma.

20.2.4 Spinal Cord Trauma

A. Pediatric spinal cord injuries are unusual.
   1. Such accidents are most commonly seen following motor vehicle accidents in children <10 years of age.
   2. In children >10 years of age, motor vehicle accidents, as well as recreational and organized sporting accidents, account for the majority of spinal cord injuries.

B. Evaluation
   1. History. A spinal injury should be assumed until proven otherwise in any comatose child. Children who are awake and complaining of neck, back or radicular pain, numbness, or dysesthesias are possible candidates for a spinal injury.
   2. Examination.
      a. Palpate for tenderness of the neck or spine in awake, older children.
      b. A careful evaluation of extremity movement, sensation, and reflexes in the awake child should be done.
      c. Any child who is awake and flaccid has a spinal cord injury until proven otherwise.
      d. Hypotension can result from loss of vasomotor tone due to a cervical cord injury.

C. Management
   1. Immobilization should be maintained until the child is alert enough to cooperate with the examination and diagnostic testing is accomplished to rule out spinal injury.
   2. Protect and maintain a patent airway.
   3. Provide blood pressure support if needed.
   4. The early use of relatively high-dose steroids is advocated for some spinal cord injuries. Prompt neurosurgical intervention should be obtained when these patients are encountered.

20.2.6 Acute Renal Failure (See Section 14.2.1H)

20.2.7 Hypertensive Crisis

A. Hypertension in children is rare, but should not be missed.
   1. It is defined as systolic, diastolic, or mean arterial pressures that falls above the upper limit of normal (>95%) for the patient's age.
   2. Careful attention must be given to the proper technique used to obtain blood pressure, especially in infants and small children.

B. Classification
   1. Hypertensive Emergency
      a. This condition has life-threatening end-organ (central nervous system, cardiac, renal) involvement and needs to be corrected within minutes to hours.
      b. Hypertensive encephalopathy, cerebrovascular

accidents with hemorrhage or infarction, seizures, and pulmonary hypertension are complications.
   c. Examples include eclampsia and pheochromocytoma.
2. Hypertensive Urgency
   a. There is no evidence of life-threatening end-organ involvement.
   b. The condition needs to be corrected in hours to days.
   c. Examples include renal failure or impairment, acute glomerulonephritis, preeclampsia, and newly diagnosed hypertension.

C. Assessment
1. Do not use too small a blood pressure cuff. The bladder width on the blood pressure cuff should be at least 2/3 the length of the upper arm.
2. Obtain a history to uncover possible underlying etiologies of the hypertension (renal disease, coarctation, pheochromocytoma, Cushing's disease, drug effect, neurofibromatosis).
3. Physical exam should include four-extremity blood pressures, evaluation for end-organ injury (retinal change, decreased visual acuity), congestive heart failure, abdominal bruits, motor or sensory disturbances, and cutaneous markers of systemic disease (café au lait spots, tubers, fibromas).
4. Obtain a urinalysis, serum electrolytes, blood urea nitrogen, serum creatinine, a chest x-ray, an electrocardiogram, and a computed tomography scan of the head (if the central nervous system is involved) as baseline studies. Specialized testing such as serum markers of disease, angiography, renin levels, etc. can be obtained as indicated by results of the preliminary evaluation.

D. Etiology (Common Causes By Age)
1. Neonates: coarctation of the aorta, renovascular disease, and intracranial hemorrhage.
2. Infants ≤ 2 years of age: renovascular disease, intrinsic renal disease, coarctation of the aorta, and neuroblastoma.
3. Children 2 to 8 years of age: renovascular disease and intrinsic renal disorders.
4. Children >8 years of age: renovascular disease, intrinsic renal disease, and essential hypertension.

E. Treatment
1. Blood pressure should not be decreased by greater than one third of the total goal over the first 4 to 6 hours.
2. Patients with underlying chronic hypertension may have a shifted autoregulatory curve and require increased blood pressures to maintain normal cerebral perfusion. Elevated pressure should be lowered more slowly in these patients.
3. Numerous drugs are available for treatment. Drug classes used include calcium channel blockers (nifedipine), arteriole vasodilators (diazoxide, hydralazine), alpha- and beta-blockers (labetalol), and combined arteriolar and venous dilators (nitroprusside). Nifedipine can be given sublingually to vomiting patients.
4. Whenever possible, secure intravenous access before beginning therapy.
5. When a patient presents with hypertension and an alteration in mental status, the hypertension workup and emergent control should take precedent over the evaluation for the change in mental status.

20.2.8 Electrolyte Disturbances (Section 15.2)

20.2.9 Gastrointestinal Hemorrhage (Section 13.4.5)

20.2.10 Compartment Syndrome

A. This syndrome develops because of increased compartment contents in a limiting fascial envelope.
1. Increased contents can be from hemorrhage, infection, or cellular swelling from ischemia or blunt trauma.
2. When compartment pressure is greater than capillary perfusion pressure, ischemia further exacerbates compartment swelling.

B. Obvious sequelae include distal vascular compromise, limb loss, or neurologic dysfunction.

C. Evaluation. Clinical signs ("5 Ps") of compartment syndrome include:
1. *P*ain is out of proportion to that expected. The most sensitive finding in the physical exam is exquisite pain with passive stretch of the involved muscles.
2. *P*aresthesia arises from sensory nerves contained in the compartment.
3. *P*allor occurs in the distal part of the extremity due to poor capillary refill (>3 seconds).
4. *P*ulselessness in the distal extremity is a very late sign.
5. *P*aralysis is also a late sign. Early weakness should be sought instead.
6. Compartment syndrome is suspected even if only one of the above findings is present.

D. Treatment is fasciotomy.

20.2.11 Open Fractures

A. Cultures should be obtained from the wound as soon as possible.

B. Antibiotic Therapy
1. Coverage should include antistaphylococcal antibiotics.
2. For severely contaminated, massive crush, or farm injuries add gentamicin and penicillin for gram-negative rod and streptococcal coverage.
3. Early operative debridement and irrigation is indicated in most cases.
4. Provide tetanus prophylaxis.

462. When should the triple airway maneuver of airway control be avoided A 20.1.2

A. cervical spine injury
B. aspirated foreign body
C. vomiting
D. macroglossia
E. seizure

463. Which of the following is a relative contraindication to nasogastric tube placement B 20.1.2

A. cervical spine injury
B. facial trauma
C. vomiting
D. airway foreign body
E. abdominal trauma

464. During the evaluation of a 6-year-old with abdominal trauma sustained in a car accident, blood is noted at the urethral meatus. Which procedure is contraindicated C 20.1.2

A. rectal exam
B. rectal temperature probe
C. Foley catheter placement
D. retrograde urethrogram

465. A child victim of trauma opens his eyes to voice, localizes painful stimuli, and has disoriented speech. His Glasgow coma score is C 20.1.4

A. 3
B. 10
C. 12
D. 14
E. 15

466. A 12-year-old child presents to the emergency department after an accidental injury. He has a pulse of 125 breaths per minute, mild tachypnea, a capillary refill time of 5 seconds, a narrowed pulse pressure, and he is anxious. What is his estimated blood volume deficit B 20.1.4

A. 10 to 15%
B. 15 to 30%
C. 30 to 40%
D. >40%

467. What procedure performed in adult cardiopulmonary resuscitation is not recommended in child cardiopulmonary resuscitation B 20.1.4

A. chest compressions
B. blind oral finger sweep
C. mouth to mouth ventilation
D. palpation of central pulses

468. A 12-year-old girl dives into a shallow swimming pool. She does not return to the surface on her own. When you examine her, you note that she is awake and alert, but is paralyzed from the level of C5 down. What intervention should be performed with the goal of preserving neurologic function B 20.2.5

A. computed tomography scan of the cervical spine
B. administer high dose intravenous steroids
C. remove the cervical collar to improve comfort
D. administer intravenous immunoglobulin
E. give antibiotics

469. What are appropriate methods for assessing endotracheal tube placement after intubation — D 20.1.4

A. check breath sounds
B. anterior-posterior and lateral chest x-ray
C. end tidal CO_2 monitor
D. all of the above
E. B and C

470. Which of the following conditions can present as coma in infants and children — E 20.1.4

A. shaken baby syndrome
B. hyperglycemia
C. isopropyl alcohol toxicity
D. uremia
E. all of the above

471. An infant presents after a fall from a moving vehicle. He opens his eyes to pain, cries with pain, and withdraws to pain. What is his Glasgow coma score — D 20.1.4

A. 6
B. 7
C. 8
D. 9
E. 10

472. Which of the following parameters is indicative of acute respiratory failure — A 20.2.1

A. $PCO_2 > 65$
B. respiratory rate of 70 breaths per minute in a 9-month-old
C. cyanosis on room air
D. respiratory rate of 50 breaths per minute in a 14-month-old
E. $PCO_2 = 50$

473. What is the most common cause of congestive heart failure in childhood — C 20.2.3

A. myocarditis
B. hypertension
C. congenital defects
D. anemia
E. hemangioma

474. All of the following are indications for endotracheal intubation except — A 20.1.4

A. Glasgow coma score of 10
B. hypoxemia despite supplemental oxygen
C. impending brainstem herniation
D. hypoventilation
E. absent gag reflex

475. A child presents with an apparent cellulitis of the forearm and hand. On exam, his digits are dusky, his radial pulse is diminished, and he experiences severe pain on flexion of the fingers. What is the appropriate intervention for this condition — C 20.2.10

A. intravenous antibiotics
B. intravenous fluid
C. emergent fasciotomy
D. amputation
E. limb elevation

476. What is the most common cause of nonessential hypertension in infants and children — A 20.2.7

A. renal disease
B. congestive heart failure
C. coarctation of the aorta
D. intracranial hemorrhage
E. central nervous system tumor

477. All of the following are components of the AMPLE history except — C 20.1.2

A. allergies
B. medication
C. pain
D. last meal
E. events surrounding illness

478. A 15-year-old presents to the emergency department with a crush injury from a farm accident. Appropriate drug management would include — D 20.2.11

A. tetanus prophylaxis
B. antistaphylococcal antibiotics
C. gentamicin and penicillin
D. all of the above
E. A and C

21 CHILDHOOD POISONINGS

21.1 GENERAL CONSIDERATIONS

21.1.1 Epidemiology

A. Approximately 1.5 to 3 million poisonings occur in the United States per year.

B. Half of these poisonings occur in children under 5 years of age.

C. Most (90%) of all poisonings occur in the home.

D. Most poisonings result from ingestion of nonpharmaceutical products.

E. Death from accidental poisoning is infrequent. The majority of exposures can be managed at home without direct medical supervision.

21.1.2 Diagnostic Modalities

A. Patient Evaluation

1. A majority of patients will present for evaluation or treatment with the ingestion of a known toxic substance. For these patients the identification of the toxin and suggested management strategies may be found in numerous texts and widely available computer-based systems.
2. For those patients presenting with an unknown ingestion or toxic exposure, the history, physical examination, and proper laboratory tests frequently enable the physician to correctly identify the substance and provide necessary medical treatment.

B. Historical Information

1. If the patient is able to answer questions, the physician should direct the history toward the identification of the ingested substance.
2. An attempt to quantify the amount of toxic exposure, the elapsed time since exposure, and the development of symptoms since exposure should be elicited.
3. For pediatric patients, available caretakers should be questioned. Questions should address the presence of household medications (prescription, over-the-counter, elicit drugs), other potential household toxins (cleaning compounds, plants), and possible environmental exposures (insecticides, herbicides, fertilizers).

C. Laboratory Studies

1. Urine drug screening is often a useful tool in determining the presence of an ingested substance. Many authorities believe that the routine use of these screens without regard to available clinical and historical patient information is an inefficient method of patient management.
2. Toxidrome-oriented drug screening is a more cost-effective and time-efficient utilization of toxicologic testing. See section 21.1.3.
3. **Anion Gap**
   a. The anion gap is another laboratory measurement utilized in the evaluation of poisoned patients. A normal anion gap is 8 to 12. It is calculated as follows:

$$\text{Anion Gap} = \left[Na^{+}\right] - \left(\left[HCO_3^{-}\right] + \left[Cl^{-}\right]\right)$$

   b. The anion gap is a method of quantifying the presence of anions not measured by routine laboratory tests. A patient with metabolic acidosis may therefore be further described as having an elevated, normal, or reduced anion gap.
   c. A simple way of remembering the common drugs or poisons causing an elevated anion gap is using the phrase AT MUD PILES.

A	*A*lcohols
T	*T*oluene
M	*M*ethanol
U	*U*remia
D	*D*KA
P	*P*araldehyde
I	*I*soniazid, *I*ron, *I*buprofen
L	*L*actic acid
E	*E*thylene glycol
S	*S*alicylates

4. **Osmolar Gap.**

$$\text{Osmolar Gap} = \text{Measured Omsomality} - \text{Calculated Omsomality}$$

   a. Serum osmolality may be measured in the laboratory by one of two methods. The first method utilizes the freezing point depression osmometer and the second method uses a heat of vaporization method to determine osmolality.
   b. When measuring serum osmolality in the poisoned patient, it is advisable to utilize the freezing point method because alcohols may "boil off" before the serum osmolality is determined if the heat of vaporization method is used. This gives a falsely normal osmolar gap.
   c. A simple way of remembering the common causes of an elevated osmolar gap is using the phrase **MEAN PIE**.

M	*M*annitol, *M*ethanol
E	*E*thanol, *E*thyl ether
A	*A*cetone
N	"*N*o Kidneys"
P	*P*ropylene glycol
I	*I*sopropyl alcohol
E	*E*thylene glycol

5. X-Ray Identification
   a. Abdominal x-rays may reveal radiopaque ingested substances. For example, recently ingested iron-containing tablets may be seen on

plain x-rays.

b. The sensitivity of this method for determining the presence of ingested materials is too low to make this a routine part of the poisoned patient's evaluation.

D. Odor Identification

1. Occasionally the identification of an ingested toxic substance is facilitated by the characteristic odor associated with the substance.
2. The sensitivity of this method of toxin identification is very dependent on the observer.
3. Common odors caused by toxins and drugs include:
   a. Acetone (chloroform, diabetic ketoacidosis)
   b. Bitter almonds (cyanide)
   c. Garlic (arsenic, organophosphates)
   d. Mothballs (naphthalene)
   e. Wintergreen (methyl salicylate)

21.1.3 Toxidromes

A. A combination of findings from a careful history and physical examination may allow physicians to clinically classify toxic ingestions into one of the common autonomic syndromes (toxidromes).

B. These toxidromes may be used as a basis for empiric treatment of ingestions prior to laboratory identification of specific toxins.

C. **Sympathomimetic Syndrome**

1. Physical examination findings and symptoms include elevated blood pressure, tachycardia (except with severe hypertension), mydriasis, sweating, mental status changes (confusion, anxiety, agitation), and hyperthermia.
2. Examples of common substance ingestions that present with this syndrome are cocaine, amphetamines, phencyclidine, and phenylpropanolamine.

D. **Sympatholytic Syndrome**

1. Physical examination findings and symptoms include hypertension, bradycardia, miosis, mental status changes (obtundation, coma), hypothermia, and decreased intestinal peristalsis.
2. Examples of common substances presenting with these symptoms are ethanol, barbiturates, sedative-hypnotics, opioids, and clonidine.

E. **Anticholinergic Syndrome**

1. Physical examination findings and symptoms include tachycardia, hypertension, hyperthermia, mydriasis, flushed, hot, dry, skin, decreased intestinal peristalsis, urinary retention, myoclonic jerks, choreoathetoid movements, and mental status changes (agitated delirium).
2. Symptoms can be remembered by the phrase "dry as a bone, blind as a bat, mad as a hatter, red as a beet, and hot as a hare."
3. Examples of common substances causing this syndrome are antihistamines, tricyclic antidepressants, atropine, scopolamine, and phenothiazine.

F. **Cholinergic Syndrome**

1. Physical examination findings and symptoms associated with nicotinic receptor stimulation are initial hypertension, tachycardia, fasciculations, and weakness.
2. Physical examination findings and symptoms associated with muscarinic receptor stimulation can be remembered by using the phrase SLUDGED:

S	*S*alivation and bronchorrhea
L	*L*acrimation
U	*U*rination
D	*D*iaphoresis
G	*G*astrointestinal hyperperistalsis
E	*E*xcitement of the central nervous system
D	*D*ecreased pupils and pulse rate

21.1.4 Therapeutic Considerations

A. The optimum management of the poisoned or overdosed patient requires an organized approach of evaluation and treatment.

1. This management should always focus on the patient first and the poison second.
2. The stabilization of vital signs, including the establishment and maintenance of the airway, breathing, and circulation (ABC's), is the first priority in all poisoned patients.
3. This should be followed by an attempt to identify the responsible toxin, institute specific therapy if warranted, performing decontamination if indicated, and providing appropriate ongoing treatment or observation.

B. Decontamination

1. Skin Decontamination
   a. Because many toxins are rapidly absorbed through the skin (organophosphates) the removal of these substances from the skin surface should be undertaken expeditiously.
   b. Contaminated clothing should be removed and the contaminated skin flushed with large amounts of water or saline.
   c. Care must be taken to avoid exposure of health care personnel during the decontamination process.
2. Eye Decontamination. Large volumes of warm water or saline should be used to flush the eyes of persons with toxic exposure of the eyes.
3. Gastrointestinal Decontamination by Induced Emesis
   a. Gastric emptying by inducing emesis only removes a small portion of the ingested substance. It is losing favor in the medical community as an approach to poisoning.

b. It should never be performed in infants under 6 months of age.
c. The most common method of inducing emesis in the poisoned patient is the administration of syrup of ipecac. This medication acts by both direct gastric mucosal irritation and by effects on the central nervous system.
d. Contraindications for inducing emesis in poisoned patients include altered mental status, risk of altered mental status, depressed gag reflex, seizures, hydrocarbon ingestion, and caustic ingestion.

4. Gastrointestinal Decontamination by Lavage
   a. Gastric lavage with a large-bore nasogastric or orogastric tube is only slightly more effective at removing ingested substances than induced emesis.
   b. The complications associated with this method of decontamination include perforation of the stomach or esophagus, aspiration, inadvertent tracheal intubation with the gastric tube, trauma to the nose or mouth, and discomfort.
   c. Lavage should be used only in older children when the potential benefit outweighs the risk of the procedure.
   d. Contraindications are the same as with induced emesis.
5. Gastrointestinal Decontamination with Activated Charcoal
   a. The administration of activated charcoal as a liquid slurry is an effective method of intestinal decontamination.
   b. It is very absorbent of most common poisons and drugs. The large surface area produced in the activation process allows the charcoal to absorb significant amounts of ingested substances.
   c. Charcoal is indicated in almost all ingestions.
   d. Some toxins are poorly adsorbed by activated charcoal (iron, lead, lithium, cyanide, alcohols, acids, bases).
   e. The contraindications for the administration of charcoal include patients who will undergo endoscopy or patients with ileus or obstruction.
6. Gastrointestinal Decontamination by Cathartics
   a. Cathartics are used to hasten the elimination of poisons or ingested substances from the gastrointestinal tract.
   b. Substances used to decrease gastrointestinal transit time include magnesium citrate, sorbitol, and polyethylene glycol solutions.
   c. The contraindications for cathartic administration include patients with ileus or intestinal obstruction, altered sensorium, and seizure activity.

C. Hemodialysis is effective in the removal of certain toxins. It is most commonly used with toxic levels of lithium, salicylates, methanol, and ethylene glycol.

D. **Antidotes**. Table 21.1.4 lists a number of specific antidotes which are available for the treatment of selected toxins.

Table 21.1.4 Antidotes for treatment of selected toxins

TOXIN	ANTIDOTE
Acetaminophen	N-acetylcysteine
Atropine	Physostigmine
Arsenic	Dimercaprol
Benzodiazepines	Flumazenil
Carbon monoxide	Oxygen
Digoxin	Digitalis antibodies
Ethylene glycol	Ethanol
Heparin	Protamine
Iron	Deferoxamine mesylate
Lead	Dimercaprol, Edetate calcium-disodium (EDTA)
Mercury	Dimercaprol
Methanol	Ethanol
Nitrates	Methylene blue
Opiates	Naloxone
Organophosphates	Pralidoxime
Zinc	Edetate calcium-disodium (EDTA)

21.2 DISEASE PROFILES

21.2.1 Acetaminophen Poisoning

A. Acute ingestion of greater than 140 mg/kg of acetaminophen or chronic ingestion of greater than 150 mg/kg/day of acetaminophen on 2 or more consecutive days can cause toxicity.

B. Stages of Poisoning

C. Laboratory Findings. The Rumack-Matthew nomogram can be used to predict risk for hepatic failure using timed serum acetaminophen levels.

D. Therapeutic Plan
1. Consider gastric decontamination with activated charcoal if patient presents within 1 hour of ingestion.
2. Draw an acetaminophen level 4 hours after ingestion or at the time of presentation if later than 4 hours.
3. Treatment with N-acetylcysteine should be started if over 4 hours has lapsed since ingestion or the acetaminophen plasma toxicity level places the patient at risk for hepatotoxicity. Administer an initial loading dose of N-acetylcysteine at 140 mg/kg followed by 17 doses at 70 mg/kg/dose every 4 hours (3 days of therapy).
   a. Ideally, administration of activated charcoal and N-acetylcysteine should be separated by at least 1 hour because the charcoal adsorbs N-

acetylcysteine.

b. If necessary, they may be administered together without significant difference in effect.

E. Prognosis depends on the presence of hepatic toxicity.

21.2.2 Aspirin Poisoning (Salicylism)

A. Aspirin toxicity may be evident with acute ingestion of 150 to 300 mg/kg (mild symptoms), 300 to 500 mg/kg (moderate symptoms), or >500 mg/kg (severe symptoms or death).

B. Pathophysiologic Abnormality.

1. Aspirin stimulates the respiratory center resulting in an initial alkalosis. As the poisoning progresses, a metabolic acidosis predominates.
2. Aspirin inhibits the Kreb's cycle and uncouples oxidative phosphorylation.
3. Coagulation disorders also occur due to inhibited platelet function and disturbances in vitamin K-dependent clotting factors.
4. Hypoglycemia may also occur.

C. Symptoms include fever, nausea, vomiting, tachypnea, lethargy, slurred speech, seizures, tinnitus, and diaphoresis.

D. Physical findings include Kussmaul's respirations, central nervous system depression, agitation, coma, seizures, and cardiovascular collapse.

E. Laboratory studies may reveal hyperglycemia, hypoglycemia, hypokalemia, coagulation abnormalities, and metabolic acidosis with an increased anion gap.

F. Chronologic Sequence of Events. Tachypnea with respiratory alkalosis followed by metabolic acidosis, central nervous system depression, and cardiovascular collapse.

G. Differential diagnosis includes other causes of anion gap metabolic acidosis.

H. Therapeutic Plan

1. Obtain a serum salicylate level, chemistries, an arterial blood gas, and a complete blood count.
2. After initial decontamination, provide supportive care.
3. Alkalinize the urine with sodium bicarbonate.
4. Correct electrolyte abnormalities.
5. Dialyze if aspirin level is >100 mg/dl.

I. Prognosis. The serum aspirin levels above 500 mg/dl often result in death despite treatment.

21.2.3 Methanol Poisoning

A. Methanol can be found in antifreeze, windshield deicers, solvents, stove fuels, and paint removers.

B. Pathophysiologic Abnormality

1. Methanol is toxic when metabolized to formaldehyde and formic acid. This occurs over several hours (giving a latent period of 8 to 24 hours).
2. Severe metabolic acidosis with anion and osmolar gaps occur.
3. Amounts greater than 0.5 ml/kg can be fatal.

C. Symptoms include headache, malaise, dizziness, paresthesia, blindness, central nervous system depression, and abdominal pain.

D. Physical findings include cardiac arrhythmias, seizures, reduced visual acuity, and retinal hyperemia progressing to a pale, avascular retina.

E. Laboratory Findings

1. Metabolic acidosis. carbon dioxide content may approach zero.
2. Methanol levels above 20 mg/dl are associated with toxicity.
3. Methanol levels can be estimated by the formula:

$$\text{Methanol level} = \text{Osmolar gap} \times 3$$

F. Potential complications include blindness and death.

G. The differential diagnosis includes other etiologies of an anion gap acidosis.

H. Therapeutic Plan

1. Check chemistries, freezing point osmolality, methanol level, and arterial blood gas values.
2. Gastric decontamination is not useful.
3. Sodium bicarbonate is administered to reverse the metabolic acidosis. Alkalinization of the urine also enhances excretion.
4. Formic acid administration may help correct acidosis.
5. Ethanol and 4-methylpyrazole can be used to competitively bind alcohol dehydrogenase sites, pre-

Table 21.2.1 Stages of acetaminophen poisening

STAGE	TIME AFTER INGESTION	FINDINGS
I	<24 hours	Anorexia, nausea, vomiting, malaise, pallor, diaphoresis
II	24 to 48 hours	Abdominal pain, liver tenderness, elevated hepatic transaminases, oliguria
III	72 to 96 hours	Peak hepatic transaminases elevation, hyperbilirubinemia, prolonged prothrombin time
IV	4 days to 2 weeks	Resolution of hepatic toxicity or progressive hepatic failure

venting methanol metabolism.
6. Use hemodialysis if the serum methanol level >50 mg/dl.

I. Prognosis. Permanent blindness correlates with the severity of metabolic acidosis.

21.2.4 Ethylene Glycol Poisoning

A. Ethylene glycol is found in antifreeze, radiator fluid, and windshield deicers.

B. Pathophysiologic Abnormality
1. The parent state is nontoxic.
2. Metabolism by alcohol dehydrogenase produces toxic intermediates including glycoaldehyde, glycolic acid (causing metabolic acidosis), and calcium oxalate crystals (damaging to all vital organs).
3. Toxicity appears within hours of ingestion.

C. Laboratory studies reveal hypocalcemia, severe metabolic acidosis, and oxalate crystals in the urine. The urine may fluoresce under Wood's lamp if the poisoning is due to radiator antifreeze.

D. The differential diagnosis includes diabetic ketoacidosis and other alcohol poisonings.

E. **Table 21.2.5** Signs and symptoms

STAGE	FINDINGS	MECHANISM
I	Central nervous system changes, coma, seizure, nausea, vomiting, hypercalcemia, crystalluria, tetany, dysrhythmia	Profound metabolic acidosis, formation of calcium oxalate
II	Coma, cardiopulmonary failure	Metabolic acidosis, hypocalcemia
III	Renal failure (24 to 72 hours after ingestion)	Acute tubular necrosis

F. Therapeutic plan is the same as in methanol poisoning.

G. Prognosis depends upon the degree of end-organ injury.

21.2.5 Isopropyl Alcohol Poisoning

A. Poisoning can occur by ingestion or dermal absorption.

B. Pathophysiologic Abnormality
1. Isopropyl alcohol is metabolized to acetone.
2. It does not cause metabolic acidosis.
3. It does cause myocardial depression, hypotension, and shock.
4. Cardiovascular collapse can occur.

C. Symptoms include intoxication and gastritis.

D. Physical findings are the result of central nervous system depression.

E. Laboratory testing reveals an osmolar gap.

F. Coma, ketonuria, and the absence of metabolic acidosis strongly suggest the diagnosis.

G. Therapeutic Plan
1. Check a serum osmolarity, arterial blood gas levels, and urinalysis.
2. Employ hemodialysis if severe toxicity is clinically evident.

H. Prognosis. Death can occur at blood levels above 400 to 500 mg/dl.

21.2.6 Ethanol Poisoning

A. Ethanol is the most frequently ingested alcohol.

B. Alcohol Levels
1. In adolescents, levels of 100 to 150 mg/dl cause intoxication and mild neurologic symptoms. Levels above 500 mg/dl may be lethal.
2. In children, levels of 50 to 100 mg/dl cause coma, hypoglycemia, and hypothermia.
3. Blood alcohol levels of 100 mg/dl result from 10 to 15 ml/kg of beer (5% alcohol), 4 to 6 ml/kg of wine (14% alcohol), and 1 to 2 ml/kg of 80 proof liquor (40% alcohol).
4. Alcohol is metabolized at about 10 to 25 mg/dl/hour.

C. Signs and symptoms include nausea, vomiting, stupor, coma, ataxia, seizures, nystagmus, and apnea.

D. Laboratory studies reveal elevated serum ethanol levels and possibly hypoglycemia.

E. The differential diagnosis includes ingestion of other alcohols.

F. Therapeutic Plan
1. Obtain an ethanol level and serum chemistries.
2. Ethanol is not absorbed by activated charcoal.
3. Institute supportive measures including airway and ventilatory support.
4. Consider hemodialysis if serum alcohol levels are above 450 to 500 mg/dl.

21.2.7 Iron Poisoning

A. This is the most common cause of childhood death from ingestion (1995).

B. Multivitamins with iron, including prenatal vitamins and postnatal iron tablets, are the usual source.

C. Pathophysiologic Abnormality
1. Ingestion of greater than 50 mg/kg of elemental iron causes toxicity.
2. Iron causes caustic damage to gastrointestinal mucosa, and at elevated levels, is a mitochondrial poison.

D. Phases of Injury (Table 21.2.7)

E. Potential Complications
1. Phase I may be associated with shock and coma.
2. Phase III may be associated with seizures, coma, and intractable shock.

F. Therapeutic Plan
1. Collect serum iron levels, an iron-binding capacity, a complete blood count, chemistries, and type and crossmatch blood.
2. Consider gastrointestinal decontamination with induced emesis if the child presents within 30 minutes of ingestion. Activated charcoal is not effective.
3. Oral bicarbonate, magnesium hydroxide, and oral deferoxamine are of questionable benefit and may produce toxicity, therefore they are not generally recommended.
4. Intravenous deferoxamine is indicated for the child with moderate to severe symptoms or a serum iron level >500 mcg/dl. The iron-deferoxamine complex may give the urine a red color (vin rosé).
5. Whole bowel lavage and endoscopic removal of large pill fragments have been tried. No definite benefit has been demonstrated.

G. Prognosis
1. Vomiting, diarrhea, serum glucose greater than 150 mg/dl, white blood cell count greater than 15,000 cells/mm^3, and radiopaque material on abdominal x-rays all correlate with serious toxicity risk.
2. Children who are completely asymptomatic 6 hours postingestion are not at risk for toxicity.

Table 21.2.7 Phase of injury

PHASE	TIME PERIOD	MECHANISM	MANIFESTATIONS
I	<6 hours	Direct mucosal injury	Diarrhea, gastrointestinal bleeding
II	2 to 24 hours	"Latent period"	Diminished gastrointestinal symptoms
III	24 hours	Hepatocellular injury	Cyanosis, profound meatbolic acidosis
IV	Days to weeks	Mucosal scarring	Pyloric stenosis, intestinal scarring

21.2.8 Organophosphate Poisoning

A. The usual source of organophosphate poisoning are lipid soluble insecticides found in the home or in agricultural use. Organophosphates can be absorbed by inhalation, ingestion, and through the skin.

B. Pathophysiologic Abnormality
1. Organophosphates irreversibly phosphorylate acetylcholinesterase resulting in accumulation of acetylcholine at cholinergic receptor sites.
2. Symptoms usually develop within 12 hours of a significant exposure.

C. Symptoms include dizziness, headache, convulsions, ataxia, coma, sweating, tremors, muscle twitching, weakness, paralysis, gastrointestinal cramps, increased urinary frequency, salivation, and vomiting.

D. Physical findings include miosis, bradycardia, bronchorrhea, wheezing, lacrimation, and accelerated peristalsis.

E. Laboratory evaluation reveals decreased plasma or red blood cell cholinesterase activity. This test is confirmatory but not usually available on an immediate (STAT) basis.

F. Potential complications include pulmonary edema and respiratory failure secondary to paralysis.

G. Differential Diagnosis. Carbamates cause reversible carbamylation of acetylcholinesterase and produce the same symptom complex.

H. Diagnosis is made based on clinical findings and a history of exposure.

I. Therapeutic Plan
1. Remove clothing and wash the skin.
2. Protect staff from exposure.
3. Administer atropine until bronchorrhea abates (may require high doses).
4. Severe poisoning is also treated with pralidoxime.
5. Avoid aminophylline and phenothiazine because of their effect on acetylcholine.
6. Carbamates respond to atropine but not to pralidoxime.

21.2.9 Tricyclic Antidepressant Poisoning

A. This is a particularly dangerous ingestion.

B. Pathophysiologic Abnormality
1. Some symptoms are due to the anticholinergic effect of these agents.
2. The more life-threatening effects are due to alteration of the cellular membrane potential which may result in ventricular tachycardia, hypotension, and torsades de pointes.
3. Seizures and coma may occur in severe overdoses.

C. Symptoms include altered sensorium (lethargy, hallucinations, coma), seizures, and urinary retention.

D. Physical findings include evidence of seizure activity, hypotension, ataxia, and dilated pupils that react to light.

E. Diagnostic testing may reveal ventricular dysrhythmias on electrocardiogram and a prolonged QRS interval which may progress to complete heart block and asystole.

F. Therapeutic Plan
1. Symptomatic patients should be monitored for 48 hours.
2. Serum levels are not helpful.
3. Consider gastrointestinal decontamination.

4. Administer sodium bicarbonate to raise the pH between 7.45 and 7.5 to help prevent dysrhythmia.
5. Start antiarrhythmic therapy with magnesium, lidocaine, or phenytoin if indicated. Quinidine and procainamide should be avoided.
6. Prognosis. A QRS interval over 0.1 second on the electrocardiogram is associated with significant morbidity and mortality.

21.2.10 Mushroom Poisoning

A. Mushrooms produce several toxins: muscarine, coprine, cyclopeptides, monomethylhydrazine, psilocybin, and ibotenic acid.

B. Gastrointestinal Symptoms (Rapid Onset)

1. Within an hour of poisonous mushroom ingestion, children complain of abdominal pain and nausea. They also have diarrhea and vomiting.
2. Etiologic toxin is unknown.
3. Treatment is primarily supportive for the duration of the symptoms. Children may be ill for several days.

C. Central Nervous System Symptoms

1. Symptoms are attributed to ingestion of ibotenic acid and muscimol in *Amanita* species of mushrooms.
2. These toxins cause agitation or lethargy, obtundation, and seizures.
3. Patients may have other anticholinergic effects, or if large amounts of muscarine are present in the ingested mushrooms, may experience effects similar to those seen in organophosphate poisoning.
4. In *Psilocybe* mushroom ingestion, psilocybin and psilocin cause hallucination, euphoria, fever, and seizures.
5. Treatment is primarily supportive.

D. Autonomic Nervous System Symptoms

1. Muscarine poisoning produces a rapid onset of diaphoresis, lacrimation, vomiting, miosis, diarrhea, and excessive urination. Respiratory distress may occur secondary to increased airway secretions. Atropine may be effective in relieving more severe symptoms.
2. Coprine poisoning causes inhibition of acetaldehyde metabolism. If affected individuals consume alcohol within days of ingestion, they develop vomiting, tachycardia, hyperemia, and tingling of the hands. The effect is similar to that of disulfiram.

E. Gastrointestinal Symptoms (Delayed Onset)

1. Most of the fatalities (95%) from mushroom poisoning are due to ingestion of *Amanita* and *Galerina* species.
2. After 6 to 24 hours, children experience nausea, vomiting, profuse diarrhea, and abdominal pain attributable to phalloidin (cyclopeptide toxin).
3. After 1 to 2 days, liver transaminases rise, hyperbilirubinemia occurs, as does renal failure, followed by coma. These effects are due to amanitotoxin (inhibits ribonucleic acid polymerase).
4. Death occurs within a week.
5. Treatment
   a. Supportive care for replacement of fluid losses early in the poisoning is necessary.
   b. Manage hepatic and renal failure as they occur.
   c. Prevent binding of toxins by administration of activated charcoal and lactulose early in the disease course.
   d. Continuous infusion of penicillin and silibinin inhibit toxin binding and enterohepatic circulation.
   e. Hemodialysis is recommended.

479. Where do the majority of all accidental poisonings occur — A 21.1.1

A. home
B. daycare
C. school
D. work

480. All of the following cause an elevated anion gap except — C 21.1.2

A. methanol
B. diabetic ketoacidosis
C. vomiting
D. salicylates
E. ibuprofen

481. Which poison smells of bitter almonds — B 21.1.2

A. arsenic
B. cyanide
C. naphthalene
D. methyl salicylate
E. chloroform

482. Which toxidrome is characterized by the saying "dry as a bone, blind as a bat, mad as a hatter, red as a beet, and hot as a hare" — C 21.1.3

A. sympathomimetic syndrome
B. sympatholytic syndrome
C. anticholinergic syndrome
D. cholinergic syndrome

483. A 15-year-old presents with excessive salivation, diarrhea, sweating, miosis, and tachycardia. He is agitated. His mother states that he was acting this way when he came home from his job at a lawn service company. Which toxidrome does his symptom complex represent — D 21.1.3

A. sympathomimetic syndrome
B. sympatholytic syndrome
C. anticholinergic syndrome
D. cholinergic syndrome

484. What is the first priority in the management of any poisoned patient — A 21.1.4

A. airway
B. breathing
C. circulation
D. establish disability
E. exposure

485. Which of the following substances is not adsorbed to activated charcoal — B 21.1.4

A. acetaminophen
B. lithium
C. diphenhydramine
D. warfarin

486. What intervention may help to prevent arrhythmia in tricyclic antidepressant overdose — B 21.2.9

A. glucose and insulin administration
B. sodium bicarbonate drip
C. antiepileptic administration
D. sodium polystyrene sulfonate therapy

487. What is the antidote for heparin — C 21.1.4

- **A.** flumazenil
- **B.** physostigmine
- **C.** protamine
- **D.** pralidoxime

488. How long after acute overdose of acetaminophen do hepatic transaminase levels peak — C 21.2.1

- **A.** 1 to 24 hours
- **B.** 24 to 48 hours
- **C.** 72 to 96 hours
- **D.** 96 hours to 2 weeks

489. What is the antidote for acetaminophen poisoning — D 21.2.1

- **A.** flumazenil
- **B.** pralidoxime
- **C.** naloxone
- **D.** N-acetylcysteine

490. A 6-year-old child with a history of recent Kawasaki disease presents to the emergency department with altered mental status, slurred speech, and vomiting. He complains of "buzzing" in his head. On evaluation, you note agitation, Kussmaul respirations, and an anion gap acidosis. What has he ingested — E 21.2.2

- **A.** acetaminophen
- **B.** meperidine
- **C.** phenobarbital
- **D.** rat poisoning
- **E.** baby aspirin

491. A child presents with altered mental status and vomiting. His urine fluoresces under the Wood's lamp. The best treatment is — A 21.2.4

- **A.** ethanol
- **B.** methanol
- **C.** glucose
- **D.** intravenous fluids
- **E.** there is no effective treatment

492. Which of the following is a potentially lethal ethanol level in an adolescent — B 21.2.6

- **A.** 100 mg/dl
- **B.** 550 mg/dl
- **C.** 200 mg/dl
- **D.** 50 mg/dl

493. What is the most important intervention in acute ethanol poisoning — A 21.2.6

- **A.** establish a definitive airway
- **B.** place an intravenous catheter
- **C.** give activated charcoal
- **D.** start hemodialysis
- **E.** evaluate the cervical spine for injury

494. What is the life-threatening effect of tricyclic antidepressant overdose — A 21.2.9

- **A.** cardiac arrhythmia
- **B.** seizure
- **C.** hypotension
- **D.** ataxia

495. When does the latent period occur in iron toxicity — B 21.2.7

A. phase I (0 to 6 hours)
B. phase II (2 to 24 hours)
C. phase III (>24 hours)
D. phase IV (days to weeks)

496. Which of the following therapies is indicated for the child with a moderate to severe iron ingestion — C 21.2.7

A. oral bicarbonate
B. oral deferoxamine
C. magnesium hydroxide
D. intravenous deferoxamine
E. whole bowel lavage

497. What is the treatment of organophosphate poisoning — E 21.2.8

A. pralidoxime
B. aminophylline
C. atropine
D. all of the above
E. A and C

498. What is the treatment of carbamate poisoning — C 21.2.8

A. pralidoxime
B. aminophylline
C. atropine
D. all of the above
E. A and C

499. Which mushroom species is responsible for the majority of the fatalities associated with mushroom ingestion — E 21.2.10

A. *Psilocybe*
B. *Amanita*
C. *Galleria*
D. all of the above
E. B and C only

22 CHILD ABUSE AND NEGLECT

22.1 GENERAL CONCEPTS

22.1.1 Demographics

A. The abuse of children certainly is not unique to this age or to our society.
   1. In ancient times, infanticide was practiced by both the Greeks and Romans.
   2. Children have been sexually "used" and physically abused throughout history.
   3. Societies' recognition of child abuse and neglect, and attempts to prevent or treat this malady, are fairly recent.

B. In the USA, there are approximately 3 million reports of suspected abuse annually. About 1 million cases are confirmed as being abuse or neglect on an annual basis.
   1. Nationally, about half of child abuse cases are neglect.
   2. One fourth of the cases are physical abuse and slightly less than that are sexual abuse.
   3. The remainder of the cases are made up of psychological maltreatment and Munchausen by proxy Syndrome.

C. Death from child abuse deserves special mention.
   1. Child abuse deaths nationally are on the rise. They now number about 1,300 a year (this number is likely a gross underestimation).
   2. About 40% of child abuse deaths are from neglect and 60% are from abuse.
   3. The single most common cause of child abuse death is head trauma (blunt trauma to the head plus shaken baby accounts for more than 40% of all child abuse deaths).
   4. Of children who die, more than 40% are less than one year of age and 65% are less than 3 years of age. More than 90% of all child abuse death victims are less than 5 years of age.
   5. The majority of the perpetrators of child abuse deaths are the natural parents. Approximately 40% of the families of child abuse death victims have a history of prior involvement with Child Protective Services.
   6. Child abuse has now surpassed falls, drowning, and fires as the leading cause of death of children age 1 to 4.

22.1.2 Legal Issues

A. All fifty states and the District of Columbia have mandatory reporting laws. A mandatory reporting law essentially requires that any person who has or should have reasonable suspicion that a child has been injured or neglected must report that suspicion to the appropriate authorities.

B. All reported suspected cases are investigated and ruled as confirmed, unconfirmed, or uncertain (unable to determine).

C. Physicians who care for children have a particular obligation to be aware of the forms of child abuse, the historical and physical indicators of abuse, the physical findings (or probable lack thereof in sexual abuse), and the appropriate diagnostic tests.

22.2 ABUSE CLASSIFICATION

22.2.1 Munchausen by Proxy Syndrome

A. This is a situation in which a parent or caretaker persistently fabricates information about a child's health or induces illness in a child in order to seek medical attention.
   1. Munchausen by proxy syndrome is a bizarre form of abuse in which the perpetrator uses a child so that they can establish a relationship with a medical system.
   2. Usually one child at a time in a family is the victim, but perpetrators may injure or kill multiple children over the course of their disease.

B. Etiology
   1. The condition evolves from severe poorly understood psychopathology in the perpetrator.
   2. The perpetrator is most often the mother.
   3. Many people doubt that the perpetrator's illness is "curable," and feel that terminating their contact with children is the only solution.

C. Presentation
   1. The child with Munchausen by proxy syndrome is usually "presented" to the medical system by the mother either with a history of significant medical problems or with actual symptoms of a disease.
   2. Perpetrators are generally either "fabricators." individuals who make up medical history about their child, or "inducers," individuals who actually injure their child or give their child medications, infections, poisonings, etc., to create an illness in the child.
   3. The parent will repeatedly seek medical attention for the child and generally becomes very involved in the child's medical support system.
   4. The medical community generally adds to the child's ills by doing a long evaluation and many diagnostic tests in an effort to address the "illness."
   5. It is only when the child repeatedly comes to medical attention with "disease" which does not make sense that the medical community begins to suspect the diagnosis of Munchausen by proxy syndrome.
   6. It is not reasonable to think that medical personnel should suspect every parent who seeks medical attention of creating illness in their child, however it is critically important to realize if a child's history or presentation is not usual or typical, the possibil-

ity that the child's illness has been fabricated should be entertained.

D. Differential Diagnosis

1. The differential diagnosis for Munchausen by proxy syndrome is true disease in the child.
2. Most illnesses that a child could truly have can be fabricated by a parent or caretaker. Some of the more common presentations of Munchausen by proxy syndrome include:
   a. Apneic episodes. Events occur only when the perpetrator is alone with the child.
   b. Seizures.
   c. Recurrent vomiting induced by the administration of emetics.
   d. Chronic diarrhea induced by laxatives.
   e. Sepsis created by injecting children with feces or other contaminated material.

E. Management

1. The medical system should make note of the circumstances surrounding the child's presentation. Provide very careful documentation of historical information, complaints, examination findings, and parent's behavior.
2. Early identification of the child at risk with removal from the home is imperative.

22.2.2 Emotional or Psychological Maltreatment

A. Emotional and psychological maltreatment are grouped together.

1. **Emotional maltreatment** is a situation in which a child is not provided with appropriate support, attention, or affection.
2. **Psychological maltreatment** is generally considered a chronic pattern of behavior, such as humiliating, ridiculing, or belittling a child.
3. Both of these forms of maltreatment may result in impaired psychological growth and development of the child.

B. To define a child as emotionally or psychologically maltreated is very difficult as many children in our society have inadequate parenting.

1. Child victims of other forms of abuse have a degree of psychological or emotional maltreatment.
2. Children who have sleep disturbances or sleep disorders, encopresis, developmental delays, speech disorders, habit disorders, or behavioral extremes should be considered as possibly psychologically or emotionally maltreated.

C. Any physician who truly feels that a child is being emotionally or psychologically maltreated should refer the situation to the juvenile justice system. Referral should also be made to appropriate mental health professionals.

22.2.3 Sexual Abuse

A. Sexual abuse is generally considered to be sexual activity that is inappropriate to the child's developmental level, does not have the child's informed consent, and violates societal taboos.

1. As a general rule, there is a discrepant age between the child and the perpetrator, but now many juveniles are also perpetrating against other children.
2. Sexual abuse does not include the concept of sexual play, sexual exploration, or other sexual activity that is appropriate to the child. Abuse is sexual activity that is inappropriate for the child and is performed for the gratification of the perpetrator.
3. Most sexual abuse is nonviolent and does not cause physical harm to the child.
4. The vast majority of children who are abused know their assailant.
5. Many of them are molested on a chronic basis in their home environment.

B. Terminology of Sexual Abuse

1. Fondling. This is inappropriate touching directly or through the clothes.
2. Oral sex.
3. Simulated intercourse, also called vulvar intercourse. It does not involve vaginal penetration.
4. Intercourse.
5. Sodomy.

C. It is estimated that 1 in 4 females and 1 in 6 males will be sexually abused by the time they reach their 18th birthday.

D. Presentation. Children who have been the victims of sexual abuse present to the medical system in many ways.

1. Children may have spontaneous disclosure of their abuse to medical personnel or to someone else. It is important to remember that when children spontaneously disclose abuse in age-appropriate language and with developmentally appropriate historical description, such history is almost never fabricated.
2. Children may not have direct disclosure of sexual abuse, but may have inappropriate sexual activity, inappropriate sexual knowledge, have a sexually transmitted disease, or be pregnant.
3. Many children present with very indirect indicators of sexual abuse.
   a. They may have nonspecific genital, urinary, or anal complaints. They may have frequent urinary tract infections, vaginal concerns (discharge, pain, irritation), recurrent abdominal pain, headaches, dizziness or weakness, chest pain, behavioral changes, eating disorders, school problems, or social problems (hyperactivity, sexualized behavior, acting out behavior).
   b. In the older child, behavioral sequelae of sexual abuse including depression, suicidal gestures, running away, substance abuse, prostitution, or sexual promiscuity may be indicators of abuse.

E. Evaluation
  1. A complete medical and social history is imperative in evaluating the child for sexual abuse.
    a. Questions about a history of sexual abuse must be asked without embarrassment.
    b. The interview should be conducted using developmentally appropriate nonleading questions. Let the child describe what has happened to them in their own way, time, and words.
    c. Realize that children frequently feel guilty about what has happened and are likely to blame themselves.
  2. A complete physical exam is performed to insure the child's well being.
    a. The vast majority of physical exams done on children who have been the victims of sexual abuse are normal.
    b. It is important to be familiar with the normal anatomy of the prepubertal child so that a description of genital anatomy beyond sexual maturity rating (Tanner) stage I can be documented. In general, the physician should "say what you see" on the genital examination of the child.
  3. Documentation of findings should include a description of the size, shape and color of the hymen, any scars, synechia, healed lacerations, and bruising that might be present. On males, describe the penis and scrotum, and the presence or absence of testicles. A general description of the anus on all children is appropriate.
  4. Diagnostic testing for sexually transmitted diseases is reasonable in many children who are the victims of sexual abuse.
    a. The general recommendation is that testing be done for an individual child based on their exam, sexual abuse history, and known risk factors in the perpetrator.
    b. Any sexually transmitted diseases that are found in the child should be treated.

F. Management. The single most important part of the management of the sexually abused child is providing reassurances.
  1. They should be told that what has happened to them is in no way their fault.
  2. They do not have to continue to live in an abusive situation.
  3. They are medically okay and that they will grow up "normal."
  4. Dispel their belief that they are no longer sexually "good," that they will never be able to have children, or have a normal sexual relationship with another person.
  5. Consider mental health counseling in children who have a significant history of sexual abuse and evidence of associated behavioral disturbance.

G. Points to Remember
  1. Females have persistence of maternal estrogen effect for up to 2 years of age and may have fimbriated estrogenized hymens until 2 years of age.
  2. All females with normal genital anatomy are born with a hymen.
  3. Hymens in the prepubertal child without estrogen effect are usually either annular or crescentic in shape and are sensitive to touch.
  4. Most child sexual abuse is nonviolent and the question "Has anyone ever hurt you down there?" is an inadequate attempt to obtain a history of sexual abuse from a child.
  5. Many sexually promiscuous adolescents were introduced to sexual activity through sexual abuse.
  6. Partly because there is a delay in disclosure of sexual abuse, any injuries that might have occurred at the time of the abuse are usually resolved by the time the child is examined.
  7. *Neisseria gonorrhea* grows well in the oral pharynx, *Chlamydia* does not.
  8. A nontraumatic medical exam is critical. Children who are sexually abused have already been traumatized.
  9. Usually children do not have hemorrhoids and the presence of these in a child should lead one to think about the possibility of sexual abuse.
  10. As a general rule, children do not lie about sexual abuse. A well documented history remains the single most important tool in the evaluation of the sexually abused child.

22.2.4 Neglect

A. Neglect is generally considered to be the failure of a parent or caretaker to provide a child under the age of 18 with basic needs such as appropriate shelter, food, clothing, supervision, and protection. It also includes failure to provide medical care when the absence of such medical care might endanger the child's well-being.

B. Neglect is the most common form of child abuse.
  1. It is estimated that the vast majority of neglected children are not identified.
  2. Most cases of child neglect in our society are identified by family, neighbors, and family contacts. They are evaluated by Child Protective Services and may never encounter the medical community.

C. Patient presentation varies greatly. The two areas of neglect where physicians most commonly have input is in growth failure and medical neglect.
  1. Growth deficiency, also called failure to thrive, is a situation in which a young child fails to follow their growth curve, fails to have adequate increase in height and weight over time, or falls across mul-

500. What is the most common lesion seen in nonaccidental blunt abdominal trauma in children — A 22.2.5

A. duodenal hematoma
B. splenic rupture
C. intestinal perforation
D. liver laceration
E. pancreatitis

Index

A

α1-antitrypsin deficiency 51, 164
Abdominal pain 160
  recurrent 45
Abnormal head shapes 197
Acanthosis nigricans 225
Accommodative esotropia 239
Achondroplasia 51, 213
Acid-Base disturbances
  metabolic acidosis 189
  metabolic alkalosis 189
  respiratory acidosis 189
  respiratory alkalosis 189
Acid-Base rules of thumb 188
Acne vulgaris 229
Acrodermatitis enteropathica 230
Acromegaly 55
Acute interstitial nephritis 179
Acute necrotizing ulcerative gingivitis 75
Acute otitis media 76
Acute phase reactants 87
Acute respiratory failure 251
Adolescence 29
Adrenal biosynthetic pathways 53, 54
Adrenal disorders 54
  Addison's disease 54
  adrenal hyperplasia 54
  congenital adrenal hyperplasia 54
Adrenoleukodystrophy 200
Agenesis of the corpus callosum 196
Agglutination tests 69
Airway obstruction 93
Alacrima 240
Albers-Schönberg disease 213
Albinism 223
Alopecia 227
  toxic alopecia 227
  traction alopecia 227
Altered mental status 252
Amaurosis 238
Ambiguous genitalia 56
Amblyopia 237
Amenorrhea 30, 31
AMPLE history 248
Amputations 213
Anagen effluvium 227
Andersen's disease 58
Anemia 127
  α-thalassemias 134
  acquired pure red blood cell anemia 127
  anemia of chronic disease 128
  β-thalassemias 134
  congenital pure red blood cell anemia 127
  Diamond-Blackfan syndrome 127
  folic acid deficiency 128
  hemoglobin C disorders 133
  hemolytic anemia
    autoimmune hemolytic anemia 132
    glucose-6-phosphate dehydrogenase deficiency 131
    hemolytic disease of the newborn 132
    hemolytic-uremic syndrome 177
    pyruvate kinase deficiency 131
  iron deficiency 129
  physiologic anemia of infancy 128
  sickle cell disease 132
  sideroblastic anemia 129
  transient erythroblastopenia of childhood 127
  vitamin B_{12} deficiency 128
Anencephaly 196
Angiokeratoma corporis 222
Anion gap 185, 257
Aniridia 238
Anisocoria 238
Anisometropia 237
Anticipatory guidance 15
Antidiuretic hormone 185
Aortic stenosis 114
Apgar score 19, 20
Aphthous stomatitis 226
Aplasia cutis congenita 229
Apnea 94, 96
Appendicitis 165
Appendix testis 34
  blue dot sign 34
Arrhythmias 117
  atrioventricular block 117
Arterial blood gas analysis 93
Arterial thrombosis 201
Arteriosclerosis 116
Arthritis 213
  juvenile ankylosing spondylitis 88
  juvenile rheumatoid arthritis 87
  reactive arthritis 88
  septic arthritis 79, 212
Arthrogryposis multiplex congenita 213
Asthma 97
Astigmatism 237
Astrocytoma 148
Ataxia-telangiectasia 65, 199, 222
Athlete's foot 228
Attention deficit disorder 47
Autoimmune diseases 66
  autoimmune hemolytic anemia 132
  systemic lupus erythematosus 88
Autoimmunity 87
Autosomal dominant 49
Autosomal recessive 49

B

Balloon angioplasty 109
Bartter's syndrome 179
Bell's palsy 202
Benign migratory glossitis 226
Benign myoclonus of infancy 198
Best vitelliform degeneration 241
Biliary atresia 166
Black hairy tongue 226
Blepharitis 239
Blepharospasm 239
Blistering distal dactylitis 228
Blood pressure screening 13
Blount's disease 214
Blue dot sign 34
Bone marrow transplant 146
Bone tumors 148
Bourneville's disease 199
Bowlegs 211
Brain abscess 73
Brain growth 193
Breast
  development 29
  fibroadenomas 32
  fibrocystic disease 32
  masses 32
Breast-feeding 20
  colostrum 20
Breath sounds 94
Bronchiolitis 77
Bronchopulmonary dysplasia 95
Bronchoscopy 94
Brown's syndrome 239
Brudzinski's sign 71
Bruton agammaglobulinemia 51, 65
Buccal cellulitis 75

C

Café au lait 223
Canker sores 226
Cardiac catheterization 106

Cardiac surgical repair
  Blalock-Hanlon procedure 109
  Blalock-Taussig shunt 109
  Glenn shunt 109
  heart transplant 110
  Jatene procedure 110
  modified Blalock-Taussig shunt 109
  Mustard procedure 110
  Norwood procedure 110
  pulmonary artery banding 109
  Rashkind procedure 109
  Waterston shunt 109
Cardiomyopathies 117
Cardiopulmonary resuscitation 249
Cataract 240
Cavovarus foot 213
Cell-mediated immunity 63
Central nervous system tumors 148
Cerebral palsy 200
Charcot-Marie-Tooth disease 200
Cheilitis 226
Chemotherapeutic agents 145
Cherry red spot 241
Chest pain 94
Chickenpox 74
Child abuse 267
  emotional maltreatment 268
  medical neglect 270
  Munchausen by proxy syndrome 267
  neglect 269
  physical abuse 270
  psychological maltreatment 268
  sexual abuse 268
Childhood cancers 145
Childhood exanthems 73
Cholesterol
  screening 13
Chondrodystrophy 213
Chondroectodermal dysplasia 213
Chromosome complement 49
Chronic granulomatous disease 65
Citrullinemia 58
Cleft lip 157
Cleft palate 157
  Pierre Robin sequence 158
Clinical manifestations of cancer 145
Clubbing 94
Clubfoot 214
Coagulation disorders 135
  disseminated intravascular coagulation 136
  factor IX deficiency 135
  factor VIII deficiency 135
  hemophilia 51
  von Willebrand's disease 136
Cobb's syndrome 221
Collodion baby 226
Coloboma 238
Color blindness 51
Coma 250
  Glasgow Coma Scale 251
Compartment syndrome 253
Complement defects 64
  C1 inhibitor deficiency 65
Complement system 63
Complications of cancer treatment 146
Congenital heart disease 109
  acyanotic congenital heart lesions 110
  aortic stenosis 114
  atrial septal defect 112
  atrioventricular canal defect 112
  coarctation of the aorta 114
  congenital mitral stenosis 113
  cyanotic congenital heart lesions 110
  endocardial cushion defect 112
  heart embryology 105
  hypoplastic left heart syndrome 111
  hypoplastic right heart syndrome 111
  mitral stenosis 113
  partial anomalous pulmonary venous return 115
  patent ductus arteriosus 113
  persistent truncus arteriosus 115
  pyloric stenosis 164
  Tetralogy of Fallot 115
  total anomalous pulmonary venous return 115
  transposition of the great arteries 115
Congenital mydriasis 238
Congenital oculomotor apraxia 239
Congestive heart failure 252
Conjunctivitis 240
Constipation 160
Contact dermatitis 224
Contraception 34
  barrier methods 36
  injectable progesterone 36
  oral contraceptive pills 34
Corectopia 238
Corneal ulcers 240
Cough 94, 95
Coxsackievirus infections 75
Cranial nerves 194
Craniosynostosis 197
Cri du chat syndrome 50
Crohn's disease 162
Croup (laryngotracheobronchitis) 77
Cryptorchidism 34
Cushing's disease 54
Cushing's syndrome 54
Cutis aplasia 229
Cutis marmorata 229
Cyanosis 94, 106
Cystic fibrosis 97
Cystic hygromas 150
Cystitis 79
Cytotoxic T cells 63

D

Dacryoadenitis 240
Dacryostenosis 240
Dandy-Walker malformation 196
Deformations 49
Degenerative central nervous system diseases 199
Dehydration 188
Delayed puberty 56
Dendritic keratitis 240
Depression 37
Dermatomyositis 89
  heliotrope 90
Dermoid cysts 240
Development
  developmental milestones 11, 12, 13
  growth curve 11
  intrauterine 19
Developmental dysplasia of the hip 214
Diabetes insipidus 55
Diabetes mellitus 51, 52
Diabetic ketoacidosis 52
Diabetic retinopathy 241
Diamond-Blackfan syndrome 127
Diaper dermatitis 228
Diarrhea 160
  acute 161
  chronic 161
Diastematomyelia 196, 215
DiGeorge's syndrome 65
Diplomyelia 196
Diplopia 238
Disorders of keratin formation 225
Disruption 49
Disseminated gonococcemia 74
Disseminated intravascular coagulation 136
Double vision 238
Down's syndrome 49

Duane's syndrome 239
Duodenal obstruction 158
Dyscoria 238
Dysmenorrhea 31
Dysmorphisms 49
Dystonia musculorum deformans 200

E

Echocardiography 106
Ecthyma 228
Ecthyma gangrenosum 228
Ectopia lentis 240
Ectropion 239
Eczema 224
  nummular eczema 224
Edema 174
Edwards' syndrome 50
Ehlers-Danlos syndrome 226
Electrocardiogram 106
Ellis-van Creveld syndrome 213
Emancipated minors 37
Embolism 201
Encephalitis 72
Encephalocele 196
Encopresis 44
Endocarditis 78
Endotracheal intubation 249
Enterovirus 73
Entropion 239
Enuresis 175
  diurnal enuresis 43
  nocturnal enuresis 44
  primary 43
  secondary 43
Enzyme-linked immunosorbent assay 69
Eosinophilic granuloma 150
Eosinophils 63
Epicanthal folds 239
Epidermolysis bullosa 224
Epididymitis 34
Epiglottitis 76
Erythema infectiosum (fifth disease) 73
Erythema multiforme 224
Erythema nodosum 90
Erythema toxicum 229
Esophageal atresia 158
Esotropia 239
Ewing's sarcoma 148
Exanthema subitum 73
Exchange transfusion 23
Exercise testing 106
Extracellular fluid 185
Eye development 237
Eye injury 242

F

Fabry's disease 222
Failure to thrive 47, 269
Familial dysautonomia 202
  Riley-Day syndrome 202
Fanconi's syndrome 180
Fatty acid deficiency 230
Fetal circulation 105
Fever and temperature regulation 69
Flat feet 211
Folic acid deficiency 128
Folliculitis 228
Fontan procedure 110
Fontanelle
  anterior 11
  posterior 13
Forbes' disease 58
Fordyce spots 226
Foreign body aspiration 96
Formula-feeding 20
Fracture 211, 215, 253
Fragile X 51
Freckles (ephelids) 223
Friedreich's ataxia 199
Fungal infections (dermatophytosis) 228
  candidal gingivostomatitis 75
  dermatophytid ("id") reaction 228
  jock itch 228
  tinea capitis 228
  tinea corporis 228
  tinea cruris 228
  tinea pedis 228
  tinea versicolor 228

G

Galactokinase 23
Galactorrhea 33
Galactose-1-phosphate uridyl transferase 23
Galactosemia 23, 51
Gas exchange 93
Gastroesophageal reflux 160
Gastrointestinal bleeding 163
Gastrointestinal tumors 150
Gastroschisis 158
Gaucher's disease 200
Genu valgum (knock-knees) 211
Genu varum (bowlegs) 211
Geographic tongue (benign migratory glossitis) 226
Germ cell tumors 149
German measles 73
Gianotti-Crosti syndrome 225
Gigantism 55
Glaucoma 241
Glomerular disorders 176
  Henoch-Schönlein purpura glomerulonephritis 179
  hereditary glomerulonephritis 178
  lupus nephritis 178
  membranoproliferative glomerulonephritis 178
  mesangial proliferative glomerulonephritis 177
  postinfectious nonstreptococcal glomerulonephritis 178
  poststreptococcal glomerulonephritis 178
  rapidly progressive glomerulonephritis 178
Glomerular filtration rate 173
Glomerular function tests 173
Glucose-6-phosphate dehydrogenase deficiency 131
Glycogen storage disease 58
  Cori's disease 58
  Forbes' disease 58
  McCune-Albright syndrome 223
  Pompe's disease 58
  Tarui's disease 58
  von Gierke's disease 58
Gonadoblastoma 149
Granuloma annulare 226
Growth hormone deficiency 55, 57
Grunting 94
Guillain-Barré syndrome 200
Gynecomastia 32

H

Hair disorders 227
  alopecia 227
  anagen effluvium 227
  hypotrichosis 227
  telogen effluvium 227
Halo nevus 222
Hamartomas 222
Hand, foot, and mouth disease 74, 75
Hand-Schüller-Christian disease 150
Harlequin color change 229
Harlequin fetus 226
Headache 45
  migraine 45
    classic 45
    common 45
    complicated 45

nonmigraine headache 46
tension 46
traction 46
Heart failure 110
Heart murmurs 107
diastolic 107
peripheral pulmonic stenosis 108
pulmonary bifurcation turbulence murmur 108
Still's murmur 108
systolic murmurs 107
venous hum 108
Helper T cells 63
Hemangiomas 150
capillary 221
cavernous 221
disseminated hemangiomatosis 221
Hand-Schüller-Christian disease 150
Kasabach-Merritt syndrome 136, 221
Klippel-Trenaunay-Weber syndrome 221
nevus simplex 229
port wine stain 221
strawberry nevus 221
Sturge-Weber syndrome 199, 221
Hematopoiesis 125
Hematuria 175
Hemoglobinopathies 132
α-thalassemias 134
β-thalassemias 134
Hgb C disorders 133
sickle cell disease 132
sickle cell trait 133
Hemolytic disease of the newborn 132
Hemolytic-uremic syndrome 177
Hemophilia 51, 135
hemophilia A 135
hemophilia B 135
Hemorrhagic disease of the newborn 24
Henoch-Schönlein purpura 89
Hepatitis 25, 78, 79
hepatitis A 78
hepatitis B 79
infectious 78
neonatal hepatitis 25
Hepatolenticular degeneration 51, 199
Hereditary angioedema 65
Hereditary elliptocytosis 130
Hereditary fructose intolerance 58
Hereditary hemorrhagic telangiectasia 221
Hereditary spherocytosis 130
Hermansky-Pudlak syndrome 223
Herpangina 75
Herpes zoster 74
Herpetic gingivostomatitis 75
Hers' disease 58
Heterochromia 238
Hidradenitis suppurativa 227
Hip problems 214
Hirschsprung's disease 165
Histiocytosis X 150
Histocompatibility antigens 87
Hodgkin's disease 147
Hordeolum 240
Horner's syndrome 238
Human papilloma virus 228
Humoral immunity 63
Hyaline membrane disease 21
Hydrencephaly 196
Hydrocele 33
Hydrocephalus 196
11β-hydroxylase deficiency 54
21-hydroxylase deficiency 54
Hyper IgE (Job's) syndrome 65
Hyperbilirubinemia 22
biliary atresia 166
breast milk jaundice 22
breast-feeding associated jaundice 22
conjugated (direct) bilirubin 22
neonatal hepatitis 25
pathologic (nonphysiologic) jaundice 22
phototherapy 23
physiologic jaundice 22
unconjugated (indirect) bilirubin 22
Hyperkalemia 188
Hypernatremia 185, 187
Hyperopia 237
Hyperparathyroidism 56
Hypersensitivity reactions 66
Hypertension 116, 175, 252
hypertensive crisis 252
Hyperthyroidism 55
Graves' disease 55
thyrotoxicosis 55
Hyphema 238
Hypoglycemia 23, 52
recurrent 52
Hypokalemia 188
Hypomelanosis of Ito 224
Hyponatremia 186, 187
Hypoparathyroidism 56
idiopathic thrombocytopenic purpura 136
pseudohypoparathyroidism 57
Hypopyon 238
Hypothyroidism 55, 57

I

Ichthyosis 225
ichthyosis vulgaris 226
X-linked ichthyosis 226
Idiopathic thrombocytopenic purpura 136
Immune deficiency
acquired immunodeficiency syndrome 65
B cell defects 64
Bruton agammaglobulinemia 51, 65
chronic granulomatous disease 65
common variable immunodeficiency 65
DiGeorge's syndrome 65
dysgammaglobulinemia 65
immunoglobulin A deficiency 65
immunoglobulin G deficiency 65
immunoglobulin M deficiency 65
phagocytic defects 64
severe combined immunodeficiency 65
T cell defects 64
Immunizations 14
conjugated vaccines 14
contraindications 14
live attenuated viral vaccines 14
recombinant vaccines 14
toxoid vaccines 14
tuberculin skin testing 14
vaccine schedules 14
Immunofluorescence 69
Immunoglobulin (Ig)
Ig A 63
Ig D 63
Ig E 63
Ig G 63
Ig M 63
Impetigo 74, 227
Inborn errors of metabolism 57
Incontinentia pigmenti 223
Infantile spasm 198
Infectious mononucleosis 76
Inflammatory bowel disease 162
Crohn's disease 162
ulcerative colitis 162
Inguinal hernia 34
Insect bites 74
Insulin-dependent diabetes mellitus

51
Interstitial disorders 179
Intoeing 211, 214
Intracellular fluid 185
Intussusception 165

J

Jejunal obstruction 158
Joint pain 213
Juvenile rheumatoid arthritis 87
  pauciarticular juvenile rheumatoid arthritis 88
  polyarticular juvenile rheumatoid arthritis 87, 88
  systemic onset juvenile rheumatoid arthritis 88
Juxtaglomerular disorders 179

K

Kasabach-Merritt syndrome 136, 221
Kawasaki disease 116
Keloid 226
Kerion formation 228
Kernicterus 23
Kernig sign 71
Klinefelter's syndrome 50
Klippel-Feil anomaly 215
Klippel-Trenaunay-Weber syndrome 221
Knock-knee 211
Kwashiorkor 230

L

Lagophthalmos 239
LAMB syndrome 223
Lamellar ichthyosis 226
Langerhans' cell histiocytosis 150
Laryngomalacia 95
Laryngotracheobronchitis 77
Lead screening 14
Leg length discrepancies 214
Legal issues of adolescence 37
Legg-Calvé-Perthes disease 214
Lentigines 223
LEOPARD syndrome 223
Lesch-Nyhan syndrome 200
Letterer-Siwe disease 150
Leukemia 146
  acute lymphocytic leukemia 146
  acute myelogenous leukemia 147
  chronic lymphocytic leukemia 147
  chronic myelogenous leukemia 147
Leukocoria 238
Lice 229
  pediculosis capitis 229
  pediculosis corporis 229
  pediculosis pubis 229
Lichen striatus 225
Limping 212
Lisch nodules 238
Liver tumor 150
Louis-Bar syndrome 199, 222
Lower airway disease 94
Lower motor unit disease 195
Lung biopsy 94
Lymphokines 63
Lymphoma 147

M

Macrocephaly 196
Maffucci's syndrome 221
Maintenance fluids 186
Malabsorptive disorders 163
Malformations 49
Malignant hyperthermia 202
Malrotation 159
Marble bone disease 213
Marcus Gunn pupil 238
Marfan's syndrome 51, 213
Mast cells 63
Mastocytosis 227
Mature minor 37
McArdle disease 58
McCune-Albright syndrome 223
Measles 73
Mechanical ventilation 250
Meckel's diverticulum 159
Medulloblastoma 148
Melanoma 222
Membranous glomerulopathy 178
Meningitis 71
  aseptic 71
  bacterial meningitis 71
  Brudzinski's sign 71
  Kernig's sign 71
Meningocele 196
Meningococcemia 80
Menkes' kinky hair syndrome 200
Menstrual disorders 29
  amenorrhea 30
  dysfunctional uterine bleeding 31
  dysmenorrhea 31
Metabolic
  screening 14
Metabolic myopathy 202
Metachromatic leukodystrophy 199
Metatarsus adductus 214
Metatarsus varus 214
Microcephaly 196
Microcoria 238
Milia 229
Miliaria 227
Mitral stenosis 113
Mixed gonadal dysgenesis 56
Möbius' syndrome 239
Molluscum contagiosum 228
Mongolian spots 229
Mononucleosis 76
Morphogenesis 49
Morquio's disease 213
Mucoceles 226
Mucocutaneous lymph node syndrome 116
Multiple endocrine neoplasia 54
Muscular dystrophy 201
  Becker's muscular dystrophy 201
  Duchenne's muscular dystrophy 201
  Emery-Dreifuss muscular dystrophy 201
  facioscapulohumeral syndrome 202
  limb-girdle muscular dystrophy 202
  myotonic muscular dystrophy 202
  scapulohumeral muscular dystrophy 201
Musculoskeletal disorders 211
Myasthenia gravis 200
Mycoplasma pneumonia 78
Myelomeningocele 196
Myocarditis 78
Myopia (nearsightedness) 237

N

Natural killer cells 63
Nearsightedness 237
Necrotizing enterocolitis 24
  pneumatosis intestinalis 24
Nephrotic syndrome 175
  idiopathic nephrotic syndrome of childhood 177
  immunoglobulin A nephropathy 178
  membranous glomerulopathy 178
  sickle cell nephropathy 179
Neural tube defects 195
Neuroblastoma 54, 149
Neurocutaneous syndromes 199
  neurofibromatosis 51, 199, 223
  tuberous sclerosis 199, 224
Neurodermal sinus 196

Neurofibromatosis (von Recklinghausen's disease) 51, 199, 223
Neuropathy 202
Nevi
- acquired melanocytic nevus 222
- congenital melanocytic nevus 222
- epidermal nevi 222
- nevus of Ito 222
- nevus of Ota 222
- nevus sebaceous of Jadassohn 222

Nevoxanthoendothelioma 238
Newborn
- apnea of infancy 96
- colic 46
- fetal circulation 19
- lupus 89
- Mongolian spots 229
- nevus simplex 229
- rashes
  - infantile acropustulosis 229
  - milia 229
  - miliaria 227
  - seborrheic dermatitis 225
- seizures 21
- sepsis 21
- transient neonatal pustular melanosis 229

Niemann-Pick disease 200
Night blindness 238
Non-Hodgkin's lymphoma 147
Non-insulin-dependent diabetes mellitus 52
Nursemaid's elbow (subluxation of the radial head) 215
Nutritional dermatoses 230
- acrodermatitis enteropathica 230
- kwashiorkor 230
- pellagra 230
- scurvy 230

Nyctalopia (night blindness) 238
Nystagmus 239

O

Occult bacteremia 70
Ocular albinism 223
Oculocutaneous albinism 223
Oculosympathetic paresis 238
Oliguria 174
Omphalocele 158
Open fractures 253
Ophthalmia neonatorum 240
Opsoclonus 239
Optic glioma 241
Optic nerve hypoplasia 241
Orbital cellulitis 75
Orotic aciduria 129
Osgood-Schlatter disease 214
Osler-Weber-Rendu disease 221
Osmolality 185
Osmolar gap 185, 257
Osteochondritis desiccans 214
Osteochondrodystrophy 213
Osteodystrophy 57
Osteogenesis imperfecta 51, 213
Osteomyelitis 80, 212
Osteopetrosis 213
Osteosarcoma 148

P

Pancreatitis 164
Pancytopenias 126
Papilledema 241
Papular acrodermatitis of childhood 225
Parinaud's syndrome 239
Paroxysmal nocturnal hemoglobinuria 130
Partial albinism 223
Parvovirus B19 73
Patau's syndrome 50
Pellagra 230
Pemphigus vulgaris 224
Pericarditis 78
Periorbital (preseptal) cellulitis 74
Persistent fetal circulation 111
Pes planus (flat feet) 213
Pharyngitis 76
- streptococcal 76

Phenylketonuria 58
Pheochromocytoma 54
Piebaldism 223
Pierre Robin sequence 158
Pityriasis alba 225
Pityriasis rosea 225
Placental function 19
Pleurisy 94
Pleurodynia 75
Pneumonia 77
- bacterial 77
- *Pneumocystis carinii* 78
- viral 78

Poisonings
- acetaminophen poisoning 259
- anticholinergic syndrome 258
- antidotes 259
- aspirin poisoning 260
- cholinergic syndrome 258
- ethanol poisoning 261
- ethylene glycol poisoning 261
- iron poisoning 261
- isopropyl alcohol poisoning 261
- lead poisoning 129
- methanol poisoning 260
- mushroom poisoning 263
- organophosphate poisoning 262
- salicylism 260
- sympatholytic syndrome 258
- sympathomimetic syndrome 258
- toxidromes 258
- tricyclic antidepressant poisoning 262

Polycythemia 135
Polymerase chain reaction 69
Polyposis 150
Polyuria 175
Pompe's disease 58
Potassium related periodic paralysis 202
Potter's syndrome 173
Prader-Willi syndrome 50
Precocious puberty 56
- isosexual precocious puberty 56
- premature adrenarche 56
- premature thelarche 56

Presbyopia (farsightedness) 237
Primitive reflexes 195
Prostaglandin E_1 110
Proteinuria 175
Pseudohermaphrodism 56
Pseudoseizure 198
Psoriasis 225
Pterygium 240
Ptosis 239
Puberty 29
- Tanner stages 29

Pulmonary function tests 93
Pulmonary stenosis 114
Pulse oximetry 93, 251
Puncture wounds 212
Pyelonephritis 79
Pyloric stenosis 164
Pyogenic granuloma 221
Pyruvate kinase deficiency 131

R

Radionuclide studies 106
Ramsay Hunt syndrome 199
Ranulas 226
Rasmussen's encephalitis 197
Raynaud phenomenon 90
Reiter's disease 88
Renal failure 176
- acute 252
- dialysis 174

Renal tubular acidosis 179
Renal tubular function tests 174
Respiration
fetal 19
respiratory distress 20
respiratory distress in infancy 93
Retinitis pigmentosa 241
Retinoblastoma 149, 241
Retinopathy of prematurity 241
Rett's syndrome 200
Reye's syndrome 201
Rhabdomyosarcoma 149
Rheumatic fever 116
Jones criteria 116
Rickets 57, 213
idiopathic hypoparathyroidism 57
nutritional rickets 57
primary hyperparathyroidism 56
pseudohypoparathyroidism 57
renal rickets 57
rickets of prematurity 57
vitamin D-dependent rickets 57
X-linked hypophosphatemia 57
Riley-Day syndrome 202
Rocky Mountain spotted fever 80
Roseola 73
Rubella (German measles, three-day measles) 73
Rubeola (measles) 73

S

Sacral dysgenesis 196
Salter-Harris classification 211
Sandifer's syndrome 161
Scabies 229
Scarlet fever 73
Scleroderma 90
Scoliosis 215
Scurvy 230
Seabather's eruption 229
Sebaceous hyperplasia 229
Seborrheic dermatitis 225
Seizure disorders 197
benign rolandic epilepsy of childhood 197
clonic seizures 21
febrile seizures 198
focal seizures 21
infantile spasm 198
juvenile myoclonic epilepsy 198
myoclonic seizures 21
neonatal seizures 21
progressive myoclonic epilepsy 198
Rasmussen's encephalitis 197
tonic seizures 21
Sensory screening 13
Sensory testing 195
Sepsis 71
Sexually transmitted diseases 37
chancroid 36
gonorrhea 35
herpes simplex virus 36
human papillomavirus 35
molluscum contagiosum 36
mucopurulent cervicitis 35
nongonococcal urethritis 35
pediculosis 36
pelvic inflammatory disease 35
syphilis 36
Shingles 74
Shock 251
Short stature 57
constitutional growth delay 57
genetic short stature 57
growth hormone deficiency 55, 57
Sickle cell disease 132
Sickle cell trait 133
Sinusitis 75
Slipped capital femoral epiphysis 214
Spermatocele 33
Spina bifida occulta 196
Spinal cord trauma 252
Spinal muscular atrophy 200
Sprains 212
Staphylococcal scalded skin syndrome 228
Stargardt's disease 241
Steeple sign 77
Steinert's disease 202
Stem cell replacement 146
Stomatocytosis 131
Strabismus 238
accomodative esotropia 239
Duane's syndrome 239
pseudostrabismus 239
Stridor 95
Stroke 201
Sturge-Weber syndrome 199, 221
Subconjunctival hemorrhages 240
Subluxation of the radial head 215
Substance abuse 37
Sucking blisters 229
Suicide 37
Supernumerary nipples 229
Supraventricular tachycardia 117
Surfactant 21
Sweat chloride 94
Sweat glands 227
Syndrome of inappropriate secretion of antidiuretic hormone 56
Syringomyelia 196
Systemic lupus erythematosus 88
neonatal lupus 89

T

Tachypnea 94
Talipes calcaneovalgus 214
Talipes equinovarus 214
Tarui's disease 58
Tay-Sachs disease 51, 200
Teeth eruption 13
Telogen effluvium 227
Teratogens 49
Teratoma 149
Testicular enlargement 29
Testicular torsion 34
Testicular tumors 34
Thrombocytopenia absent radius (TAR) syndrome 136
Thrush 75, 228
Thumbprint sign 77
Tibial torsion 214
Tonic pupil 238
TORCH infections 21, 80
Torsion of the appendix testis 34
Torticollis 215
Total body water 185
Transcobalamin II deficiency 65
Transient (toxic) synovitis 212
Transient erythroblastopenia of childhood 127
Trichotillomania 227
Trisomy 13 (Patau's syndrome) 50
Trisomy 18 (Edward's syndrome) 50
Trisomy 21 (Down's syndrome) 49
Tuberous sclerosis 199, 224
Turner's syndrome 50

U

Ulcerative colitis 162
Umbilical hernia 158
Upper airway disease 94
Upper motor neuron disease 195
Urinary tract infections 79
Urine electrolytes 173

V

Varicella 74
shingles (varicella zoster) 74
Varicocele 33
Vascular malformations 221
Vasculitis 89

Venous sinus thrombosis 201
Ventricular septal defect 112
Vernal conjunctivitis 240
Visual acuity 237
Vitamin A deficiency 230
Vitamin B_{12} deficiency 128
Vitamin E deficiency myopathy 202
Vitiligo 224
Volvulus 159
von Gierke's disease 58
von Recklinghausen's disease 51, 199, 223
von Willebrand's disease 136

W

Waardenburg's syndrome 223
Warts 228
Waterhouse-Friderichsen syndrome 54
Werdnig-Hoffman disease 200
Wheezing 95
Wilms' tumor 148
Wilson's disease 51, 199
Wiskott-Aldrich syndrome 65, 136

X

X-linked (Bruton) agammaglobulinemia 65
X-linked hypophosphatemia 57
X-linked ichthyosis 226
X-linked inheritance 49